Current concepts in
CLINICAL NURSING

Edited by

EDITH H. ANDERSON, R.N., Ph.D.

BETTY S. BERGERSEN, R.N., Ed.D.

MARGERY DUFFEY, R.N., Ph.D.

MARY LOHR, R.N., Ed.D.

MARION H. ROSE, R.N., Ph.D.

Volume IV

With 37 illustrations

5892

THE C. V. MOSBY COMPANY

Saint Louis   1973

Volume IV

Copyright © 1973 by The C. V. Mosby Company

All rights reserved. No part of this book may be reproduced in any manner without written permission of the publisher.

Volume I copyrighted 1967; volume II copyrighted 1969; volume III copyrighted 1971

Printed in the United States of America

International Standard Book Number 0-8016-0178-9

Library of Congress Catalog Card Number 67-30797

Distributed in Great Britain by Henry Kimpton, London

Current concepts in
CLINICAL NURSING

Volume IV

Contributors

Dyanne Affonso, R.N., M.S.

Instructor, Department of Professional Nursing, School of Nursing, University of Hawaii, Honolulu, Hawaii

Edith H. Anderson, R.N., Ph.D.

Dean, School of Nursing, University of Hawaii, Honolulu, Hawaii

Patricia M. Baren, R.N., B.S.N., M.S.

Graduate Student, College of Nursing, Arizona State University, Tempe, Ariz.

Lorna M. Barrell, R.N., B.S., M.S.N.

Assistant Professor, Psychiatric–Mental Health Nursing, College of Nursing, University of Illinois, Chicago, Ill.

Betty S. Bergersen, R.N., Ed.D.

Chairman of Graduate Medical-Surgical Nursing and Professor of Nursing, School of Nursing, University of Colorado, Denver, Colo.

James E. Bock, R.N., B.S.

Orthopedic Staff Nurse, Porter Memorial Hospital, Denver, Colo.

Judith Ann Buten, R.N., B.S., M.S.

Head Nurse, Labor/Delivery Suite, University of California at Los Angeles, Los Angeles, Calif.

F. Ann Day, R.N., M.S.

Assistant Director of Nursing, Richmond General Hospital, Richmond, B. C., Canada

Margery Duffey, R.N., Ph.D.

Professor of Nursing and Assistant Chairman, Graduate Education, Department of Nursing Education, University of Kansas, Kansas City, Kan.

Claire M. Fagin, R.N., B.S.N., M.A., Ph.D.

Director, Department of Nursing, Herbert H. Lehman College of the City University of New York, Bronx, N. Y.

Mary M. Fowler, R.N., M.S., COL, ANC

Nurse Clinician, Department of Obstetrics and Gynecology, Trippler Army Medical Center, Honolulu, Hawaii

Katherine F. Galloway, LTC, ANC

U. S. Army Institute of Surgical Research, Brooke Medical Center, Fort Sam Houston, Texas

Helen K. Grace, R.N., B.S.N., M.S.N., Ph.D.

Associate Professor, Psychiatric–Mental Health Nursing, College of Nursing, University of Illinois, Chicago, Ill.

Sara Hammes, R.N., B.S.N., M.S.N.

Instructor, Department of Nursing Education, University of Kansas Medical Center, Kansas City, Kan.

Cheryl Hall Harris, R.N., B.S.

Infant Care Coordinator, The Children's Mercy Hospital, Kansas City, Mo.

Helen Huber, R.N., M.S.N.

Director of Nursing Service, Fort Logan Mental Health Center, Denver, Colo.

Lois A. Johns, Ph.D., LTC, ANC

U. S. Army Institute of Surgical Research, Brooke Army Medical Center, Fort Sam Houston, Texas

Joan M. King, R.N., B.S.N., M.A., D.Sc.N.

Professor, Psychiatric–Mental Health Nursing, and Assistant Dean for Graduate Study, College of Nursing, University of Illinois, Chicago, Ill.

Mary Lohr, R.N., Ed.D.

Dean, College of Nursing, University of Illinois, Chicago, Ill.

Kleia Raubitschek Luckner, R.N., B.S.N., M.S.N., C.N.M.

Clinical Director, Obstetrical, Gynecological, and Neonatal Nursing, and Assistant Director, Perinatal Research, The Toledo Hospital, Toledo, Ohio

Nancy A. Lytle, R.N., Ed.D.

Professor and Director, Maternity and Gynecological Nursing, Case Western Reserve University, Cleveland, Ohio

Nancy Malcolm, R.N., M.P.H.

Assistant Professor, School of Nursing, University of Minnesota, Minneapolis, Minn.

Elizabeth M. Maloney, R.N., B.S., M.A., Ed.D.

Assistant Professor, Mental Health–Psychiatric Nursing, Department of Nursing Education, Teachers College, Columbia University, New York, N. Y.

Betty G. McGranahan, LTC, ANC

U. S. Army Institute of Surgical Research, Brooke Army Medical Center, Fort Sam Houston, Texas

Anne Lally Milhaven, R.N., M.S.N.

Assistant Director of Nursing, Rhode Island Hospital, Providence, R. I.

John Giles Milhaven, Lic. Theol., Ph.D.

Associate Professor, Department of Religious Studies, Brown University, Providence, R. I.

Irene Murchison, R.N., B.S., M.A.

Nursing Consultant, Legal Areas of Nursing Practice

Eileen Gallagher Nahigian, R.N., M.S.N.

Formerly Instructor, Department of Nursing, Morris Harvey College; Pediatric Clinical Nurse Specialist, Memorial Division, Charleston Area Medical Center, Charleston, W. Va.

Thomas S. Nichols, L.L.B., M.S., A.B.

Partner in Davis, Graham and Stubbs, Attorneys and Counselors at Law, Denver, Colo.

Patsy A. Perry, R.N., M.S.

Senior Instructor in Nursing, School of Nursing, University of Colorado, Denver, Colo.

Jeanne N. Quesenbury, R.N., B.S.N., M.N.

Formerly Associate Professor, Department of Nursing Education, University of Kansas Medical Center, Kansas City, Kan.

Julina P. Rhymes, R.N., Ph.D.

Assistant Professor of Nursing, Yale University School of Nursing and Child Study Center, New Haven, Conn.

Irene Riddle, R.N., Ph.D.

Associate Professor, Director of the Graduate Major in the Nursing of Children, Department of Nursing, St. Louis University, St. Louis, Mo.

Paulette Robischon, R.N., Ph.D.

Associate Professor, Department of Nursing, Herbert H. Lehman College of the City University of New York, Bronx, N. Y.

Marion H. Rose, R.N., Ph.D.

Professor of Nursing and Director of Graduate Program in Family-Child Nursing, College of Nursing, Arizona State University, Tempe, Ariz.

Jean Shannon, R.N., B.S.N., M.S.

Graduate Student, College of Nursing, Arizona State University, Tempe, Ariz.

Beverly Shea, R.N., M.S.

Clinical Instructor, School of Nursing, Baylor University, Dallas, Texas

Paul Silverstein, M.D., MAJ, MC

U. S. Army Institute of Surgical Research, Brooke Army Medical Center, Fort Sam Houston, Texas

Marie D. Strickland, R.N., M.Ed.

Assistant Professor, Cornell University–New York Hospital School of Nursing; Head of Department of Obstetrics and Gynecology, The New York Hospital–Cornell Medical Center, New York, N. Y.

Lorraine Struempler, R.N., B.S., M.N.Ed.

Assistant Professor in Pediatrics and Chief Project Nurse of the Children and Youth Project, College of Medicine, University of Nebraska, Omaha, Neb.

Leonide M. Tanner, R.N., M.S.

Assistant Professor of Nursing, School of Nursing, University of California at Los Angeles, Los Angeles, Calif.

Edith G. Walker, R.N., M.A.

Associate Professor, Maternal-Child Nursing, School of Nursing, University of Massachusetts, Amherst, Mass.

Gwen T. Will, R.N., B.S.N., M.A.

Psychiatric Nurse Clinician and author, Austen Riggs Center, Inc., Stockbridge, Mass.

Preface

More than a hundred nurses engaged in a variety of thoughtful approaches to clinical practice have contributed to the first three volumes of *Current Concepts in Clinical Nursing* since the inception of the series in 1967. The editors are proud of the response of the authors who were willing to share with colleagues their ideas and concerns about new modes of practice. Contributing to the literature is one way to refine the concepts on which practice is built.

The reception of the previous volumes has been most gratifying to the editors and authors. This fourth volume is presented with enthusiasm and with the hope that it too will serve the nurse practitioners toward whom it is aimed. Bringing together in one volume new concepts in practice gives nurses a view not only of their own clinical areas of interest but of other areas as well.

A new section on an excursion into the law of nursing practice has been added to the sections on psychiatric, pediatric, maternity, and medical-surgical nursing. Many of the concepts dealt with in each chapter cut across sections and the traditional nursing practice fields, a pleasant reflection on the advances nursing has made in developing its science. In the next volume we will make further changes in the organizational framework of the sections.

We hope that this volume will help to advance nursing practice and the care of people. We trust that our readers will find the new ideas it contains stimulating and that more authors will join us in describing excellence in practice.

Edith H. Anderson

Contents

Psychiatric nursing

with an introduction by
Mary Lohr

The psychiatric nursing section of this volume is composed of selected clinical material illustrating application of principles that have relevance for the practice of psychiatric nursing.

Major problems confronting persons concerned with prevention and treatment of psychiatric disorders are identified and approaches to solutions offered. Illustrations are derived from nurse-patient interaction in hospital, clinic, and community settings. Clinical descriptions include individual and group treatment with acute as well as chronic patients.

Clinical data are presented to illustrate the role of the nurse as a therapeutic agent working as a leader and collaborator with persons in other health disciplines. Theory guiding therapeutic intervention is made explicit and amply illustrated with verbal as well as other descriptive data.

1

Developmental concepts relating to psychiatric nursing practice

Gwen T. Will

The practice of psychiatric nursing deals with a transactional field composed of persons from whom certain things can be expected. This field is complex, and, because of the past experience of those in it, predictability cannot be precise; the field is in a constant state of flux. However, in a practical sense it is this field or transaction that can be observed, studied, and at times altered therapeutically.

In a discussion of psychiatric nursing, it is important to distinguish the *concept of the profession* (its ideals and traditions) from the *practice of the profession* (the formulated technical procedures). In making such a distinction one may discover that there may or may not be a close correlation between the two; that is, there may be advances in theory not widely reflected in practice, and there may be excellent practices that have not as yet been incorporated into known and accepted theory or have not been formulated so that they can be communicated to others.

The word "nurse" has meanings such as to rear, to foster, to take care of, and to nourish. The variety of meanings is indicative of shifts in the concept of nursing. It is notable that the concept of nursing—expressed as the "role" of the nurse—is not always defined with precision. For example, nurse, physician, psychoanalyst, hospital administrator, and patient may give different definitions of the role, suggesting that each has different needs of the nurse and that each sees the person in a certain way, depending on his past experience and current needs.

Psychiatric nursing has certain techniques and practices, which are applicable to a considerable degree to all branches of nursing. The reason for this is that the focus of professional attention has been placed on the transaction between patient and nurse—the interpersonal field. This field—the interpersonal relationship—is characteristic of all medical and nursing activities, although it may at times seem to be greatly minimized by the use of technical procedures and equipment. Prior to a discussion of certain relationships between theory and practice, it may be helpful to outline the trend of psychiatric nursing toward the operational and *interpersonal* approach.

The concept of psychiatric nursing has meaning in terms of the patient and of psychiatry. Also it should be noted that to some extent psychiatric and nursing theory (and, to a possibly lesser extent, practice) reflect current cultural and scientific beliefs and values. This is to say that medicine and nursing are not somehow "professional entities" of themselves but are outgrowths and reflections of the culture in which they exist and to some extent are influential in molding aspects of the culture —its beliefs, practices, and values.

Following are examples of changes in scientific ideas, psychiatric theory, and conceptions of psychiatric nursing:

1. Once those now called mentally disordered were not looked on as ill but were thought to be accursed or sacred. At such a time the afflicted person was thought of as being "wicked" or "possessed"; his care was often turned over to the clergy or the law; he often did not have full human status; he was not hospitalized; and he was not a subject for the attention of physician or nurse.

2. When the mentally disordered came to be designated as sick, the physician and

nurse had roles to play in respect to them. The roles of physician and nurse were somewhat defined, as was that of patient. The concept of disease was undergoing considerable refinement in the nineteenth century. Thus the psychiatric patient and his disorder were quickly fitted into the nineteenth century concept of the doctor-patient-nurse-disease relationships. The characteristics of these concepts were as follows:

a. The disease might be the result of an invasion of the person (as by bacteria), an injury to tissues (trauma), a hereditary-constitutional defect, or a physiological malfunction.

b. The patient was the person who "had" a disease and, as a result, was sick, that is, was removed from a former state of more or less "good health."

c. The physician was required to diagnose and take action for its relief, removing (if possible) the disease from the patient through the application of certain remedies by the use of various techniques.

d. The nurse aided the physician and also took action against disease but was permitted "less professional and more personal" interest. (The last unfortunately was often considered as not satisfactorily scientific; hence it was less highly valued.)

3. Notice in the foregoing that the emphasis in Western European culture is on clearly specified dichotomies and separations of subjects and objects. For example, an attempt was made to clearly distinguish between such concepts as the disease and the person—the one being "inside" or "outside" the other—sickness and health, sane and insane, the person and the environment, the organic and the functional; emphasis was also placed on a clear separation of roles—physician, nurse, patient, and family.

Note also that such attempts at clear-cut separation are not made in all cultures (such as Far Eastern) or even considered to be desirable. This emphasis on dichotomy—on object-subject—was also in keeping with the Newtonian physics of the seven-

teenth century—the concept of energy transmitted from one object to another in clearly comprehended ways and with clearly predictable results. Medicine, including psychiatry, attempted to duplicate such precision and predictability and to a certain degree was successful, but, in all this emphasis on objectivity and precision and scientific method, the patient was at times rendered less human, that is, he might be referred to as "a tubercular" or "a schizophrenic." The *disease* became the subject of interest, or the professional techniques were of greater concern than the person to whom they were applied. For example, a patient might feel abandoned, as his physician and nurse labored to apply *techniques* to "his" disease.

4. A more recent interest in physics has been in such concepts as the "field" (of Einstein and, in addition, Lewin in the behavioral field), a conception of a dynamic interaction of forces in which predictability may not be precise for a particle in the field and in which the observer of the field and his methods of observation are influential in altering the field characteristics. With this trend the emphasis on precise boundaries has diminished, it being increasingly recognized that the boundaries between self and nonself, sane and insane, organic and functional, and person and environment are often tenuous, shifting, and difficult to define. Also the observer, recognizing that his act of observing alters the characteristics of the behavioral field, must then attend to what he does, that is, he is *more* than his role (as physician, nurse, patient); he is not a fixed and static entity in contact or out of contact with other entities but a factor in a dynamic transaction, what he does (and is) being of importance in the character of the transaction.

5. These shifts have led to certain alterations in concepts that are relevant to psychiatric nursing theory and practice. For example:

a. The roles of physician, nurse, and patient are recognized as *not* being static but dynamic, somewhat fluid, reflective of the culture, and to some extent dependent on each other for refinements of definition.

b. The concepts of health and disease are more precisely defined but not so clearly distinguished, and the relationship between disorder, the person, and the environment is more clearly seen.

c. No longer can one clearly separate the patient from his environment; thus the patient's behavior (sick or otherwise) is thought of as depicting or characterizing in a symbolic fashion the family from which he comes and the larger culture of which the family is a part; one can no longer think with assurance that a sick patient comes from a well family.

d. Distinctions between organic and functional or emotional are not emphasized to such an extent, bridging this gap by use of the awkward term "psychosomatic."

e. *Mental disease* is no longer spoken of with enthusiasm, if by that term is meant a disease *within the mind,* since behavior is no longer considered purely a function of the central nervous system. Thus behavior is thought of as having meaning and relevance to past experience and current impinging events; that is, one seeks a greater comprehension of behavior by viewing the field in which it exists.

f. No longer does one think of the nurse's applying a treatment via techniques to remove a disease; the idea that the interpersonal field in which the behavior occurs is of itself significant must be included.

g. It has been observed that the concepts of psychiatry, nursing, and patient are bound by tradition but also are subject to alteration and reflect to a great extent the culture in which they exist and the current scientific ideology. Thus definitions of such concepts will alter with the times and, more importantly, will alter with changing concepts of the human being.

h. Note also that the roles of physician, nurse, and patient cannot be defined apart from each other or from the culture in which they are operative; that is, a nurse *is* such only in terms of a concept of a patient, of psychiatry, and of humanity. The term in and by itself is of no significance. In other words, the term suggests an interpersonal relationship and is best defined operationally in terms of what the nurse does and the image created of self, patient, humanity, and job.

i. Last, the object of our study no longer is the nursing role, technique, the patient, his disease, or the social field, but the interaction characterized as being composed of, in part, nurse-patient-illness-family. In a very practical sense *this field or interaction is what can be observed, defined, and at times altered* "therapeutically."

From a careful consideration of these shifts in psychiatric etiology, it becomes clear that certain available theory and knowledge are relevant to the practice of psychiatric nursing, and from the exploration of this knowledge one can begin to identify and distinguish certain concepts of our profession and in turn see the relationship between these concepts and nursing practice.

As previously stated, the practice of psychiatric nursing deals with a transactional field, composed of persons from whom certain things may be expected. However, because of the past experience of each, predictability cannot be precise, and the interaction is in a state of constant change. This interaction must be continuously observed and evaluated if nurses are to constructively intervene and in doing so develop certain skills.

These skills are the interpersonal skills that are learned in relation to other persons in the developmental process. Further understanding and refinement of these may come through the study of interpersonal theory. Such refinement is essential to psychiatric nursing because the primary focus is the patient—a person who has defects and distortions in his interpersonal skill as a result of his past living. Whether these defects continue, become more deviant, or can be altered constructively will depend to a great extent on his current experience, in which the nurse plays an integral role.

Theoretically, interpersonal skill develops as the result of the timely matching of biological potential and cultural opportunity. This development is a result of the experience the individual has with others in a social field.

The following material will include a synthesis of the important interpersonal skills that evolve in developmental sequence in this process and psychiatric nursing skills as they relate to and are formulated from the conceptual data.

ONE-TO-ONE SKILL—DEPENDENCY

The person, in growing up, first has an interpersonal experience in which he relates in a dependent mode and hopefully does this in relative comfort. He is dependent on others for survival, and out of this experience are developed skills that are basic for his later development. Defects or distortion in dependency skill makes subsequent and more advanced learning difficult if not impossible. Thus it is important to examine carefully what goes on with the infant and his mother during this period when the skill of being *dependent* on someone is fostered and to look carefully at the infant as he gradually moves toward becoming, little by little, separated from his mother, tolerating interference to his wishes with comfort, and struggling to express his need. Herein lie concepts that are relevant to psychiatric nursing practice; out of the understanding of the concepts of these first five brief years of development, when the primary mode of relationships is dependency, comes an important nursing skill—the one-to-one skill.

The patient needs to learn to be dependent in comfort—to learn to count on someone. The nurse needs skill in a one-to-one relationship that allows a dependent mode of interaction and to do this with comfort and alertness that will enable recognition of cues indicating that the patient may be moving toward a less dependent integration. The nurse also needs to have a good understanding of the subtleties involved in the field in which this occurs. Such concepts as empathy, the satisfaction response, se-

curity, and *anxiety,* as it is expressed in the total field, are all in need of particular attention and scrutiny.

To be more specific, many techniques are available to the nurse in developing one-to-one relationships such as unconditional care and acceptance, being with the patient with no expectations, and accepting and responding to communications at the level expressed. These are techniques that are also used by a mother with her infant. One important concept relevant to these mother-infant techniques is the satisfaction response, meaning that the infant has need for care, nourishment, and comfort and the mother has need to give these to the infant in a warm and loving manner. Here is already an interaction—a mutual process. Only then is there a satisfaction response. If this care is given by an anxious mother or as a routine (as with some institutionalized infants), the infant, although cared for, has no satisfaction or comfort from this. In other words, his dependency need is not satisfied in the interpersonal sense, and out of this comes distorted or defective dependency skill. The need not satisfied may be distorted into a longing, and the child continues to attempt only dependent integration long after this has ceased to be acceptable to those in the situation and constructive to his further development.

In nursing a very sick patient (a withdrawn schizophrenic), one who needs a relationship in the dependent mode, it is essential that here, *too,* a satisfaction response be realized. This requirement is a difficult one because of the complexities of the field. First, dependency in our culture is at best discouraged, if not completely rejected, in the adult person. The patient is an adult, having had the range of adult experiences, and to ignore this will be a threat to his already shaky self-esteem (causing anxiety). It is therefore not a matter of assigning a nurse to give care to a patient on a one-to-one basis but of providing a situation in which one-to-one skill can be utilized in a mutually effective way acceptable for both patient and nurse and for the situation in which this care is given. This implies that (1) the concepts relating to dependency are understood by the total staff and that they are aware of the reasons for and values in this care, (2) the nurse's own feelings regarding dependency are considered, and (3) there is an appreciation of the type of anxiety that may be stirred up in the situation and expressed in various ways, such as hostility, resentment, envy, and jealousy. This further implies that acceptable forms of nursing action, which consider the patient and his self-esteem, are employed. As with the infant, much of the interaction and communication is on a nonverbal level, with physical contact, closeness, and tenderness being paramount. Giving physical care is a traditional and extremely acceptable role for the nurse, and it will afford contact with and show concern for the patient. Nurses too often overlook the interpersonal aspects of bathing, dressing, feeding, and attention to bodily complaints of the patient. These situations provide some of the best opportunities for using one-to-one skill in a way that may be mutually satisfying, that is, a satisfaction response is experienced. The nurse who is made anxious in the one-to-one relationship, whether because of personal feelings or because of tension in the ward, cannot be effective with the patient. This anxiety does not escape the patient, and, although he may continue to be dependent, he experiences no comfort or satisfaction but only a further repetition of previous interactions out of which his pathological behavior was patterned. In addition, his doubts regarding the possibility of a useful human relationship are increased.

If the infant has had a good experience with the mothering person, he as a young child begins to reach out on his own a bit and be separate from her for at least short periods of time. In other words, although he still relates in a dependent mode for the most part, he is beginning to see himself as separate from others. Some of this learning comes about when the mother no longer gives unconditional care, that is, distinctions between him and his environment center around indulgence and deprivation. Therefore some deprivation is necessary. It is the extreme of either indulgence or deprivation that is to be avoided. The child also is increasingly able to tolerate interference with his wishes in relation to another person.

The relevance for these concepts in nursing practice can be recognized. The patient, now having some mutual trust and some experience in counting on another person, will be able to move into experiences in which he can learn something about (1) tolerating frustrations with less anxiety and (2) beginning to see himself as a separate person. The nurse does not need to look for or set up elaborate experiences, since they are constantly available in the day-to-day nursing situation. First, the patient must become aware of and accept the limits set for him in the ward situation. This whole area of limit setting is a vital and necessary part of psychiatric nursing. An extensive exploration of this is outside the realm of this discussion. However, the intensive study of the concepts found in interpersonal theory relating to child training and its developmental implications will shed much light on the complexities involved in limit setting and will give some insights on which to base principles for determining the type of limits to be set and techniques involved in their presentation and follow-through. Following is an example: some of the limits that are set for the young child are imposed because of the mother's need or limitations (deprivation). Yet nurses are frequently reluctant to impose limits on patients because it is advantageous for the staff—or at least to give this as the reason for the limit. A mother comfortable as a result of the limit on her child is preferable to an anxious and resentful one and no limit. The important principle here is that the child understands that it is "because I want you to or say so" and not because "it is good for you." When my daughter was nine, she was a very able bicycle rider. She repeatedly asked to ride to the village with her friend. However, the highway was dangerous, and I did not permit her to go, saying: "You're too young," or "It's not safe," always implying that she was not responsible or capable. The requests and refusals to go were repeated daily until I became aware of the real reason: my own discomfort and anxiety. My daughter was able to manage the trip, but I would be too uneasy and worried. When I explained that this was my problem and I was sure she was capable and responsible, she accepted this. The limit was set because of me—not her—and we both understood this. Also, before the summer was over, she was making frequent bicycle trips to the village.

The same clarity should exist in the nursing situation and should be available to both patient and staff. However, the increase in emphasis placed on the therapeutic value of patients being encouraged to make their own decisions, to take increasing responsibility for their own lives, and often to live in an unrestricted (open) setting has created even greater problems in limit setting. Nurses functioning in situations where some limits are inherent in the structure (locked doors or physicians' orders) are less anxious and therefore better able to observe and evaluate their ongoing relationships with patients and to be more aware of the total field of interaction. It is necessary, however, that nurses be aware of this and become more free to set limits because of their own needs and anxieties so that they may be increasingly effective in functioning in a less structured setting. This implies the need for group and individual supervision for nurses, available conference time for planning and evaluating patient care, the opportunity to formulate reasonable nursing goals for patients, and freedom to make decisions and to take action in their implementation. This does not negate the importance of close collaboration with all other members of the therapeutic team but implies that nurses should take increasing responsibility for nursing care and make explicit not only their goals for patients but also the limits that are necessary for constructive patient care and for more effective functioning on the part of the nurse.

In addition to the value of limit setting in effective nursing, limits are essential experiences for the patient in his struggle to identify and accept himself. Out of this one can readily see the destructive influence of rigid rules for all patients or a consistent approach to one patient by all staff members (even were this possible). The patient needs experiences in which he will learn that different persons react in different ways and are treated in different ways. He can then begin to take a look at the behavior

that may elecit these varying responses. A common problem faced in working with patients is that of "splitting" the staff, or playing one staff member against the other. In confronting a patient with a limit a struggle often occurs in which the theme is stated thus: "I can't see why you won't allow this. Miss Jones says it is all right. I guess she is more understanding." The nurse involved may at this point become anxious and attempt to justify her decision by such statements as "It's for your own good" or "I'll talk with your doctor." Another alternative is simply to say, "I'm not Miss Jones and I see we do think differently about this. It may be helpful to both of us to discuss my reasons for this decision." In this there is mutual learning for both the patient and the nurse. It also may discourage the type of splitting that patients are often successful in accomplishing, having had much experience with this in their earlier relationship with their parents.

With the use of techniques other than limit setting, for example, helping a patient to see you as a separate person and then others as separate people, a nurse can help the patient to see himself more clearly as separate. The infant at first sees himself and his mother as one. Gradually he begins to make a distinction, as he becomes aware that at times his mother is apart from him. The cosmic nature of his early perceptions gradually changes; time and space, as well as people, take on different perspective. The schizophrenic patient also has a cosmic type of perception. Straightening out time and space, as well as people, can be done consistently through everyday experiences by way of verbal explanations as to roles, time commitments and schedules, and careful orientations.

GROUP SKILLS—INDEPENDENCE

The child who for the most part is dependent does not engage to any extent in group interactions; although he plays with other children, for the most part this is parallel play up to school age. He then begins to develop more complicated interpersonal skills that will enable him to participate in a group. This transition from dependency to beginning independence is crucial to the child but, if all has gone well, comes about smoothly. In our culture, with the advent of school, the child moves into a group situation with his peers and in this situation begins to develop group skills essential to the second interpersonal learning—learning to become independent.

The transition for the patient is not always so clearly distinguished. Because he has had most of the experiences leading to becoming an adult, he has some group skill or at least can go through the motions of participating in a group. It is therefore important in nursing to have some insight regarding the interpersonal skills of the juvenile and preadolescent developmental periods, during which the person struggles with the task of learning to become independent. Out of these concepts the second important psychiatric nursing skill can be identified and formulated. I refer here to the group skills.

The child learns to become independent through his experiences in the group situation—the family, school, and community setting. He will also use other interpersonal skills of the dependency period to establish further one-to-one relationships but hopefully on a different level of maturity. There will be a real give-and-take relationship first with his peers and later the development of chum relationships with the first beginning of the capacity to love, that is, show the same respect and concern for another as he has for himself.

When the child moves into group experience, he will gradually develop certain interpersonal skills directly concerned with maintaining his security (self-esteem in relation to others) in a group situation.

The first of these is *competition*. The child competes for things, for persons, and for activities or accomplishments. Through this competitive skill he learns more about himself in relation to others.

Another interpersonal skill is *compromise*. Children learn this through daily group situations such as taking turns—first play my game and then I will play yours—and exchange of toys. These early skills are learned and used throughout life in increasingly complicated experiences and in an ever-changing field.

Cooperation is another more advanced skill, the giving up of one's own wishes to enable another to realize his desires. This implies the *beginning of concern for another person*.

The nurse's need for proficiency in group skill is essential both in the care of patients and in working together with other staff members in the situation. These go hand in hand, since the working relationship of the staff is reflected in the total therapeutic program.

Traditionally, nursing was more oriented to working with patients on a one-to-one basis; it was not until a few years ago that the group experience has been recognized as important and consequently given study and consideration.

In programs that focus on the group experience, the trend has been to organize group therapy, patient government projects, and the like. Nurse participation in these endeavors has been encouraged and has proved useful. This trend, however, which has gained ground rapidly in psychiatric centers, has overlooked an extremely useful and readily available part of the patient's care and nursing practice.

It is not necessary to set up artificial situations, since the group experience has been ever present on the ward. Nurses in psychiatry have always worked with groups. It is important to recognize this and to endeavor to make explicit the nature of these group skills. Once again one can refer to the conceptual data available in normal personality growth and development, which can be readily translated into principles for nursing practice.

It is extremely useful for the patient to have experiences in which he can learn to compete, and these are readily available: the patient competes for persons (the personnel on the ward) and their time and attention. He competes for use of facilities such as the television, bathroom, radio, and food. He also competes for position in the group, as well as in organized activities. The skill with which these day-to-day happenings are handled determines their usefulness in terms of the patient's going on to learn the more refined skills of compromise and cooperation.

Many opportunities for compromise and cooperation occur in nursing practice. Compromise, like cooperation, is best handled on a verbal level with patients, as in discussion of ward problems and group participation in their solution.

The nurse's ability to recognize competition and direct it in a useful direction, her skill in assisting patients to arrive at mutually satisfying compromises regarding their daily living together, and her ability to distinguish cooperation that implies real concern for others, as against conformity, are some of the important aspects of group skill.

Little by little, as these experiences are available to the patient, he will be increasingly able to participate effectively in a group, first with anxiety (i.e., loss of self-esteem) and then with a gradual diminution of anxiety. With these experiences his chances for learning to be independent are greatly increased.

PROBLEM-SOLVING SKILLS— INTERDEPENDENCE

Learning to become interdependent is the next interpersonal task that the individual undertakes. Developmentally this struggle begins in adolescence and continues until maturity, which for most of us means for the rest of our lives. Most persons, however, manage to accomplish this to some extent in some area of their living, whether this be in their working situation or in the more intimate one of the family.

Theoretical concepts pertaining to this developmental stage, as in the earlier stages, stress certain interpersonal skills that the person needs to acquire if he is to move from an independent mode of living to becoming interdependent in relation to his fellowman. Those concepts relevant to this discussion can be explained briefly.

The adolescent, after learning to be independent to some extent through the accomplishment of certain skills, is now ready and intensely desirous of again forming one-to-one relationships, first usually with a person of his own sex. If he is successful in this, he will have experience that should give him skill in several important aspects of interpersonal relationships:

1. He will learn to use consensual validation, that is, in reciprocal exchange he will begin freely to share his ideas, attitudes, doubts, and fears with another person and to do this without threat to his own se-

curity. In this way he will come to understand much more about himself and the world and be relieved of guilt feelings and anxieties.

2. He will learn to collaborate first with one person and then later with others in a group. This means that achievement will be no longer a personal success in terms of "I" but a mutual success in terms of "we." He will move from a desire to maintain his position in the group to deriving satisfaction in terms of group accomplishment.

3. The capacity to love, as previously defined, will be further refined and developed during this time. This precedes and is a requirement for the development of the ability to form enduring, intimate relationships.

From the careful study and exploration of these theoretical concepts, the last and probably most important psychiatric nursing skill can be formulated. This is the problem-solving skill so essential in our practice. Persons who are able to develop such skill have had experience in consensual validation and can use this skill freely and tolerate with increasing comfort the fear of loss of security. They also are able to use collaboration with another person and with a group. Finally, they have come to have the same concern about the welfare of others with whom they work as they do about their own, which is, in part, the capacity to love.

The techniques of problem solving in themselves are not difficult to define. They can be as simple as (1) observation of the situation in which the problem exists, (2) discussion and evaluation of this data, (3) formulation of plans of action on the basis of evaluation, with the goal being solution of the problem, and (4) implementation of plan of action and subsequent observation, evaluation of result, and further formulation of action as indicated.

Whether the results of these techniques are a success or failure is not simple. Much depends on understanding the subtleties of the concepts of consensual validation, collaboration, and mutual respect, along with the ability to use these in nursing practice. For example, in working with a clinical problem on the ward, one might ask the following questions about this operation: (1) Does the group exchange ideas and feelings freely with a feeling of security, that is, without the threat of loss of self-esteem? (2) Is there mutual respect for persons, ideas, and opinions? (3) Does individual satisfaction come from group accomplishment or from a desire to maintain status in the group?

In a nursing situation in which the staff has come to work in an interdependent way with each other (at least to some extent), most probably valuable experience will be available to patients. They may begin to be able to share their true feelings without overwhelming anxiety; they may learn that their opinions are heard and considered worthwhile; they may begin clearly to see differences in people, attitudes, and values; they may begin to show the same concern for the welfare of those in a situation that they do for their own. And they may do this because of their everyday experiences, as well as through their therapy.

SUMMARY

Psychiatric nursing is an interaction taking place in a field that is composed of patient, nurse, physician, illness, family, hospital, culture, and other factors. *This field is what can be observed, defined, and at times altered therapeutically.* We cannot separate one part of this field from its totality. It is an ever-shifting, seldom predictable, always reciprocal interaction. The one constant phenomenon is the presence of *anxiety*, although the source, degree of intensity, and mode of expression varies from situation to situation.

The three types of skills inherent in psychiatric nursing as here defined have been formulated as (1) one-to-one skill, (2) group skill, and (3) problem-solving skill.

These skills as such are not new. However, they have been presented from an operational point of view that increases their usefulness in observing, defining, and altering the field in which they are to be used. In addition, the theoretical content from which these skills are formulated has been identified, and an attempt has been made to explicate their implementation and therapeutic usefulness.

These skills do not exist *except* in relation to another person and in an operational field. They are interpersonal skills that have a developmental sequence.

In this chapter, the skills were presented in sequence for conceptual clarity but not to infer that the nurse uses one of these skills in isolation from the others. The nurse uses these skills concomitantly. For example, in caring for a mute, withdrawn patient, one-to-one skill is used. However, this interaction is occurring in a field, the varied events in which constantly influence the interaction. The nurse, if successful in this endeavor, is required to work with the total situation, communicating her experiences with the group and using problem-solving skills in conferences with all members of the therapeutic staff.

In conclusion, historically the practice of psychiatric nursing has been greatly influenced by the etiology and philosophy relating to psychiatry, medicine, and the culture in general. As more scientific knowledge becomes available, the concepts shift and new trends in their application are evolved. Identifying these concepts and distinguishing them from the current practices of the profession and seeing the relationships and the differences that exist, are requirements that seem to have no ending. However, it is a requirement for which nurses have responsibility if they are to lessen some of the existing gap between theory and practice and participate as fully professional members in the total program of psychiatry.

Bibliography

Anderson, J.: The psychology of development and personal adjustment, New York, 1949, Henry Holt & Co.

Blos, P.: The adolescent personality, New York, 1941, D. Appleton Co.

Brill, A. A., editor: The basic writings of Sigmund Freud, New York, 1938, Modern Library, Inc.

Erikson, E. H.: Childhood and society, New York, 1950, W. W. Norton & Co.

Freud, S.: Collected papers, vols. II and V, London, 1948, The Hogarth Press and Institute of Psychoanalysis.

Havighurst, R.: Developmental tasks in education, Chicago, 1948, The University of Chicago Press.

Josselyn, I. M.: Psychosocial development of children, New York, 1949, Family Service Association.

Lief, A.: The common sense psychiatry of Dr. Adolf Meyers, New York, 1948, McGraw-Hill Book Co.

Ribble, M. A.: The rights of infants, New York, 1943, Columbia University Press.

Sullivan, H. S.: Conceptions of modern psychiatry, Washington, D. C., 1947, The William Alanson White Psychiatric Association.

2

Creating chronicity

Lorna M. Barrell

Despite progress in mental hospital care and treatment in the past quarter century, some patients reflect poorly used human resources and potential by their continued residence in institutions. Chronic patients pose special challenges for the planning of nursing care because of behavior that reflects recurring themes of loss, abandonment, and apathy.[32] The following examples of patient care data illustrate variations in planning problems presented by long-term hospitalized mental patients.

Mr. McAdam, a 48-year-old veteran of World War II hospitalized consistently for twelve years, attended a nursing care conference called to review and evaluate his progress and to plan his care and rehabilitation. He was neatly groomed and dressed in a suit; he had been accompanied by a staff member to a nearby city to purchase the suit because of his reluctance to leave the hospital grounds by himself. For the preceding ten years he had lived on an "open" ward and moved freely about the hospital grounds. He had distributed and shelved gym shoes at the hospital gymnasium for nine years as his therapeutic work assignment. In describing his contacts with patients he smiled, and his face was animated. He said the therapists had told him that he did his assignment well. He reported that they often commented on his dependability over the years.

In response to questions posed by the nursing group, he said he had no close patient peers; he felt close to the therapists at the gym. He explained that, although his siblings live in a nearby city, his brother visits only about twice each year because "the roads are bad in winter." He had not been to the city to see his family for a number of years.

His replies in the conference were straightforward. "No, I would not like to leave the hospital." "I don't know what might happen if I lived outside." "Yes, I would like to continue with my current assignment." "Yes, I am satisfied with my hospitalization." "The doctor knows what is best for me."

Mr. McAdam's demeanor was in sharp contrast to that of another patient who was oriented toward using his hospitalization to alter his behavior sufficiently to return to the community. Mr. Sterling, a 51-year-old World War II veteran, spent a total of eight years in mental hospitals. When he was seen in the nursing care conference, he had been in the hospital for three weeks, after having been out of the hospital for one year. Like Mr. McAdam, Mr. Sterling had never married. He, too, lived in the nearby city; however, he identified no close family or friendly relationships outside the hospital. During the past year he had lived in a residential hotel, eaten his meals in restaurants, and worked as a package deliveryman.

In the conference he was neatly groomed in cotton trousers and sport shirt. He responded to all questions, although his speech was somewhat slow and his voice was low. When asked how he was feeling before he decided to return to the hospital, he said, "I was feeling tense. I guess I was feeling a little depressed, too; it's pretty lonely there." Had he tried to meet people? "Yes, I went to the Sunday evening club at the church in the area and I'd go over to the YMCA. I knocked on my neighbor's door once to borrow a Band-Aid. I'd see people at work, too." Did he feel he had anyone to talk with or a consistent place for socializing? "No."

Unlike Mr. McAdam, Mr. Sterling did

not know what he would like to do in the hospital; he would like to get back to his job as soon as possible.

Although Mr. McAdam and Mr. Sterling reflect different orientations to hospitalization, the critical issues for each include how he sees himself as a patient, how he perceives the hospital, what he wants and expects from the hospital, and how he feels he will have to change to be mentally well. The range of potential meaning of the mental hospital for patients such as these two gentlemen is limitless. In one sense the patient is a client seeking the services that will restore his mental health, or he may see himself as imprisoned, an inmate, deprived of rights and privileges, with restoration of his mental health not high in priority.[13] The mental patient becomes a part of the professional organization in which he seeks treatment. As a hospitalized patient he holds a kind of membership or position in the organization structure. He is provided with services, but claims are made on him. Thus he is accorded limited rights that are defined in relation to the hospital's authority.

Being a patient further carries a wide range of meanings not only for the patient, the occupant of the role position, but also for others who are in contact with him. Whether the patient sees himself as a client, prisoner, or student, his point of view is a major determining factor in his movement toward achieving health. Because of his ascribed position in the total organization, the work of the patient toward self-change may be facilitated or hindered by the role expectation of the patient himself, of his family, of staff members, or of other patients.[13]

The need exists for the individual to come to terms with himself and with the hospital in molding his role. Mr. McAdam's resolution was to stay in the hospital beyond the period of acute illness; Mr. Sterling, on the other hand, used the hospital for self-change and return to the community. Facilitating the patient's work toward recovery, whatever his motivation, is the formal obligation of the mental hospital to society.

The philosophies and goals of mental hospitals began to change some years ago. They now emphasize intensive treatment and the ward milieu. Previously the mental hospital was a catchall, accepting society's casualties. Patients given no responsibility became more dependent and lethargic and lost hope and initiative. Estrangement from family and the outside world was fostered by long absences. To some degree times have changed, although reversing the effects of institutionalization is more difficult than preventing the situation in the first place. Hospitalization is a social as well as a medical experience in which the milieu can help or hinder the recovery of the patient. The process of change is slow because the existing order is challenged and because of the complementarity of the roles of staff and patients. A shift in one has impact on the other.[20]

A hard-core group of chronically ill mental patients still occupies most mental hospital beds. They are not participants in the current upsurge of discharge rates and currently constitute about two thirds of the resident hospital population.[21]

The responsibility for the care of these long-term hospitalized mental patients is in large measure that of the nursing staff. Holmes[8] defines therapy as the process of interaction with patients as well as the mutual study of the interaction. In this way it is possible to help the patient see himself in relationship to the staff and to other significant people in his life outside the hospital. Therefore the hospitalization can be used to help the patient learn to live more effectively with other people. The patient's job or work role in the psychiatric hospital is to gain some understanding of what his personality is like and what changes in that personality will make for a more adequate personal adjustment. The staff are responsible for assisting the patient in accepting his work role and for helping him to accomplish his task, since whatever changes occur in the patient's adjustment must come from within himself.[8] Identification of patients' role conceptions, therefore, helps nurses and other caregivers develop more constructive plans for intervention to contribute more effectively to the modification of role expectation and to the reduction of the patients' length of hospital stay.

CONCEPTS EXPLAINING THE CHRONICITY PROCESS

Analysis of the concepts of role, socialization, psychiatric nursing, and therapeutic milieu relates directly to the process of institutionalization of patients. For example, the role that patients assume and perform, their learned adjustment to the hospital social system, their relationships with psychiatric nurses, and the meaning of the hospital world and the therapeutic milieu comprise the critical components of patients' hospitalization experiences.

Socialization

Socialization is simply the process by which an individual learns to adjust to a group by acquiring social behavior of which the group approves.[6] This concept is used primarily in the fields of child development and social psychology. Its meaning in the two fields coincides.

Socialization begins at birth and continues in the family with the child's behavior becoming similar to that of family members and socially appropriate for that group.[3,28] For example, the child learns about orderliness according to the norm of neatness that is required in his home, he learns eating habits and table manners, and he learns to interact with his parents and other adults.

According to Brown,[2] socialization includes selectivity, which is determined by the child's experiences and intellect at a given point in time. Furthermore, the child processes what he perceives to be the behavior of mature members of his society. This extends the process beyond one generation's giving the next generation an encapsulated, static system of norms, or lessons for behavior. Socialization does not end with childhood.[12] Whereas some of the early socializing experiences are lasting, others are short lived and are overlaid with new learnings because of new life requirements.

The use of the concept of socialization in social psychology continues along Lambert's[12] line of thought that socialization does not end with childhood. Similarly socialization is described by Clausen[3] as a process of learning, beginning at birth and continuing throughout life, including the acquisition of personal and group loyalties and the knowledge, skills, and feelings necessary for adult role performance in the private and public life of an individual. Socialization for some individuals is an active process in which they work with their experience to influence their destinies. For others, socialization is an ongoing process of which they are passive recipients. This point is illustrated by the following examples: A young woman entering a collegiate nursing program is socialized into both the role of college student and the role of the nurse. In both instances she acquires knowledge, skills, and feelings necessary for appropriate adult role performance. As a college student she learns values of study, of social life, of school loyalty, and how to relate to faculty, housemothers, and peers. As a result, in or out of the college setting she behaves unmistakably as a college student. At the same time she is learning to be a nurse. Here the socialization includes recognizing her feelings about herself as a caregiver and learning how she feels about patients, physicians, and other persons, as well as her knowledge and feelings about health and illness, birth and death, her skills as a practitioner, and loyalties to the profession, to nurses, and to other persons. These two role situations reflect active commitment and participation in the socializing process. The socialization of a patient in a mental hospital illustrates the passive process.

The individual admitted to a psychiatric unit for treatment has limited ideas of what it means to be a patient, what he needs, what help is available, who gives it, and what the signs of progress are. However, in that setting he learns that he is told what to eat, when to sleep, when medicines are given, what activities are good for him, to whom he may talk, and when he may visit with his family and make phone calls. Thus socialization leads into a more helpless and dependent state, in which, if he complies, he is regarded as a cooperative patient and soon fits into the system. He, too, has acquired the loyalties, knowledge, skills, and feelings necessary for acceptable, albeit immature, role performance in a setting, although he has not actively invested in the process of his socialization.

In summary, the concept of socialization describes a process beginning at birth and continuing throughout life, in which the individual learns social behavior appropriate to a given situation or group setting, personal and group loyalties, and knowledge, skills, and behavior that coincide with those of the family or group of which he is a member.

Role

A further elaboration of the concept of socialization, especially that of an individual into the role of patient, leads to consideration of the result of the process—the acceptance and performance of the patient role. The following discussion of the concept of role focuses on these attributes: Role is learned behavior[26] and is the end product of socialization.[5] Roles do not occur in isolation but are the result of interactional, reciprocal, complementary processes.[25,26] Role performances and their interdependence contribute to the stability of a social system.[9,19]

Role, a concept found in the fields of sociology, social psychology, and anthropology, is a metaphor borrowed from the theater; it suggests that public conduct is associated with certain "parts" or statuses.[25] Role enactment occurs in social situations with others.[5] Human beings, Sarbin[25] explains, acting to locate themselves accurately in their environments, make choices among behavior alternatives. Using available knowledge and cues, the individual, locating himself in a social system, infers the role of others and concurrently his own role. The individual identifies his place in the social system through a reciprocal process that implies relationships and complementarity. For example, the following roles are complementary: mother-child, teacher-student, and nurse-patient. Mead[17] proposed that both members of the interacting pair learn both roles. When a nurse and patient are together, the nurse gives cues about the kinds of behavior she considers appropriate for the patient; simultaneously, the patient must learn about her motives and feelings to respond appropriately. The patient's ability to perceive what

the nurse expects of him in a situation means he has learned something of the nurse's role. In the course of their interaction the two come to understand each other and to act in their own roles, while understanding the role and anticipating the behavior of the other.

According to Sarbin,[25] status, or position, is an abstraction or set of beliefs defined by the expectations held by members of the relevant society; role, on the other hand, is a set of public modes of behavior enacted by an individual to make good his occupancy of a particular status, or position. Role includes the cultural patterns associated with a particular status, including attitudes, values, and behavior ascribed by the society to all persons occupying the status.[14] The role of patient is the patterning of behaviors and attitudes that patients are expected to show in the hospital in their status as patients.[25] The status of mental patients is an abstraction defined by the mental hospital community, both patients and staff, and by the general public.

The example of the individual in the learned role of mental patient, performed on the basis of the patient status, provides an additional illustration. During the time the individual is in the active status of patient, his statuses as worker, father, husband, adult male, and friend are latent. The roles associated with these latent statuses temporarily recede and are held in abeyance, although they continue to be integral parts of the individual's cultural equipment.[14] The individual unconsciously adjusts the roles associated with each of these statuses, and normally no conflict results. To have a role means establishing one's relationship with others and having an established place in the social scheme of things. This outer structuring provides essential continuing support for inner structuring, or personality integration.[24]

Social systems require members to play certain roles; the systems will not produce the intended results unless roles are adequately played.[9] A social system may foster the individual's playing a role well and may regard the individual as normal but be contributing to an unhealthy personality. The hospital system requires participants (staff and patients) to play certain roles. For example, the hospital social system is in the business of giving care and delivering health services. Therefore for the system to work, certain members of the system must give care and others, receive it. An individual patient, then, may play his patient role satisfactorily and meet all the requirements of the patient role but not be regarded as healthy or be contributing to the restoration of his health by the acting of the patient role. Likewise a staff member may administer care and be regarded as expert in its delivery but be jeopardizing the patient's restoration of health by not permitting independent action by the patient in his own behalf. The system, therefore, is in some ways self-limiting and self-defeating. If the fit, or complementarity, is so adequate, with the patient playing the patient role and the staff playing staff role, the system leaves little room for growth, and groups will maintain stable characteristics because of the regularities of the members' behavior toward one another.[19]

In a study of institutional dependency, Lipsitt[15] describes the reciprocal nature of the roles of the long-term hospitalized patient and the staff. He suggests that patients and staff enter into a contractual agreement that requires each to fulfill the role ascribed to him by the others, whether that role be fact or fantasy. For example, he suggests that the patient forfeits individuality, initiative, and self-esteem, whereas the institution guarantees protection, food, and shelter.

Expansion of the concept of role, including that of the hospitalized mental patient, leads to exploration of the concept of patienthood as it ties into the role. Levinson and Gallagher[13] studied the efforts of the patient to deal with his situation in the hospital: the actual situation of the patient within the hospital system, his adaptation to his hospital life, and his personality. Role in their study is the linking concept between the individual's personality and the hospital social structure. The patient, as a member of the hospital world and as an occupant of a defined position, progresses through formation and enactment of a social role.

The work of patienthood in accomplishing the organizational role and career is adaptation to problematic role issues. The work includes adapting to role issues such as the following: What is the way to recovery? What constitutes an ideal mental patient and hospital? In what way is the hospital good or bad for me? What is wrong with me? What are other patients like? What do I need in my everyday hospital life? The task of working on role issues is problematic for both patients and staff and is dependent on the patient's needs and investment, as well as on the staff's availability, skills, and investment. For the patient, every role issue presents a task, in that he must adapt to it in some way. His personal role definition, including both internal and external influences, determines how he adapts. External demands and opportunities, as well as intrapersonal determinants, influence the patients' conceptions of patienthood and the uses they make of it.

In summary, to aid in explaining the behavior of patients in mental hospitals, it is useful to consider the concept of role. Referring to the simple economic principle of division of labor within an organization, a task is to be accomplished; in the mental hospital, this task is giving care, which is distributed among members of the system. For staff members the mental hospital is a place of work, where they learn and ply their trade, perform useful services, and make a living. On the other hand, for patients the mental hospital is a setting in which they learn and perform their role as clients and recipients of the services and ministrations of the staff. The resulting interactive adjustment leads to more or less stable behavior patterns. Roles of staff and patients consequently are interdependent, and the extent to which stability is maintained in the system limits the growth potential for both.

The role of the patient is the patterning of behaviors and attitudes that patients are expected to show in the hospital in their status. The patient's role conception, that is, his view of himself as a patient, his reaction to the role issues or tasks on which he must work, and his enduring personality traits are the significant aspects of patienthood that influence his use of hospitalization.

Psychiatric nursing

Discussion of the concepts of role, especially the role of hospitalized patients and their patienthood, and socialization in the hospital setting leads to consideration of the complementary concept of psychiatric nursing. To establish a framework for developing this concept, a broad definition of nursing is included. The distinctive feature of nursing practice is the doing for or along with a person that which he or his family would but are unable to do for a time or for all time. The nurse, Kreuter[11] continues, identifies and meets, in varying degrees, needs of the person, so that he may achieve or resume his position in society, function within the limitations imposed by his illness, or comfortably conclude his lifespan. The unique function of the nurse is to assist the individual in the performance of activities contributing to health or its recovery that he would perform unaided if he had the necessary strength, will, or knowledge and to do so in such a way as to help him gain independence as rapidly as possible.[7] To do for someone something he might learn to do for himself is to keep him weak, disabled, and dependent and consequently results in a waste of potential human resources.[10]

Furthermore, nursing is an interpersonal process in which the professional nurse practitioner assists an individual or family to prevent or cope with the experience of illness and suffering and, if necessary, assists the individual or family to find meaning in these experiences.[31] Additionally nursing's concern is sustaining the patient in his experience of struggle in overcoming his illness and in dealing with life issues, such as making the best of his personality, finding a place for himself in the community, being a good parent, and living within the confines of his handicap. The nurse's intervention may help the patient go beyond tolerating the experience into examining, understanding, and integrating the experience into his life.[32]

From the general reference point in which nursing provides care for patients, to the degree they are unable to care for themselves, the concept of psychiatric nursing may be viewed on a continuum that extends from simply helping patients accept themselves and improve their relationships with other persons[18] to more sophisticated psychotherapeutic counseling with patients.[22] Psychiatric nursing is service to people with pathological thought processes or personality disorders that interfere with healthy living.[30] The goals of psychiatric nursing include prevention of mental illness and detection, treatment, and rehabilitation of persons with psychiatric disorders.[16] The essence of psychiatric nursing is the therapeutic use of self. The main focus of psychiatric nursing is on developing a beneficial relationship with the patient to effect improvement in his competence in living with himself and others.[8,30] Through the process of communication between nurse and patient, the latter acquires better understanding of the consequences of his behavior. This psychiatric nursing process includes the following steps: observing behavior, evaluating the patient's needs, intervening based on the identified needs and behavior, and appraising the results of intervention in view of subsequent nursing.[27] In addition to the psychotherapeutic counseling of patients and customary nursing functions, psychiatric nursing includes managing, teaching, and socializing activities with patients.[23]

In summary, psychiatric nursing, as a part of the broader concept of general nursing, is distinguished by the nurses' therapeutic use of self, helping patients cope more effectively with life problems and relate more effectively to other people. This communication process is characterized by shared problem solving, which continues until the patient is able to function independently.

Therapeutic milieu

The conceptual focus to this point has been on the individual as he is socialized into the patient role in a mental hospital and on the complementary concept of psychiatric nursing. As previously described, a patient enters a mental hospital and adapts to and is integrated into the social structure. The concept of therapeutic milieu is presented because of its unifying characteristics in this process. Simply, the therapeutic milieu includes the aspects of the society and culture of the ward or hospital that may be influential in reducing behavioral disturbances of patients.[29] Furthermore, it involves the scientific manipulation of the environment to produce changes in patients' personalities.[4] As a small segment of society that resembles the larger social system, the distinctive features include (1) patients' inclusion in information-sharing processes, (2) patients' participation in decisions about one another, and (3) patients' participation in the democratic community process, which is regarded as treatment. In the therapeutic milieu all forces are deemed relevant, and treatment is the responsibility of everyone.[8]

Ideally, the environment offers to patients practice areas for learning more adaptive patterns of behavior: crisis resolution (problem solving) and role performance for functioning in society. Involvement in the ward provides an array of experiences for problem resolution and role enactment. For example, a patient may work on the problem of developing social skills by relating first with one staff member and then with small groups of staff and patients in a setting that offers familiarity and support; opportunity for role-repertoire expansion is provided in the same setting, in which the individual may move from the role of isolate to one of active participation in leadership in a patient group. The milieu provides information, facilities, support, freedom of action, and protection against too severe consequences of failure.[4]

According to Cumming and Cumming,[4] in the therapeutic milieu the patient is defined as actor, initiator, cooperator, and manager of his own affairs; others assist him in this process. This differs from the caregiver-care recipient arrangement of traditional settings. Staff in this setting contribute a wider variety of roles and models of more integrated functioning. For example, when a patient observes a nurse participating constructively in her work role, the patient is learning her attitude and her commitment to the world of work. Nurses can use their skills in cooperation with patients rather than on them. To be of enduring value, hospitalization must be used by patients, staff, and families to work on the problems that interfere with the patients' leading useful, enjoyable lives.[8]

The therapeutic milieu includes forces that provide patients with opportunities to practice more adaptive patterns of behavior in a protected setting. Since the staff invests time and effort in the patients' behalf, the two groups are collaborators. Therapeutic milieu, therefore, is a prime determining factor in the patients' use of hospitalization and consequently contributes to patients' progress and reduced length of hospital stay.

In the foregoing analyses of the concepts of socialization, role, psychiatric nursing, and therapeutic milieu, the following potential sources of difficulty for institutionalized mental patients are recognizable: the learning, over time, in personal interaction the norms, knowledge, skills, and feelings for the role, the performance as a mental patient. The societal norms accepted are those of a deviant population—the care receiver in a mental hospital. Furthermore, the individual acquires his role in relation to others; his career, or occupation, of patienthood is taught by others in the hospital setting. The reciprocal process that occurs between staff and patients has potential for helping or harming patients, depending on the investment the patient makes and is permitted to make in learning more adaptive patterns of behavior relevant to healthy coping in modern society. The patients' learning is also dependent on the skill and commitment of the caregivers.

How effectively an individual patient uses his hospitalization depends on many factors, including the patient's fundamental capacity for growth, learning a role, and development of a healthy mature personality; the nature of the role that is deemed appropriate for the patient in the hospital into which he is socialized; and the nature and effectiveness of the process of his socialization into that patient role.

Summary of the process

An individual enters a mental hospital because of personal discomfort or disequilibrium. As the individual enters the mental hospital, he must learn about a new social system. Through interaction with patients and staff he learns group attitudes, expectations, and norms. He reacts in the setting and gets feedback from the group. He synthesizes the information and integrates it with present and past experiences; he makes further judgments about what is regarded as appropriate behavior in the setting. He learns to achieve the aim of appropriate behavior and to demonstrate loyalty to the hospital society's group norms. At this point he has been socialized into the patient role.

In this role he acquires the attitudes and learns behaviors that are ascribed by patients, staff, and the community to the position, or status, of mental patient. During his hospitalization, other life roles are held in abeyance and not enacted. Assumption of the patient role leads in some ways to greater comfort for him and for the hospital system. The patient enacts his role, and the staff surrounding him enact their roles; thus the care-receiving and care-giving complementarity lend stability to the social system. This stability may, however, limit the usefulness of hospitalization for the patients' healthy growth.

Among the caregivers in the mental hospital system are psychiatric nurses. Their role is to give care to the patient that he and his family are unable to give, toward the goal of helping him resume his position in society. Through the development of a helpful relationship and the process of communication, the nurse assists the patient to acquire better understanding of his behavior and skills in coping more effectively with life problems.

All forces in the mental hospital are relevant to the patient's care; in a therapeutic milieu the environment is structured and manipulated to produce changes in patients. Essentially the therapeutic milieu provides patients with opportunities to practice more adaptive patterns of behavior: problem solving and role performance for more constructive functioning in society.

Why some patients use their hospitalization in their own behalf whereas others do not continues to be a key issue in hospital psychiatry. To be of lasting value, patients, staff, and families must work on problems that interfere with the patient's leading a useful, enjoyable life. To utilize his patienthood he needs to come to terms with problematic role issues that stem from the institutional structure, his situation in it, and his needs as an individual.

IMPACT OF CONCEPTUAL KNOWLEDGE ON CLINICAL PRACTICE

Understanding the process of creating chronicity contributes to rational clinical practice. The major role task of patienthood is self-change, for which staff and patients bear joint responsibility. Nursing bears major responsibility for the care of long-term mental patients, since in most hospital settings the nursing personnel provide the continuing care. Nursing shares with all caregivers the obligation to help patients develop more fully as persons.

Two broad principles for practice are generated from knowledge of the development of chronicity. It is the joint task of patients and staff to work toward a consensus of the goals of hospitalization as a growth experience for both patients and staff. The ease and danger of falling into an intuitive, assumed, and therefore routinized approach to working with patients is acknowledged. An all-giving, all-caring helping experience locks patients as well as staff into producing in the patient a helpless dependency. The first principle is that conscious and continuous assessment of the patient's present level of functioning, of his progress, and of the milieu by all (patients and staff), as well as constant encouragement of the patient's active achievement, can lead to the development of the hospital experience as a constructive, active force in the treatment process.

The second general principle is that of the necessity of conscious awareness of the socialization process and of the power of reciprocity and complementarity in a social system. Intervention or disruption of the socialization process can potentially and legitimately occur at any point in the process. Therefore it should be possible for treatment of patients in mental hospitals to occur without leading to their deep and enduring commitment to the passive-dependent patient role. This more active approach, however, requires the shared responsibility, active investment by both staff and patients, and constant change and evaluation of approach for the patients' continuous growth. This potentially involves experiences for both patients and staff of not knowing and consequently of anxiety. But it does achieve more constructive life roles. Changes in existing hospital systems are slow to occur because a change in one part of the system (staff or patients) has impact on all other areas of the system. The broadest implication from this knowledge then is that to endeavor to avoid having patients reach long-term patienthood and to have staff avoid reaching the steady state of automatic care giving is indispensable.

Three specific principles for nursing intervention are indicated from the knowledge of the chronicity process. Good patient care is the aim of all nursing, which provides care for a patient as long as he is unable to provide care for himself; the goal of nursing is to assist the patient to resume his place in society and to function at the highest level possible within the limitations of his illness. Therefore nurses need to assess intelligently the needs of patients at the time of admission and throughout hospitalization and constantly to seek to answer the following questions: (1) Is care being provided for the patient that he could provide for himself? (2) In view of the patient's current needs, what is the next reasonable learning step for him in his move toward health and greater active mastery of his experiences?

In addition to assessment, the second principle for nursing is the establishment of therapeutic relationships with psychiatric patients aimed at reversal or avoidance of chronicity and dependency. Since the essence of psychiatric nursing is the therapeutic use of self through the development of a relationship and through the communication process, the patient can be expected to acquire better understanding of himself and his behavior. Furthermore, he can learn to cope more effectively with life problems and relate more effectively to other people by moving in the relationship from shared to independent problem solving.

The work of the patient is to learn more adaptive patterns of behavior, and the work of the nurse is to help him in his effort; however, it is the patient's right and obligation to assume large measures of responsibility for his treatment. The third nursing principle, then, is for nurses consciously to expect patients to maintain their responsibility and active involvement from the day of admission. Too few demands are placed on patients. Patients need to be asked to identify immediate and long-range personal goals for their hospitalization that are commensurate with their present level of mastery. Nursing can contribute to the disruption of the stable state of noninvestment and relative contentment in the institution by expecting patients to share in the establishment of nursing care goals for themselves, as opposed to being passive recipients of a plan developed by nursing. To extend this principle for nursing in supporting patients' maintenance of responsibility is to plan to assist patients consciously to use all experiences within the life space of the hospital as learning for subsequent life outside the institution. This could be accomplished by identifying with patients the meaning and usefulness of activities for them as a part of the everyday hospital experience.

SUMMARY

Mental hospitals over time have become human warehouses, containing individuals who have handled their patienthood in passive-dependent ways, through socialization into the roles of good, compliant, conforming individuals who prefer structured environments and nonchallenging relationships with patients and staff. This routinization of life and passivity preclude their return to active work and productivity in society. The evolution of this process of chronicity and institutionalization can be understood through inspection and integration of the concepts of socialization, role, psychiatric nursing, and therapeutic milieu. Ayllon[1] suggests, "The major objective of the hospital of tomorrow should be to generate in the patients a desire to rejoin the human family by way of acquiring skills with which to maintain themselves after their release." Conscious and explicit clinical practice can contribute to more thoughtful rational care of hospitalized mentally ill individuals. It is essential for good patient care and generally for a healthy society that persons refine their capacity and habit of engaging their fellow men in active decision making and in interactive processes that lead to continuous personality growth and independence.

References

1. Ayllon, T.: Toward a new hospital psychiatry. In Abroms, G. M., and Greenfield, N. S., editors: The new hospital psychiatry, New York, 1971, Academic Press.
2. Brown, R.: Social psychology, New York, 1965, The Free Press.
3. Clausen, J. A., editor: Socialization and society, Boston, 1968, Little Brown & Co.
4. Cumming, J., and Cumming, E.: Ego and milieu, New York, 1962, Atherton Press.
5. Goffman, E.: Encounters, Indianapolis, 1961, The Bobbs-Merrill Co., Inc.
6. Gould, J., and Kolb, W. L.: A dictionary of the social sciences, New York, 1964, The Free Press.
7. Henderson, V.: Nature of nursing, New York, 1966, The Macmillan Co.
8. Holmes, M. J., and Werner, J. A.: Psychiatric nursing in a therapeutic community, New York, 1966, The Macmillan Co.
9. Jourard, S. M.: The transparent self, Princeton, 1964, D. Van Nostrand Co., Inc.
10. Kennedy, J. F.: The role of the university in the building of a flexible world order, Charter Day address, University of California, Berkeley, March 23, 1962, Department of State Bulletin 46:615, 1962.
11. Kreuter, F. R.: What is good nursing care? In Viewpoints on curriculum development, New York, 1957, National League for Nursing.
12. Lambert, W. W., and Lambert, W. E.: Social psychology, Englewood Cliffs, N. J., 1964, Prentice-Hall, Inc.
13. Levinson, D. J., and Gallagher, E. B.: Patienthood in the mental hospital, Boston, 1964, Houghton Mifflin Co.
14. Linton, R.: Concept of role and status. In Newcomb, T. M., and Hartley, E. L., editors: Readings in social psychology, New York, 1947, Henry Holt & Co.
15. Lipsitt, D. R.: Institutional dependency—a rehabilitation problem. In Greenblatt, M., Levinson, D. J., and Klerman, G. L., editors: Mental patients in transition, Springfield, Ill., 1961, Charles C Thomas, Publisher.
16. Matheney, R., and Topalis, M.: Psychiatric nursing, ed. 5, St. Louis, 1970, The C. V. Mosby Co.
17. Mead, G. H.: Mind, self, and society, Chicago, 1934, University of Chicago Press.
18. Mereness, D., and Karnosh, L.: Essentials of psychiatric nursing, St. Louis, 1966, The C. V. Mosby Co.
19. Newcomb, T. M., Turner, R. H., and Converse, P. E.: Social psychology, the study of human interaction, New York, 1965, Holt, Rinehart & Winston, Inc.
20. Padula, H.: Approaches to the care of long-term mental patients, Washington, D. C., 1968, The Joint Information Service of the American Psychiatric Association and the National Association for Mental Health.
21. Paul, G. L.: Chronic mental patient: current status—future direction, Psychol. Bull. 71:81, 1969.
22. Peplau, H. E.: Interpersonal techniques: the crux of psychiatric nursing practice, Am. J. Nurs. 62:50, 1962.
23. Peplau, H. E.: Therapeutic functions. Presented at Eastern Regional Conference of National League for Nursing Project, Washington, D. C., April 16-20, 1956.
24. Polansky, N. A., White, R. B., and Miller, S. C.: Determinants of the role image of the patient in a psychiatric hospital. In Greenblatt, M., Levinson, D. J., and Williams, R. H.: The patient and the mental hospital, Glencoe, Ill., 1957, The Free Press.
25. Sarbin, T. R.: The scientific status of the mental illness metaphor. In Plog, S. C., and Edgerton, R. B., editors: Changing perspectives in mental illness, New York, 1969, Holt, Rinehart & Winston, Inc.
26. Sarbin, T. R., and Allen, L.: Role theory. In Lindzey, G., and Aronson, E., editors: The handbook of social psychology, Reading, Mass., 1968, Addison-Wesley Publishing Co., Inc.
27. Schwartz, M. S., and Shockley, E. L.: The nurse and the mental patient, New York, 1956, John Wiley & Sons, Inc.
28. Sears, R. R., Maccoby, E. E., and Levin, H.: Patterns of childrearing, Evanston, 1957, Row, Peterson & Co.
29. Stainbrook, E.: Milieu therapy. In Freedman, A. M., and Kaplan, H. I., editors: Comprehensive textbook of psychiatry, Baltimore, 1967, The Williams & Wilkins Co.
30. Statement on psychiatric nursing practice, New York, 1967, American Nurses' Association.
31. Travelbee, J.: Interpersonal aspects of nursing, Philadelphia, 1966, F. A. Davis Co.
32. Ujhely, G.: Determinants of the nurse-patient relationship, New York, 1968, Springer Publishing Co., Inc.

3

Jean: a clinical case study

Patricia M. Baren

Jean, 31 years of age, was admitted to the state hospital in March, 1971, and discharged in February, 1972. I became involved in Jean's case in September, 1971, as a part of my clinical work in graduate school. I know little about Jean except what I learned in an eight-month period through my relationship with her. What little history I was able to obtain prior to my involvement with Jean remained unchanged with few details added.

Jean was born in Hong Kong. She was the youngest of seven children and the only child who was educated through high school. Jean is the only child by her mother's second husband, who apparently died when Jean was approximately 2 years old. After Jean completed high school, she taught kindergarten until her marriage. Jean often speaks of the fact that she was very spoiled as a child because she was able to have an education.

Twelve years before our meeting Jean married and came to this country with her husband. Their marriage had been arranged through one of Jean's cousins. Jean and her husband, Mr. M, had not known one another prior to their marriage. It is for this reason that Mr. M is unable to give any information regarding Jean's early history. Mr. M does state, however, that her adjustment to this country was minimal throughout her first year in America. She would accompany Mr. M to various places, but she often was withdrawn and preoccupied.

Approximately a year after the marriage, Jean gave birth to the couple's first child, Sara. Four months after the birth of Sara, Jean was admitted to a private psychiatric hospital in an acute psychotic episode. She was diagnosed as schizophrenic, catatonic type. She received six electroshock treatments and was discharged. In 1963 she was

readmitted to another private psychiatric hospital in an apparent psychotic episode. After a short hospitalization, she was discharged. From 1964 through 1968 Mr. M sent Jean back to Hong Kong twice, hoping this would help her. On the last visit Jean stayed for a year, and the couple's second child was born while she was there. In 1968 Mr. M sought private outpatient treatment for Jean. In a three-month period she received eleven electroshock treatments. Treatment was stopped when Mr. M went bankrupt. There was apparently no psychiatric treatment until Jean was admitted to the state hospital.

Mr. M was also born in China to Chinese parents, but he was raised by an American couple. Mr. M states that he has no family. He came to America during the revolution in China in the early fifties. In the early sixties he returned to China to marry a girl of Chinese descent. He returned to America and began his own produce business, which was quite successful until his bankruptcy in 1968. Since that time, the family has lived in very modest circumstances. Mr. M has started the business again, but the profits are small.

Mr. M has been described by people in the community and by various professional people involved in Jean's case as isolated, not only from Jean, but also from the community. Mr. M never visited Jean while she was hospitalized, and he was quite reluctant to talk with any professional person regarding her case. There appears to be a minimal relationship between Mr. M and Jean. Jean is frightened of Mr. M and will only talk with him when it is absolutely necessary. Although Jean is at home since her discharge, the couple remain isolated from one another. Mr. M spends all his available time at work.

Jean was committed to the state hospital

after she threatened her neighbors with a meat cleaver because she felt they were trying to poison her children. She was diagnosed as schizophrenic, paranoid type. When I entered the case, the staff described Jean as depressed and tearful, isolated, and suspicious. The community team to which Jean was assigned thought her isolation and regression would increase unless a relationship could be established with her. Jean's isolation from the staff and other patients was increased not only by her schizophrenic communication but also by her inability to communicate clearly in English. Jean rarely caused any trouble on the unit or even expressed her needs. In other words, she blended quietly into the ward routine. The staff was concerned about Jean, but patients with more alarming needs often received the staff's attention before Jean.

When I first met Jean, she was sitting quietly on the unit with her head down. She was dressed in clothing provided by the hospital. Her dress was long and tight; she wore what looked to be an army fatigue jacket and held a battered purse close to her. A pair of tennis shoes, tattered and full of holes, were only half on her feet. She looked up when I introduced myself and told her I would like to talk with her a while. At first she was reluctant, stating she did not speak good English and could not understand. After some persuasion she accompanied me to a small room, where our interviews were held throughout her stay at the hospital. She sat with her head down during the entire interview, only glancing at me occasionally. She continually scratched her legs. She questioned anxiously why she had been brought to "this place." When asked about her family, she stated, "I don't know about it." She talked with me for twenty minutes and then left the room. I was left staring into space, wondering who this person was who had been sitting with me only minutes earlier. She had been very difficult to understand. I had great difficulty understanding her English, let alone her manner of presenting her communication. Much time was spent trying to be sure I understood words that I then had to put into phrases. This took the utmost attention and con-

centration. In this endeavor I had forgotten the feeling tone with which the words were spoken. She had been terribly anxious—unable to sit still or to maintain any silence. I wondered if I would ever understand Jean and if she would allow me to enter a relationship with her.

Will has written as follows of the need for human relatedness for survival in whatever man does:

> The schizophrenic reaction may be looked upon as the expression of complicated patterns of behavior adopted by the organism in an effort to deal with a gross inadequacy in relating to other humans, the appearance of the clinical syndrome being a late expression of the accumulating disasters of many years.*

Will goes on to state that intimacy with others involves anxiety, but a failure to move toward intimacy brings a threat of loneliness and unrelatedness. In addition, relatedness helps to define self, and, as self is defined, the anxiety that surrounds relatedness diminishes. He states the reason as follows:

> Only as man can accept himself and his relatedness to others can he stand apart and tolerate aloneness; learning that he can be both related and lonely, he may at times embrace his loneliness, knowing that it is not cause for shame, but reflects certain personal—and perhaps situational—limitations restricting his participation and in itself may have value and offer great comfort.*

The schizophrenic has an intense need for relatedness but also an intense fear due to the overwhelming threat of loneliness and complete isolation from human contact, which implies nonbeing. Will[2] outlined several behaviors he observed in treating schizophrenics that confirm the concept of relatedness. First a mutual approach and retreat between therapist and patient will occur, so that individual selves can be identified. Second the patient will fear the relationship because of the threat of unrelatedness. Third he may need to confirm his existence in the therapist's eyes. Last the patient will communicate a need that must be identified by both therapist and patient. This requires the therapist to encourage the patient to state his needs in a clear, direct manner.

---

*From Will, O. A.: Human relatedness and the schizophrenic reaction, Psychiatry **22**:205, 1959.

From this I was able to draw some of the goals for my work with Jean. In some way I had to convey to her that my interest in her was real. I wanted to enter a relationship with her if she would allow it. Each day that I met with her, I had no particular subject I wanted to talk about with her. I let her guide the initial steps of defining and entering the relationship. I responded to her in the context of where she was at the time of our meeting. In other words, therapy was geared to a here-and-now orientation. I had no goals for where she should be in terms of her social functioning or her relationship with me or herself. This proved helpful in reducing her anxiety surrounding our relationship; however, I must admit that holding to these goals was at times difficult, as will be illustrated at points throughout this chapter.

The therapeutic process, or the process of the relationship between Jean and myself, can be somewhat divided into the initial stage of the relationship, the middle stage, which was marked by plans for discharge, and the subsequent adjustment to home and community, which terminated our relationship. It should be noted at this time that my work with Jean covered weekly sessions for approximately eight months. The changes that were noted in the relationship are small in comparison to the work done by some therapists who have spent years working with schizophrenics in daily sessions. Nevertheless, a relationship between Jean and me did develop, and a termination to that relationship was reached.

The initial stage of therapy covered approximately the first two and one-half months of therapy. During this time Jean exhibited a great deal of approach and avoidance behavior. She was aware of the time of our scheduled appointment. She often remarked whether I was a few minutes early or late. However, Jean was unable to tolerate the sessions for much longer than twenty or thirty minutes. On two occasions we simply walked around the grounds of the hospital or went to the hospital canteen for a soft drink. Many times we did not speak and when we did we simply remarked about the natural surroundings of the outdoors.

During these brief encounters I began to see Jean's confusion, helplessness, and view of the world around her and of herself. The content of the sessions was focused on Jean's feelings about hospitalization and her confusion about her current circumstances. The following excerpt from a session illustrates this point better than I can describe it:

J: I don't feel—feel very well because I can't do a lot of things . . . I don't know what to do or not. The other day I told my friend to come see me, but they go out already. They are not in this country.
T: Some friends come to see you?
J: Yeah, they come to see me, and they go back.
T: What friends, Jean?
J: I don't know.
T: You don't know what friends?
J: No. I has a lot of friends. I don't remember. They feel so suffering; that's why they . . .
T: They feel so what?
J: They feel suffering a lot.
T: They are suffering a lot, or you are suffering a lot?
J: The people and me, too. I take care of them. But this is not real hell; this is nothing. Nothing we can do about it. Not good for the people. They put the people in the place. They are poison.
T: What people are poison, Jean?
J: Those—ah—Does this place belong to the policeman? I haven't seen a policeman, but—I just don't know what to do with these policemen. I go home already. I don't feel fun to stay in here. The other day I cry a lot and I tell them about it . . . Whose idea to put the people in here? They don't feel good. They don't have good dress—only old clothes and old shoes . . .

Although I did not know who "they" were or what meaning the word "poison" had to Jean, her utter despair was apparent. In other words, even though Jean's communication was distorted, I could not help feeling the full impact of her depression and loneliness. Gradually she began talking about the loneliness she had felt since coming to this country. People and customs were strange to her. She did not relate to her husband or children and saw her task in the family as simply to clean the house and do the wash. She expressed the feeling that she had been lonely at home but the hospital was worse. It was as though at home she at least had some identity, no matter how marginal in my eyes. In addition, she was resigned to the fact that life at home was her only existence, past and future. She was not, however, resigned to the state hospital. She wanted to return home.

The environment at the hospital did not allow for a differentiation between self and others. All patients looked the same. Few personal belongings were allowed on the unit. Patients kept their belongings beside their beds in a small cabinet, which was often without a lock. Patients slept, ate, and carried out daily activities in large rooms with no private areas. Looking back, I am sure that home life, no matter how isolated it might appear to be, provided an opportunity for Jean to relate to surroundings that provided her with an identity.

In the initial sessions I found myself overwhelmed with depression in response to Jean. Often I left the hospital with tears in my eyes and found it difficult to listen to the tapes of the sessions. I picked up her feelings of hopelessness and despair. I would forget her potential for growth because it seemed almost superfluous to think about. The road ahead seemed long and demanding. I felt a need to give her something. Since Jean was unable to state her needs clearly, which is often the case in the schizophrenic, as stated by Will,[2] I found myself defining her needs for her. Usually the need was defined as help. This often fostered helplessness and a decreased sense of identity. This was clearer to me in the middle stage of therapy than in the initial stage.

As stated, Jean's communication was distorted. During the initial stage of therapy I was preoccupied with the feeling tone behind the communication, which tended to involve me more on a pure feeling level with little analysis of the communication. As I became more comfortable with Jean and her mode of communicating, I was able to define the obscure forms the communication took and how they were utilized to define Jean's experience of her surroundings. I was then able to begin to define her needs more clearly. At times this was a frightening experience to me. I was actually feeling, defining, and acting on obscure communication stated by someone I seemed to know little about. Searles has stated the following:

The obscurity of the patient's communications is such that his therapist tends to become the sole expert, or in any case the leading expert, in de-

ciphering his communications. This circumstance contributes greatly to the private aura which their relationship develops, an aura of uniquely close communion as contrasted with their subjective distance from an outer world which "does not understand." Moreover, the therapist progressively moves into a position where he translates the communication of the confused schizophrenic patient even for the latter himself; in this, as well as in other ways, he functionally does the patient's thinking and feeling for him, to a considerable degree—he comes to personify the patient's externalized ego.*

The foregoing statement by Searles was often a source of comfort to me during periods when I felt I too must be schizophrenic to understand Jean's communication. Also, the statement reflects my feelings of expertise regarding Jean. In my dealings with the community team responsible for Jean's care, I often became impatient with their lack of understanding of her behavior. I found that my supervisor was the only person I could listen to in terms of adequately dealing with the therapeutic process. In other words, only two people really understood.

Although Jean's communication was distorted throughout therapy, the middle stage marked the beginning of trying to put meaning into the words. When I was able to make associations between Jean's communication and our relationship in the context of the here and now, I found interpretation and subsequent invention much easier. It became clear that Jean displaced most of her experience to other people, times, or symbolic objects. For instance she continually referred to "they" or "the people," to "the other day," which meant either distant or recent past or the present, and to shoes, jewelry, and other articles of clothing.

> J: Afraid of everything. The people always teasing. Want to take all my things away. Why are they so cruel? I has a good time when I was so young.
> T: What things do they want to take away?
> J: Take the things of yourself.
> T: What things?
> J: My shoes, clothes—anything I have. So fantastic all the things they take. . .

Interpretation of this mode of communication was based on assumptions of Jean's experience. "The people" often referred to

*From Searles, H. F.: Collected papers on schizophrenia and other related subjects, New York, 1965, International Universities Press, p. 410.

me or persons in her immediate surroundings. "The other day" reflected Jean's inability to unify her past, present, and future experiences. Objects such as shoes reflected her experience of loss of self and others.

In addition to displacement, Jean often projected her feelings onto me. This was particularly noticeable when Jean talked about her relationship with her children.

J: They play themselves. Don't like to play with the children. They make trouble.
T: You don't like to play with the children?
J: No, don't I mean that. Some trouble. Sometimes I tell them. You really don't like the children.
T: I really don't like them.
J: Yeah. Sometimes make the trouble. They cry and make the trouble.
T: You don't like them, or I don't like them?
J: I don't know because I—you have the other children when you come here (home); you nurse the other children.

As I was able to analyse Jean's communication, I was also able to begin to clarify some of Jean's experience to her. This process seemed to bring our relationship closer because we were able to begin to understand each other through verbal behavior, no matter how obscure that behavior seemed.

The communication aspect of our relationship seemed to be a major part of the middle stage. Approach and withdrawal behavior was exhibited verbally. Jean's communication often became so distorted that I could not respond and thereby placed a distance between us. At other times I would withdraw. I would find my mind wandering, instead of focused on Jean. We approached one another by continually trying to clarify what our verbal behavior meant. Jean would try to express a concept to me in many different ways, if I stated initially that I had not understood her. It seemed to reflect a caring, that each of us was trying to understand the other.

During the middle stage of therapy Jean's need for increased relatedness was identified, and plans were made for discharge. This involved a variety of therapeutic interventions and resulted in Jean's expression of feelings of loss, ambivalence, inadequacy related to her role as a wife and mother, and fear of other people.

It was apparent that Jean was more involved in the unit. She interacted with other patients in a playful, childlike manner, she stated her need for passes off the hospital grounds in community meetings, and she attended social functions such as dances that were held on the unit. However, the longer she remained in the hospital, the more isolated she became from her family, home, and community. I felt a need to maintain her identity as a member of a social system outside the hospital rather than to encourage an identity consistent with the hospital. I began to make inquiries into the possibility of discharging Jean to her home and continuing my work with her there. This meant an investigation of the feelings of many people. I needed the support of Jean's community team at the hospital so that they could help make the arrangements, support Jean in my absence, and maintain open communication with me regarding her case. The team seemed enthusiastic with the approach and maintained contact with the case after Jean's discharge. When the end of the school year terminated my relationship with Jean, the social worker on the team, with whom Jean had numerous contacts in the hospital, picked up immediately on the case.

I then contacted Mr. M to determine his feelings about having Jean at home despite her minimal social functioning. I was somewhat concerned about this because Mr. M seemed so terribly isolated from Jean. Although he seemed not to care, he agreed that she could return home. Throughout my work with Jean after her discharge, I continually had to explain the mystical quality of her illness to him. He was ashamed of Jean because of her distorted manner of speech and her sloppy dress. For these reasons he was reluctant for her to be seen in public and for others to be involved in the family.

The most important resource seemed to be within the community itself. Prior to Jean's hospitalization, she and the children had become involved in a church that catered to the needs of the Chinese-American population in the community. Several women involved in the church took great interest in Jean and often looked after the M children during Jean's hospitalization.

These women were the only people who visited Jean throughout her stay in the hospital and at home after her discharge. I contacted the minister at the church, who was able to provide me with the names of the women who would be willing to work with Jean after she returned home. After I contacted them, they took it on themselves to talk with Jean's neighbors and to make plans for the amount of involvement they would be willing to make in their endeavor to relate to her. After discharge, the women welcomed Jean home, helped her adjust to the routine of a housewife, visited with her, and took her shopping and to church functions.

Some problems were encountered in the relationship between these representatives of the community and Mr. M. They were suspicious of his isolation and felt he resented their involvement in the family. Mr. M seemed to be reacting to having others know of Jean's condition. This involved educating these persons in the role mental illness was playing in Jean's life and by outlining how their intervention was helping Jean. However, Jean's illness was isolating her from others. Only small inroads were made prior to termination.

Prior to Jean's discharge she went home for a few hours to see her family. In addition she went home for five days over a holiday season. After these visits many of Jean's feelings of helplessness were expressed. Initially she was frightened that if she were discharged I would not see her any longer. Both of these feelings were expressed in the following excerpt from a taped session.

> J: I was alright. Everything was so new and expensive. We lost the chance. Not powerful or rich people. Don't have money buy things. I don't know what do to. Watch the children. They are so young and need a guardian to take care of them. You leave here because you are my guardian and take care of me and you do some good thing for me anyway. I couldn't let—might send another girl to see me. . .

At other times Jean was assertive as to the help she did or did not want. During a visit home, an Oriental neighbor came to help Jean clean the house. This was Jean's reaction in the session following her visit home.

> T: How did you feel about your visit at home?
> J: Yeah. I don't know about my aunt (woman who helped)—come to see me and makes the things so nervous. . .
> T: What did she do that made you nervous?
> J: I wanted to do things with myself and I don't need other people to do it. They don't know how to do it. Do it by themselves. I don't know what they do. . .

Following Jean's discharge I too tended to forget that she was able to identify what help she needed. She usually refused my help with anything! I learned that the relationship was what was important. Soon Jean and I were able to do things such as water her plants because we enjoyed doing that together rather than because Jean needed help. I then began to stop focusing on the disarray of the house and Jean's appearance and refocused my attention on the content and feelings expressed during the hour I visited her at her home.

Although Jean returned home, her isolation and loneliness continued. She remained suspicious of anyone new to her. The house was always locked with the curtains drawn closed. Jean rarely left the house alone except to water the outdoor plants or to sweep the front stoop. She appeared terribly frightened of the world outside her front door. At other times when I would accompany her to mundane places such as the health department, she would dress up and act very excited that we were going someplace. This again reflects her need for relatedness, yet her intense fear of it.

The middle stage of therapy was marked by an increased relatedness between Jean and me due to clarification of communication and by a change in Jean's immediate environment. Thus there was a refocusing of Jean's feelings from utter despair in the hospital to feelings of inadequacy coupled with an increase in identity and feelings of loneliness coupled with increased relatedness.

Termination was difficult for both of us. Although we both knew that the relationship was limited from the beginning, we did not speak of it until the last month of therapy. From the time I spoke extensively of my leaving, I wished that the time would go slowly. I wondered if I would cry when I said good-bye for the last time. I wanted to make sure that we both realized that, although we were suffering a loss, we had also gained a great deal from one another. When I initially asked Jean about her feelings related to my leaving, she stated:

> J: I think you be so happy. All the things are new. All the people come and leave and I don't know how they are feeling. Sometimes they happy to make the journey. Don't really know about them. . . Just give them good luck and enjoy their whole life. Go find a new life and do different things—find new things. . . You see any people in hospital. Miss them a lot. A lot of time real nice. Like to say hello to them, but so far from here. Sometimes it's lonely job. Don't know what to do sometimes. Can you show me what to do?

Although it is sometimes confusing to determine which of us she is actually referring to in this statement, at the time it was said, it really did not seem to matter. She spoke of feelings we both had.

Jean's helplessness was expressed many times. She also expressed loss, anger, and the fear of having someone else come talk with her because they too might leave or not understand "the things about me." She expressed her anger in relation to cats and dogs.

> J: I don't know how can talk about it. Like cat or dog. If you love them, get them a lot of food. If you don't love, you just send them away.
> T: I'm treating you like a cat or dog?
> J: Might be. If don't treat them so good—frighten them. . .

Loss was expressed as it had been throughout therapy—loss of objects. I had given Jean some flower seeds to plant soon after she returned home. One day after I arrived, she became upset that someone had taken her seeds. Later she missed other objects from her home, such as shoes and jewelry. She not only believed that I no longer loved her because I was leaving but also that I was taking things away from her when I left. I was beginning to feel horribly guilty for becoming involved with Jean. However, Jean was right that I was taking something of her away with me. She had taught me a great deal about her experience of life. She had painted picture

after picture of her feelings through her communication. I felt that Jean had expressed her feelings more clearly to me than had any "normal" person I had ever been in contact with before. Although a vast amount of her communication I simply did not understand, the feelings always had come through crystal clear. In some ways I also felt cheated. At the time I was finally beginning to clarify communication and define ego boundaries, I had to leave. Somehow it all seemed so unfinished.

During one session Jean asked me why I came to see her. We both were from different cultures, socioeconomic backgrounds, and life experiences. Why did I come? I had taken something of Jean away with me, but what had I given her? I came to give myself to Jean in a way she could relate to. From this I tried to give Jean a unified experience of our relationship. We had a past, a present, and a future.

CONCLUSION

> . . . to be sure, an ordinary passerby would think that my rose looked just like you—the rose that belongs to me. But in herself alone she is more important than all the hundreds of you other roses: because it is she that I have watered; because it is she that I have put under the glass globe; because it is she that I have sheltered behind the screen; because it is for her that I have killed the caterpillars . . . because it is she that I have listened to, when she grumbled, or boasted, or even sometimes when she said nothing. Because she is my rose!

For,

> It is only with the heart that one can see rightly; what is essential is invisible to the eye.*

---

*From de Saint-Exupéry, Antoine: The Little Prince, New York, 1943, Harcourt, Brace & World.

References

1. Searles, H. F.: Collected papers on schizophrenia and other related subjects, New York, 1965, International Universities Press.
2. Will, O. A.: Human relatedness and the schizophrenic reaction, Psychiatry 22:205, 1959.

4

Aspects of therapeutic intervention with adolescents

Claire M. Fagin

Therapeutic intervention with adolescents, emphasizing the nursing role, will be discussed in three parts. First some developmental characteristics of adolescents that have bearing on therapeutic intervention will be discussed briefly. Then, since I believe the therapeutic milieu is essential for effective therapeutic intervention with adolescents, considerable attention will be given to this treatment modality. The aspect of the therapeutic milieu that is most troublesome to "daily-living" personnel is the concept of permissiveness. Therefore this will be discussed at some length. Finally, the therapeutic relationship from the standpoint of the *special position* of the nurse vis-à-vis the adolescent, pitfalls resulting from this special position, and some recommendations for effective intervention will be considered.

Basic to therapeutic intervention with any human being is some degree of sophistication on the part of the intervenor regarding the developmental characteristics of the group. This background knowledge is implicit to understanding deviations in behavior from infancy to senescence. For successful intervention with adolescents obviously the intevenor *must* have a deep sense of and sensitivity to the normal, age-typical developmental characteristics and behavior of the adolescent group.

My experience with mental health professionals has too often indicated either our rapid forgetting of the normal, our never having learned it, or our knowing but not applying our knowledge. This is evidenced by a focus on pathology and interpretation and a propensity for labeling behavior of children, mothers, fathers, and the elderly as an aberration when often it is an age-typical indication of developmental changes or crises.

The adolescent in particular, subject to a ream of physiological, psychological, and emotional changes and so often a stranger to himself as his own moods and inclinations shift dramatically, requires of the therapist a clear starting point. Therefore some bascis regarding psychodynamic, cognitive, and physical development will be discussed first.

With regard to psychodynamics I have always found the writings of Anna Freud helpful in understanding and dealing with emotionally healthy as well as emotionally disturbed adolescents. Three related aspects of the adolescent's psychic development she identifies are narcissism, restitution relationships, and polarization of affects.[2]

More recent observers believe that the narcissism seen in earlier periods is more exaggerated or at least more openly expressed today. There is obvious self-absorption and self-gratification in many of the new freedoms and experimentation. This open narcissism poses potential therapeutic problem areas, which are dealt with later.

As the youngster moves through the phases of adolescent development, from narcissism to homosexual to heterosexual object choice, a major change occurs with respect to his childhood love objects. Typically with regard to parents significant disenchantment occurs for both rational and irrational causes. This disenchantment may be expressed behaviorally in various ways. The youngster may isolate himself and behave as though he and his family are strangers, or his devaluing his parents may temporarily affect his acceptance of their values, standards, and interests. When his peers represent a different and stronger influence or when the adolescent has contact with, to him, more admirable adults, he will find new attachments to replace the earlier ties. Sometimes the relationships that we see take the form of passionate friendships where the youngster actually believes he is in love with someone his own age, his own sex perhaps, or sometimes an older person whom he takes as a leader. These relations are exclusive and passionate, and they may be of short duration. It is important to remember that these fleeting love fixations are not really *object relations* but rather *identifications* of a primitive kind. Through these so-called restitution relationships the adolescent is trying to recover the former relation to his family or perhaps in some cases an ideal love he never experienced. The idealized friendship may look rather odd for the big fellow our adolescent now is. In many ways it resembles the infant's and the young child's feelings about the adults who surround him in terms of their omnipotence and perfection. Understanding the dynamics of these relationships hopefully makes it easier to accept and deal with them even when the particular ideal is obnoxious to the viewer or, indeed, when the ideal is delightful to the therapist, momentarily being himself.

The third characteristic Freud[2] talks about, in which the youngster varies between ego gratification and denial of instinctual impulses, she calls a polarization of affects. The conflicts and vicious circles created by the self-gratification–asceticism paradox may drive some adolescents farther from realistic adjustment. This is likely to be the case when one's need for closeness, affection, and intimacy with another person becomes essential. Any increase in intimacy demands an increased exposure to oneself and others. Through this exposure the adolescent is faced with an unpleasant, perhaps even unbearable, part of himself that threatens the self-concept he has formed as well as threatening to destroy the incipient relationship. In more healthy situations adolescents may temporarily withdraw into isolation and fantasy as a means of handling these problems.

Increased cognitive skills play a major

part in the development of the mechanism of intellectualization, which adolescents may utilize privately and interpersonally to handle their heightened emotionality. Putting feelings together with ideas helps them gain control. Psychoanalytic experts have described youngsters' delight in abstract intellectual discussions and speculations, and many of us see these characteristics in the adolescents we know. More recent psychological research[4] has indicated that a large proportion of people *never* develop the capacity for abstract thought and reasoning. As therapists we have to recognize the variation in cognitive ability with regard to particular adolescents' methods of dealing with their emotional upheavals. As described by Werner,[8] the use of creative magic with rituals and fantasies doing the work is probably just as relevant for many adolescents as the use of intellectualization. In any case, all teen-agers know they must prepare to make their own decisions. Seeing the faults in many adults does not free them from learning their own rules of living. Some individual method of preserving integrity when faced with varied views and beliefs must be found.

My more recent experiences with adolescents offer many examples of the use of rituals, fantasies, and, related to these, the mechanism of denial to handle problems of dissonance. For the youngster capable of abstract thought and intellectualization, discussions of the merits of particular systems, philosophies, and values are possible. The literature focuses on this mechanism but has few examples of denial as a dominant mechanism of adolescence, although it is mentioned in relation to specific neuroses. I have been struck recently by this phenomenon in dealing with freshman students. I would be interested in studying the uses of denial among different socioeconomic and intellectual classes of adolescents. It seems to be closely tied to both areas. It also, incidentally, is exceedingly difficult to deal with. Whereas particular ramifications of denial vary, it seems to be a frequent method of handling the reality threat, present for this age group, of looking at one's intellectual ability in light of one's close-at-hand future. In my experience it is extremely rare for students to express a realistic appraisal of their abilities. Instead they tend to deny their failures as well as the existence of objective evaluations.

All these characteristics point up sharply the discrepancy between the adolescent's biological, emotional, and cognitive maturity.

The most outstanding physiological development during adolescence is the maturing of reproductive organs, but a quick look at physical growth may be worthwhile. For example, within one year a youngster may gain 25 to 30 pounds in weight and 4 or 5 inches in height. The timing of the physical growth varies, but, whenever it occurs, it must affect the expectations of the adults in the adolescent's circle. Here is a youngster looking very like an adult himself—big, grown-up in so many ways, yet in others more like a big baby—full of questions about acceptance, achievement, identification, identity, love, and other matters important to his self-concept, questions that must be answered regardless of cognitive abilities and disparities of development. Self-identification is a task that affects adolescents of all varieties. Finding a stable belief system is difficult in today's world. Although young people have always shown rebellion against much that parents hold dear, today their uncertainties are increased by the varied meanings social phenomena have to them, their peers, parents, and other adults. Such matters as drugs, sex, concepts of family and of war and peace, and lack of common ideology generate uncertainty.

This brief summary was meant to provide a frame of reference for therapeutic intervention. It posed problems but also solutions, if we can, as the young folks say, "get it together."

The following section will consider the therapeutic milieu, a vital part of treatment with disturbed adolescents. For many reasons, adolescents seem to be particularly resistant to the traditional "therapy hour." The milieu or life situation, being more flexible and crisis geared, may be the more effective treatment methodology. Redl has commented that "even the trusted adult loses his value in a role of therapist or counselor, unless he is somewhere built in

to the normal power hierarchy in which youngsters operate and unless he is close to the scene where life events occur and available when they do."* In speculating about the reasons for the importance of the milieu, he points out the greater safety from introspection and from the emergence of transference fantasies and the degree to which the therapy hour and couch are symbols in our popular literature. He also mentions that many youngsters are afraid of the possibility for a deep commitment, which is reduced in more familiar territory. He believes the resistance that many of our adolescents have against seeking help might be "the well-known resistance not only against therapeutic change, but against the specific design of time and space and role distribution which has become part of our traditional, professional armamentarium."* Furthermore, many of the characteristics reviewed earlier, such as denial, intellectualization, and narcissism, militate against the delays of the structured confrontation, especially in the early phases of the acquaintance.

Assuming that the therapeutic milieu is an important treatment modality for adolescents, I would like to outline its basic constructs and then expand on a few particulars relevant to therapeutic intervention.

First, in terms of the social structure, the milieu may be said to be democratic rather than authoritarian, treatment oriented rather than custodial, humanitarian rather than oppressive, and flexible rather than rigid. Second, interactions may be said to be individualized and personal rather than stereotyped or routine, sympathetic and respectful rather than hostile or contemptuous,[7] and need oriented and permissive rather than neglectful and punitive. Third, philosophy carried out has to do with interest in the effect of experience on constructively changing behavior. This would imply open communication around the problems affecting the patients as well as involvement of personnel in administra-

---

*From Redl, F.: Adolescents—just how do they react? In Caplan, G., and Lebovici, S., editors: Adolescence: psychosocial perspectives, New York, 1969, Basic Books, Inc., p. 93.

tive structure similar to that described previously.

Instead of skimming over each item on this outline I would rather develop one or two in some detail. I believe the cluster of flexibility, need orientation, and permissiveness give daily-living personnel the most difficulty. Before going into examples of the possible problems with these concepts I would like to spell out to some extent how the words are being used. First of all, when related to adolescents, such a milieu would protect youngsters from traumatic handling by any personnel associated with the unit. Second, there would be a great deal in the way of gratification, love, and affectional tokens absolutely divorced from any consideration of whether the youngsters deserve them. In other words, such gratifications would be part of treatment rather than a reward for good behavior or a punishment for bad behavior. The treatment environment provides tolerance for symptoms and some leeway for regression, yet there is protective interference on the part of the staff at moments when it is necessary to protect the adolescent from his own overwhelming guilt, anxiety, or depression, as well as to protect other patients. The concepts of flexibility, need fulfillment, and permissiveness require some thought as to the best physical surroundings for adolescents, emphasizing such factors as space in which youngsters can move about without disturbing the territorial needs of others, space in which one can be noisy or alone and quiet and distributed in such a way that the patient is able to move from privacy to contact with small groups to contact with larger groups. There should be some privacy in toilet and bath facilities. Furnishings should be varied, with attention given to auditory, tactile, and visual stimulation, and wherever possible the setting should not differ sharply from that of the socioeconomic class with which the patients identify. It is important to consider here that Redl's[5] concept of the life-space interview as an integral part of the therapeutic milieu means that the setting should allow the possibility of holding such interviews, so that the daily-living personnel can exploit life issues as they occur. Where the setting permits, the possibility exists for

interviews when necessary and indicated, rather than or as well as at prescribed times during the day or week.

It is important to consider the neighborhood or social style of the youngster when examining the concept of permissiveness, since what is au courant for one group might be different from what is acceptable behavior in another. What is permitted in terms of play, fighting, language, and other manifestations must reflect the understanding of prevailing patterns. It is terribly important to convey to the group your awareness of what is age-typical, socially acceptable behavior, what are difficulties that are possible to express and live out without too severe consequences and rejection from the adult, and then again what behaviors will not be permitted. The youngster needs to recognize that there is a difference between toleration of his symptoms and either indifference to or vicarious enjoyment of his problem behavior. Unfortunately, such terms as *permissive* and *need fulfillment* sometimes evoke suggestions for actions that are impossible to carry out and that lead to the reaction of imposing excessive limits.

Some years ago I worked with a psychiatric administrator who believed that a therapeutic milieu for patients revolved around a particular philosophy of psychiatric nursing. He described the model for nurse-patient role behaviors that dealt with "interrelated behavior attitude patterns designated by the terms *permissiveness, need-fulfillment, interpersonal relatedness, and treatment of the patient as an adult person.*"[6]

"In this philosophy, permissiveness meant that patients were to be given a 'maximum amount of freedom' to behave as they wished and that the nurse was to place minimal restriction on patient behavior. Patients were free to do as they liked, e.g., eat what they liked, remain unbathed, tear up clothing, destroy furniture, to play the phonograph loudly, etc."* Nurses were told not to interfere with patient's acts either directly by verbal limits or indirectly by

---

*From Schwartz, M.: What is a therapeutic milieu? In The patient and the mental hospital, New York, 1957, The Free Press, pp. 404 and 405.

responding with displeasure or physically withdrawing from the patient. As far as possible patients were to have access to all parts of the ward and were to be permitted the free use of matches, cigarettes, mirrors, sharp things, and other potentially dangerous objects.[6] "It was specified that nurses were to gratify as many of the patients' wishes and desires as possible and patients were to be encouraged to express their needs in any way they could."* In all cases the nurse's comfort and well-being determined how far the nurse went with a particular kind of behavior, but the clearly stated ideal was for nurses to be sufficiently comfortable to behave in the "right" way to meet the patients' needs.

Schwartz's investigation of the problem indicated that the nurses had a high level of understanding of the philosophy, were highly motivated, and had a great investment in the work situation. Their acceptance of the problems they experienced was considerably below their own expectations as a result of this. The first problems that occurred had to do with heterosexual and homosexual behavior; later problems complained about were importunity, destructiveness, withdrawal, and messiness. In relation to these behaviors the requirement of permissiveness presented the most problems. "It was difficult for nurses to permit patients to do anything they wanted when such permission included . . . being kissed and fondled, watching homosexual behavior, standing by while patients destroyed furniture [burned themselves], etc."†

Permissiveness defined in this way so conflicted with their own norms that their discomfort was sometimes acute.[6] In addition to this conflict, the staff found it a fine line between permitting patients to do what they wanted and neglecting or failing to protect them. The concepts of permissiveness and need fulfillment expressed in this situation clearly conflicted with the middle-class value system of the nurses.

*From Schwartz, M.: What is a therapeutic milieu? In The patient and the mental hospital, New York, 1957, The Free Press, pp. 404 and 405.
†From Schwartz, C. G.: Problems for psychiatric nurses in playing a new role. In The patient and the mental hospital, New York, 1957, The Free Press, p. 410.

An important point of consideration was that nurses were expected to play conflicting roles in this institution, since this unit was only one of many, and nurses playing the described role successfully were in conflict with the rest of the hospital. Supervising nurses and the maintenance, housekeeping, and dietary departments, among others, were not in agreement with what went on in this ward, and the nurses for the most part were the ones in an interface situation with workers in other departments. In general, the physicians could lead their own lives on this ward without any flak from other departments or from their colleagues. The nurses were required to turn in reports on time, to protect the wards against fire, to report accidents, and to conform generally to the routines prescribed for all wards. The flexibility requirement made it difficult for them to meet the ward demands on one hand and the hospital demands on the other.

I have described this situation deliberately, even though it is an extreme example, because it points up the kinds of conflicts often overlooked when prescribing principles from one treatment mode to another. It is important to examine what one means by need fulfillment, flexibility, and permissiveness over a life-time-space situation. Implementing these concepts in the way the example described is antitherapeutic in my view. Instead of encouraging personality organization and recognizing the levels of development, responsibility, and training that each participant had reached, it abdicated responsibility, rational authority, and any autonomy for personnel or patients. Such distortions of the guidelines for the therapeutic milieu cannot help but fail and frequently lead to what is considered the alternative in the minds of many critics—an authoritarian or autocratic model. This alternative will, I believe, be totally ineffective in preparing the adolescent for today's unpredictable world, in which he requires independence, self-reliance, and adaptability.

We must strive for a rational model of permissiveness and need fulfillment in the therapeutic milieu that implies an acceptance of the young person as a human being, a recognition and acceptance of his problems and his symptoms, with a clear understanding of what limits are necessary for physical and social behavior and why, and we must be able, among ourselves and with adolescents, to articulate this. It should at the very least be clear to us that some limits are part of the treatment design and other limits are simply what people have to do to live together in a particular setting.

Earlier, in outlining the basics of the therapeutic milieu, I stated, as the second major category, the quality of interactions. It stands to reason that disturbed adolescents, in and out of residential settings, will not just naturally manage to relate constructively to peers or well-meaning adults. To put the matter somewhat simplistically as a means of summarizing, we have here a composite youngster whose appearance may be near adult but who is unable to communicate his needs to the adults or peers in his life. The fact is that the adolescent whose difficulties with parents are severe will often be unable to form successful and constructive peer relationships. Their needs for closeness, for human contact, and for expression of deeper questions and fears are often not met in the peer group when their adult relationships are poor.

Despite the emphasis on the setting or the therapeutic milieu with adolescent patients, it is of vital importance that within this setting there be some ability to develop an intimate relationship with another human being. The comforting protective presence of another person is of vital importance in developing or restoring equilibrium to the personality. The youngster must have possibilities for contact with another person—nurse, physicians' aide, or another patient, who can be a stable, well-defined supportive figure, effective in guiding him toward a higher level of maturity through closeness, affection, friendship, support, or whatever may be helpful. The human relationship is a primary and vital agent in furthering change in a favorable direction.

In terms of the therapeutic relationship I believe there are particular advantages in the position of the physician-nurse in relation to the adolescent. Many adolescents' symptoms are physiological or psychosomatic, such as acne, oily skin, blackheads, such cardiac symptoms as palpitation of

the heart with expressed fear of this type of disease, muscular pain, genital changes with questions and fears about their normalcy, upset stomachs, severe headaches, and many more. To me, the particular combination of frequent symptomatology and psychoanalytic descriptions of narcissism and restitution relationships provide more than a felicitous arena for therapeutic intervention. Some adolescent symptomatology is especially suitable to nursing intervention, since, to be more graphic, nursing suggests the mother-surrogate configuration of laying on of hands. This configuration contains an instant suggestion of help offered or provided for the many real and imagined ailments besetting adolescents. One might say that the period of adolescence is a favorable situation that provides ties between the unconscious of the health and medical worker and the unconscious of the patient. The remainder of the chapter focuses primarily on this phenomenon after a few words on some expected differences between therapeutic and other relationships with adolescents.

For a variety of reasons those with whom we work in therapy have not had normal relationships with parents and others earlier in their life, so that there is no early adjustment that can serve as a model for a particular useful restitution relationship. Therefore the responsibility for channelling this relationship falls almost entirely on the therapeutic worker. The youngster's only tendency is to transfer the attitudes he had toward his parents to the persons in authority. This can evoke one of two kinds of reactions. The first is for the worker to adopt the same attitude toward the child as did the parents, thus fostering a continuing of the reciprocal relationship, a destructive integration.

The second possibility is for the therapist to work consistently within the basic and changing psychodynamics of adolescent development. This second reaction requires two characteristics in the worker: one is extreme sophistication as to age-typical behaviors and problems of adolescents and the second is full awareness of his own needs for approval and satisfaction in the situation. For example, he will respond to the child's feeling of a need for punishment but will not satisfy this need. He will try to indicate his understanding of the rationality of the youngster's behavior to him in a particular situation. Recognizing that forming a successful enough relationship for the adolescent to begin to communicate is a slow process, we carefully select the right moments and a variety of ways to let the youngster know that we have some understanding of his difficulties. Whereas we do not respond as his mother or father did or would, we do indicate a healthy skepticism at times for the youngster's explanations and denials, still appreciating his need for telling his story in a particular way. We have to be clear that a straight story will eventually have to be told if treatment is to be successful.

It should be obvious that the therapeutic relationship must first compensate for the lack of love the youngster has perceived. Demands on them should be made only with great caution and then in a step-by-step process, bringing to bear no pressure that can be avoided. It can be expected that the behavior that brought them into the hospital will be increased after admission, through permissiveness on the part of the therapeutic staff. After all, the behavior will be saying, "If whatever bad behavior is not getting the expected reaction, I guess I'll have to be even worse."

Obviously intervention must occur at the point where the behavior is going to be harmful to them or to anyone else. However, intervention with some practical limits is not necessarily punishment, particularly when gratifications are provided in many other ways. At some point in all this, provided the therapist maintains himself as a separate person who really is adult and different from the adolescent, the youngster will begin to want to give some gratification to the adult, to impress him, to do something that will have a positive meaning for him, so that he himself can make an impression other than as a jerk or what have you. He begins to have some incentive to submit to whatever the reality expectations of the therapist are. As the youngster begins to develop some tender feelings toward the people that are working with him, he begins to get the incen-

tive to do what is expected in the reality situation.

In looking at the appropriateness of nursing, particularly at points of difficult communications, it is important to recognize again here where the youngster is really limited in his ability to relate. He may be approachable only in the most primary aspects, such as physical care, touching, dressing of wounds, and protecting from injury. Rapport may be built up in these ways before any kind of verbal communication can take place.

For the female nurse working with adolescent boys this clearly poses potential problems dealing with both the transference and countertransference situations. For the youngster a lack of clarity exists between the nurse as a romantic object, the nurse as a mother figure, and the nurse as a stranger who is trying to meet some of his needs in a rational and constructive way. Many jokes, stories, and modern films ("M.A.S.H.," "Catch 22," and—horror of all horrors—"The Nurses") that depict nurses in a frivolous, sexy, and certainly anti-feminist way will obviously contribute to such fantasies. That these films do not in too many ways ruffle the majority unconscious is evidenced by the fact that there is no significant picketing or other objections by nurses or other women in relation to the manner in which nurses are depicted. So that gives us some understanding of the youngster's own fantasies in relation to his role vis-à-vis this woman who is taking care of him and who is addressing herself to his many and varied needs.

The part of the therapeutic relationship that I now want to discuss briefly has to do with the possibilities for the nurse to become seduced into the position of friend without influence, which, I think, is an extremely common occurrence for all therapists working with adolescents. All the forces brought into play by adolescents, their particular needs, and the way the worker meets these needs makes such an occurrence almost inevitable. The youngster's seeking of restitution relationships, the combination of physical and psychological problems, the nonjudgmental giving of acceptance on the part of the therapist during the early phases of a developing relationship, the use of physical and sometimes intimate vehicles for developing this relationship in themselves can create a receptiveness for the friend relationship on the part of the worker. Furthermore, in our efforts to move into a relationship as quickly as possible we are often, unwittingly perhaps, literally seductive with the rather easily seduced adolescent. Many of us do not hesitate to use our feminine, masculine, or intellectual attributes to gain some kind of initial relationship and acceptance by the young person. It is sometimes difficult to keep in mind that the object of all this is to help the relationship move to a feeling attachment quickly but that the initial narcissistic identifications have yet to be replaced by interpersonal learning. But it is at this point in the developing relationship that we are in the most difficulty. The possibility is that many of the methods the worker has used to communicate with the adolescent have succeeded, in the sense that the young person now looks at a particular worker with something like hero worship. How many of us can resist the thought of being the one and only important person in a disturbed adolescent's life. How many of us can avoid coveting the marvelous feeling of success where others have failed and subsequently avoid being used by the adolescent as a means of replaying his scenario with a partial change of cast.

The possibility of seduction of the worker is enhanced by the natural tendency on the part of most of us in psychiatry to look about for places to cast the blame for a youngster's difficulties, most often choosing the parents. Our own superiority to these very imperfect beings is apparent; furthermore, our superiority to other people who have already tried to deal with the adolescent, be they teachers or other therapists, is also of great significance to us. This is not an uncommon occurence for nurses, since nurses in traditional and sometimes nontraditional settings have the advantage with adolescents of dealing with them in their daily living. So, in the setting where other workers use the more structured means of psychotherapy, sometimes a rather significant differ-ence appears between the youngster's communication with the nurse and with his therapist. It is difficult to avoid letting such comparisons go to one's head, but avoid it we must if we are to move to the position of being more useful to the youngster.

I have found this problem even more exaggerated when dealing with poor black teen-agers from multiproblem families. In these cases the saviour complex seems to infect even the most sophisticated therapists. Harris and Fregly have described an almost classic instance of this.[3] Here the adolescent was part of a multiproblem family with whom a variety of agencies had dealt. In all cases each worker felt she or he was the most important, insofar as the youngster was concerned. There was no coordination, cooperation, or even honest sharing of information from worker to worker. Each agency representative magnified her own relationship with the adolescent and the family so as to exclude others rather than use them as partners. It is unfortunate that this ego trap is so common with adolescents, since it cannot help but serve as a barrier to the youngsters' growth in therapy.

The problems of seduction, envy, and other countertransference symptoms give us difficulty in the area of our reactions to drug and sex behaviors. Recently, in talking with psychiatric nurses about different problems they were seeing on their adolescent unit from when I first worked with adolescents, they seemed surprised. One said, "Different, how? They've always been sex and drugs, drugs and sex." Well, always is a big word and not entirely accurate in this instance. Social acceptance of both these areas has changed markedly. These nurses were fairly close in age to their adolescent patients; at least they were under 30. The narrower the gap in age between the worker and the adolescent patient, the greater the possibility for empathy with or antagonism toward adolescent behaviors. This needs careful looking at, since we react strongly in one way or another. But in all cases it is assumed today that "the use of drugs, especially marijuana but including hallicinogens, amphetamines, barbiturates, and assorted others, by middle class youth has become normative behavior."[1]

Despite this, in each instance the use of drugs must be looked at in terms of what the disturbed youngster is trying to accomplish with them and how he is not succeeding. Unless we are very clear about the rational and irrational elements of our own reactions to drugs, our reactions to the youngsters' attempts will be far from helpful. Drug use and abuse as well as the apparent sexual freedom of our adolescent patients must be reacted to "clean" if you will, in terms of the particular adolescent and what the behavior means to him. Envy, identification, and sentimentality will not help us help anyone. Therefore, returning to the earlier statement that problems are all the same (sex and drugs), we can look at these problems from the standpoint of symptom behaviors for many of the youngsters with whom we deal, since these behaviors do not work to enhance human contact.

The attempts at closeness through sex or at relaxation and camaraderie through drinking or drugs do not work. So the young person, through one or another form of acting out or because of severe psychotic symptoms, comes to the experts for help in solving earlier problems as well as the working through of his presently exacerbated adolescent ones. Helping persons, such as physicians and nurses, are in a position in which thoughtful use of the behavioral manifestations of adolescent development can move the youngster rapidly into the first part of a therapeutic relationship. What comes next will depend to some degree on the variables discussed.

CONCLUSION

Some generalizations or principles should be drawn from the foregoing with regard to therapeutic intervention with adolescents. First is an awareness that any one of numerous behaviors observed during early adolescence may be a perfectly normal developmental phenomenon; this requires knowing what age-typical behaviors are. Second is sensitivity to one's own needs and reactions and a willingness to look at these by oneself and with others, both peers and supervisors, at various points during thera-

peutic encounters. Third is an interest in looking into the historical pattern of the youngsters' problem behaviors. Fourth is continuous, consistent, and honest use of other workers in the area and the sharing of important information concerning adolescents. I do not believe by any means that lack of sharing is a nursing phenomenon. If one accepts the fact that adolescents are difficult patients and that adolescent therapy is frequently aborted at some point, it should be clear to all workers that collaborative efforts are required to achieve some success. Fifth is a recognition of the parents' role in the problem and its solution. Parents of healthy adolescents often need some support to accept their youngster's movements away from them toward independence. Parents of disturbed children require support as well as participation in the treatment process. Sixth and perhaps most important is getting clear about where we stand and why on some adolescent behaviors that are widely discussed today.

Finally, I should like to state that I think adolescents are probably more difficult to deal with at present than at any recent historical period. Several reasons have been suggested in this chapter and by others. The adolescent's impelling need for adult clarity is unfortunately answered by adult confusion. In presenting some baseline data on developmental characteristics, I have tried to set the stage for a milieu and the relationships within it based on some understanding of the normal adolescent's needs. Recognizing that we do not have all the answers but are interested in observing and learning, being neither sentimental nor seduced by our adolescent patients, and being adult enough to handle our own lives in our arenas, not theirs, will, it is hoped, contribute to building relationships of confidence and trust.

References

1. Esman, A. H.: Consolidation of the ego ideal in contemporary adolescence. In Psychosocial process, vol. 2, No. 19, p. 51.
2. Freud, A.: The ego and the mechanisms of defense, New York, 1946, International Universities Press.
3. Harris, F., and Fregly, M.: An adolescent struggle for independence. In Fagin, C. M., editor:

Nursing in child psychiatry, St. Louis, 1972, The C. V. Mosby Co.

4. Kohlberg, L., and Gilligan, C.: The adolescent as a philosopher. The discovery of the self in a postconventional world, Daedalus, Journal of the Academy of Arts and Sciences **100:**1051, Fall, 1971.

5. Redl, F.: When we deal with children, New York, 1966, The Free Press, pp. 35-67.

6. Schwartz, C. G.: Problems for psychiatric nurses in playing a new role. In The patient and the mental hospital, New York, 1957, The Free Press.

7. Schwartz, M.: What is a therapeutic milieu? In The patient and the mental hospital, New York, 1957, The Free Press.

8. Werner, H.: Comparative psychology of mental development, New York, 1961, Science Editions.

Bibliography

Redl, F.: Adolescents—just how do they react? In Caplan, G., and Lebovici, S., editors: Adolescence: psychosocial perspectives, New York, 1969, Basic Books, Inc.

5

Rules of conduct and the mental health of a profession*

Elizabeth M. Maloney

The parameters can be set at once when the question of defining mental health arises. The most obvious one is that little agreement exists as to what constitutes mental health other than to say that it is a life state with two potentials for definition—internal and external—and even those are studied with ambiguity. It is possible to be a raving lunatic internally and to present simultaneously a facade of sweet reason to the community. When this statement is subjected to examination, the fog truly rolls in. Is the definition of mental health possible purely on an internal basis? A seriously depressed person, if he could rouse himself from his grievous ruminations long enough to argue the case, would say yes. Yet in the spirit of sophistry it could be argued that his mental health comes into question only at the point at which someone else is discomfited or inconvenienced by his dysfunction. This is when the community comes into the picture. As with the phase *mental health,* community, too, is a many splendored thing. It can be large or small, paranoid or golden age, urban ghetto or privileged suburb. Community can designate a small interpersonal system, a commune in the Idaho hills, or a community of scholars in Oxford.

It has so far been indicated that both mental health and community are elastic terms. They are essentially expansible, con-

tractible, and, up to a point, subject to eccentric definition by any group or persons. Some factor common to both might help to serve as a focal point for examination. Thus in a universe of multiple possibilities, I would like to advance the concept of rules of conduct[2] as the framework on which to base a consideration of how the identity of a health occupation, whatever its stage of evolution, is joined to its sociopsychiatric function in patient care. Partially I am talking about the rules of conduct for a professional life and, now and again, about the rules that one occupation covertly (and sometimes arrogantly) sets down for another.

In May, 1971, at Boston University, Silber[4] gave an address that was simultaneously inaugural and commencement. The title of it was "The Pollution of Time," and it contains more wisdom about mental health than most psychiatric workers have uttered in years. (This is not surprising, since many people in the psychiatric field devote at least half their waking hours to obscuring issues with language; the other half they spend attacking each other with it. Both are counts on which almost all people who wish to help change behavior could be indicted at one time or another.)

I would like to quote Silber to indicate at least a tenuous rationale for the use of three concepts as signal beacons in ordering this discussion. For mental health in any community is life itself in this, our one and only time on earth. We are time-bound and spacebound, and even the most lost among us try from time to time to elicit a modicum of meaning for their lives.

All over the nation we hear cries of alarm about the pollution of air and the pollution of water, but

---

*This discussion has been adapted from two presentations. The first was a speech sponsored by Sigma Theta Tau, Xi chapter, of the University of Pennsylvania and Alpha Nu chapter, Villanova University, May 1, 1971. The second was the keynote address on the occasion of the Festival of Life and Learning, College of Nursing, University of Manitoba, February 10, 1972.

we hear little or nothing about a pollution far more serious—that of time itself. We can, after all, recycle air and water through filters. But we cannot recycle time . . . when the structure of time is destroyed, the basis for significance in our lives is likewise destroyed. All meaning is lost in the instantaneous.*

He goes on to say that the demands of youth for relevance and of the older generation for law and order are both sides of the same coin:

> . . . The human concern for meaning, for a life that makes sense. In the search for meaning, man is essentially concerned with time, for time is the very matrix of human existence. Our overarching project becomes that of building a structure or pattern of significance into our lives.*

It can be accepted then that man structures time and space to provide some element of control over his existence and that the structure and control operations themselves are outward manifestations (or symptoms, if you will) of a value system. A value system gives meaning to life, and value systems are precisely what mental health is all about.

Again Silber makes the telling point that "the instant culture allows no time for the development of a variety of human relationships at substantially different levels of intensity"*—instant friendships, instant loves, instant demolition of these because there was no commitment to them in the first place (not even a commitment to the self—above all, not that). We have a cult (or cant) of sincerity and honesty, but, as the same source states, this is no substitute for integrity because integrity can be assessed only through the passage of time. Integrity in turn is a close relative of an unequivocal sense of identity, and an acceptable, workable sense of identity is what provides stability in an individual and, in a large sense, the occupation to which he belongs.

Perhaps a few thoughts on the search for identity in general in our culture might be appropriate here. Wheelis said that " . . . with increasing frequency in recent years a change in the character of the

American people has been described . . . "* and he cites Riesman, Glazer, and Denny as among those making the description. The change is still in progress. Whereas our grandparents were largely held to be inner directed, our fate is alleged to be that of forever having our radar tuned to the group. Wheelis says, referring to the inner-directed group, "Nobody worried about rigidity of character; it was supposed to be rigid. If it were flexible you couldn't count on it. Change of character was desirable only for the wicked."* He then concluded his remarks on a nostalgic note:

> Many of us still remember the bearded old men; the country doctor, the circuit rider, the blacksmith, the farmer. They were old when we were young, and they are dead now. . . The character that went with them is disappearing and soon even its memory will be lost.*

Societies function smoothly only when there is a reasonable consensus that established rules are to be followed. Sciologists have described whole classes of people who deviate from adherence to the established norms. Goffman states that "the psychiatric study of situational improprieties has led to studying the offender rather than the rules and social circles that are offended"† and makes the important point that, more by accident than design, psychiatrists have made us aware of an important area in social life—that of behavior in public and semipublic places. The behavior allowed is based on a set of rules.

Laing wrote, "The deeper 'social' laws are implanted; the more 'hard-programmed' or 'pickled' into us, the more like 'natural' laws they come to appear to us to be. Indeed if someone breaks such a 'deeply' implanted social law, we are inclined to say that he is 'unnatural',"‡—or, we might add, crazy, a psychiatric problem, or has lost his mental health. Whatever appellation is ap-

---

*From Silber, J. R.: The pollution of time, Bostonia 45:9, 1971.

*From Wheelis, A.: The quest for identity. In Milton, O., and Wahler, R., editors: Behavior disorders: perspectives and trends, ed. 3, Philadelphia, 1973, J. B. Lippincott Co., p. 216.
†From Goffman, E.: Behavior in public places, New York, 1963, The Free Press, p. 3.
‡From Laing, R. D.: The politics of the family and other essays, New York, 1969, Pantheon Books, a division of Random House, Inc., pp. 90, 103, 111, and 113.

plied, nine chances out of ten the person involved has broken a social rule, one relevant to a particular setting or community, and, what is more, he probably has done so, or it is feared that he will do so, in a public place.

Still, in relation to rules and rules about rules (metarules), Laing goes on, "There is said to be a *time* and place for everything. For ex: at home one must *not* put mother's pearl necklace down the W.C.,"* but more germane to the discussion of any degree of mental health is his following statement:

I have never come across anyone (including myself) who does not draw a line as to: *what may be put into words* and, *what words what may be put into*. . . . We at this moment may not know we have rules against knowing certain rules.*

As an example, Laing cites a family rule that little Johnny should not have filthy thoughts. He is a good boy and does not have to be told not to think this way, so there is no rule against this because there is no need to make a rule about something that never occurs. There is also no need to talk about this "dreary, abstract and even vaguely filthy subject,"* since it is nonexistent anyway.

That our daily lives are governed by adhering to whole networks of little and larger rules seems factual enough. Goffman makes the following point:

One of the best guides to a systematic understanding of the observable conduct of mental patients in and out of hospitals, and of others' response to this conduct, is to be found in etiquette manuals.†

And what is Emily Post but a guide to appropriate and proper social interaction? Still, not to know the finer points of when to leave a calling card will not raise any questions concerning one's mental health. Rules also govern distance and closeness in friendships, business, work, and other human interactions—unwritten but known to most adults. Refusal to follow a timetable or some failure in understanding this rule

and cue system also will not raise questions about one's mental health to the point where the alienists are sent for, but it can leave the individual lonely and thus cheated of what might be numbered among the richer experiences of life.

Community mental health is tied to the time in which patients and nurses live. Mental illness, the pathology with which psychiatric and other nurses concern themselves, is defined by a set of rules laid down by the consensus of a public or, to put it another way, by one's contemporaries. Now what of these nurses themselves? How do their dilemmas affect, even in a small way, the health picture in this country?

"PSYCHOLOGY" OF NURSING

Of course, it is patently impossible to sketch in anything but the bold outlines or the mainsprings that make an occupation move or become decadent and eventually die. The motivation behind much activity in nursing for the last 25 years has not only reflected a wider societal ferment but additionally what seems to be a slowly emerging professional identity with concomitant problems.

First and of vital importance to the discussion of nursing is that it is predominately a woman's profession. The mental health of most nurses is as good as the average citizen's, one presumes, but, if the disciplined use of one's capacities in the pursuit of excellence is necessary for mental health, three occupational factors militate against this. The first is the collective and individual nursing perception of how to act or how to view the rules of the occupational game, the second is the physician's view of how the game ought to be played, and third is the gaming rules of the patient's own Monte Carlo, the hospital, where a stay can at times be likened to a game of roulette as far as getting personal and sometimes even physical needs met.

Speaking of games, Rapoport has said that "Games ought not to be played in certain contexts, for example, where human lives and human welfare are at stake."* The argument will be advanced

---

*From Laing, R. D.: The politics of the family and other essays, New York, 1969, Pantheon Books, a division of Random House, Inc., pp. 90, 103, 111, and 113.
†From Goffman, E.: Behavior in public places, New York, 1963, The Free Press, p. 6.

*From Rapoport, A.: Fights, games and debates, Ann Arbor, 1961, University of Michigan Press, pp. viii and xiii.

that, in the largest sense of the game concept, nurses and others do engage in games that are detrimental to themselves. More important, these games are unnecessarily traumatic to patients. Rapoport indicates that the "starting point" is not so much disagreement, ". . . but on the contrary an agreement, namely an agreement of the opponents to strive for incompatible goals within the constraint of certain rules. This type of struggle is now technically called a 'game'."*

THE HOSPITAL AS A THEATER FOR GAMES

The hospital is a social system and, aside from its highly specific functions, is the universe in miniature or microcosm. Cultural factors and streams of action afoot in the broader society eventually find their way in some form into the hospital institution. Special interest groups are now developing ways to affect others. This is a fact of life that nurses (with some exceptions) appear too slow to grasp, apparently feeling that somehow a benevolent deity will lead them out of the desert into the promised land. This is a time of confrontation, accumulation of clout, and rhetoric and negotiation. Thus follows an attempt to limn interpersonal strategies and the game analogy[3] because, if nurses really mean to be patient advocates, then they must use the tools of the times.

Burnstein[1] makes the activities inherent in any simple social situation analogous to a game situation, pointing out that many daily encounters are pretty dull, as are some games. He also adds that in a simple two-person situation no realistic assumption of "complete strategies" is possible because no one person can do more than speculate on what the other one will do, since he is free to select from among many possible alternatives, or options. To the degree that all of us are neurotic, of course, we go on monotonously selecting the prototype that "done us wrong" in the first place. Logically then, if any of us are known to have limited reactive scope or a

paucity of options locked into selected areas, then the astute strategist can (to that degree) predict our behavior. For example, some people will explode with anger around such sensitive areas as politics, war, religion, and authority; next they will walk away from the situation or otherwise withdraw, frequently resorting to covert strategies to deal with the problem, so that you know, if x button is pushed, y action will follow.

The next proposition to be advanced is that generally nurses have strong positive feelings about what goes on in regard to their ability to give expert care to patients but that, when they meet obstacles, they characteristically assume an overtly docile surface response and then resort to manipulative, seductive, or covert operations to achieve goals. They are responding reflexively and in almost Pavlovian fashion to the thesis that the limits of what can happen are set by the rules of the game.

One of the significant observations that one can make about hospitals (or other institutions) is that the sociocultural rules have changed and the game has changed, but the actors in this particular plot are not wholly aware of this. Paraprofessionals are much more alert to the possibilities of power politics and probably, in the end, will provide some new rules for hospital life.

Politics is essentially the art of the possible, to paraphrase a common comment. Pressure and negotiation are the operations used in the achievement of the possible. Hospitals have been authoritarian and hierarchical institutions in a democratic society, which depends on the reconciliation of multiple points of view into a working consensus. The consensus, then, is translated into policy or action.

As an example of the newer modus operandi, a movement is now afoot or established for a nursing group to pass on nursing practice in a given institution; so one of the rules bends a little, to permit a peer group to evaluate a peer group, thus eliminating the unwritten rule that physicians and the nursing establishment shall be the sole purveyors of the accolade "good nurse." Changing rules means changing mores. If this practice should become wide-

---

*From Rapoport, A.: Fights, games and debates, Ann Arbor, 1961, University of Michigan Press, pp. viii and xiii.

spread, no longer will the practitioner sit around waiting to be anointed from on high.

Another change is apparently in process. The holders of de facto power are beginning to know they have it; possibly now they will begin to use it as a means of achieving better patient care. Not long ago, nurses in New York took an advertisement in the *New York Times* to proclaim that they wanted not only legal recognition of their independent functions but also freedom to provide better nursing care. Let us look at the operations here:

They ceased playing by the established rules by (1) summoning nurses and the public to close ranks in the common goal of better patient care, (2) going over the heads of established authorities, (3) using a somewhat sophisticated brand of rhetoric, (4) attempting to form a new power bloc, nurse-consumers, which confronted the then current position of the State Medical Society and others, and (5) ending with successfully negotiated new legislation defining nursing practice.

If this analysis is even reasonably accurate, notice how the game is played now: power blocs, support, a certain amount of rhetoric, confrontation, persuasion, and negotiation. That is "where it is at" today. The game must be altered, the players will be held to more accountability, and pressure from the consumer will eventually force change. It might be diverting to briefly examine how inevitably some will regard "outsiders" as having the right to participate in making policy for health planning in the years ahead. Michael Michaelson wrote an article called "The Failure of American Medicine" in *The American Scholar*, Autumn, 1970. The idea that either organized medicine or nursing could ever fail its clients is anathema to both groups, and predictably our medical brethren's lamentations rose to the vaults of heaven in letters to the editor in the Spring issue of the journal. Many atrocity stories were cited to illustrate what would occur if anything happened to upset the status quo, and a great many of them were probably legitimate. Statements such as the following represent, however, the philosophy by which a select group still lives.

The most offensive part of the whole article is the idea of regulation to be imposed by those of lesser mind, whether bureaucracy, hospital administrators, sociologists or politicians on physicians, who, by virtue of their inclination, perspicacity and training, are, as a group of health specialists, best suited to decide what constitutes good and adequate medical care for all.*

PSYCHOLOGICAL MALPRACTICE

Psychological malpractice is admittedly a slippery concept to examine, but it does exist—usually under other labels. However, some nursing interactions with patients border on trauma. Being charitable, one can postulate that, when an individual nurse derives no satisfaction from a situation, the satisfaction of the patient is nonexistent also. The all-too-common practice of stereotyping and scapegoating one or more patients has the result of almost painfully isolating such a patient. In addition, the consensus on a unit that an individual is difficult, neurotic, or a crank sets up a vicious action-reaction circle that sometimes the patient can escape only through dying or being discharged.

More often the nurse engages in witting or unwitting petty harassments than in larger enterprises. Withholding or delaying medication is one strategy. The following was such a recently observed maneuver:

A patient entered the ward office and asked a nurse if his medication were available, stating that he felt jumpy and tense. The nurse, who was doing nothing at that time on a small, just then quiet private unit went through the ritual of glancing at her watch and, to make sure the patient got the message, at the wall clock. Then she said, "It will be along if you wait a half hour." The tone was cool, the manner faintly contemptuous, and the dismissal absolute. The situation was, first, that the medication (a mild tranquilizer) was due and the patient was aware of that fact and, second, that the nurse never did administer it. Two hours later the night nurse gave the medication. The patient, who presumably had incurred some animus, was not physically harmed but could be viewed as a victim of some kind of psychological gamesmanship.

Such small put-downs are tension reducers and are used every day in every walk of life. They are not conducive to the mental health of either participant in the transaction, particularly the one with the power.

---

*From Letter to the editor, The American scholar, p. 529, Spring, 1970.

Hospitals are for sick people? Not entirely. They are also semibankrupt businesses, training grounds for health careerists from nutritionists to x-ray technicians, and battlegrounds for unions and management; last they are for the sick. They were pesthouses once and are in a fair way to becoming so again. In other words, it was once worth your life literally to go into a hospital; hospitals currently are becoming more oriented to the acute and lifesaving activities and thus again are, in that sense, places to go to die, as well as to live. Perhaps it is time that professional nurses abandoned these limping institutions to the physicians and the ever-burgeoning numbers of technical workers, who, realistically, cost less and ask fewer questions, and decamp to where the action really is—in prevention and perhaps rehabilitation in the community.

It would be fair to say that nurses rather consistently satisfy their own needs at the expense of patients. Aside from their selection of the nursing field in the first place, many contributory factors indicate why they do so. First, they are women, with all of the rights and wrongs that accrue to that sex in today's American cuture. Second, they are still a dependent arm of the ancient profession of medicine (ancient in more ways than one) and frequently therefore are required to exercise power covertly to achieve a sense of professional self-esteem. Third, they still work to a large degree in those status-ridden, outmoded, but necessary institutions known as hospitals. Fourth, they work with helpless and sometimes powerless people, which enhances to a degree the need to be needed, with psychiatric, medical-surgical, and public health nurses exhibiting this need in a different way and in a different setting. Most important, an effort has been made to identify some reasons why nurses satisfy their own needs, whereas those of the patients frequently wither on the vine.

If primary care or prevention is to become even more important than it is now and if nurses are to be concerned with the community's mental health, some of the unthinking psychological transactions that go on now should be subjected to appraisal. To document the disillusionment of

nurses is easy enough. It is most tellingly reflected in the rate of dropouts and in the all too frequently observed cases of copping out.

The Lysaught report,* which replaces the Brown report, which replaced the Goldmark report, not only documents our manifest failings but also provides a highly visible public pillory in which to do penance for the mess we are in. The main point here is, "Nursing is a sorely troubled profession." The first question is why we go on expending large sums of money to document this. More important, why are we such a troubled group?

SUMMARY

Obviously to talk about the mental health of such a large group of health workers as nurses is partially caricature. Equally obvious is the fact that persons are being lost to nursing at an alarming rate. Only a few of the reasons have been speculated on here. Some of the underlying psychological reasons that are never given on exit interviews have been described in the metaphor of gaming. They are destructive games in many ways and fall into the same descriptive category as not knowing that "we have rules against knowing certain rules" about conducting our lives.

Among some of the rules that we must not know are the rules that have not until recently been spoken about. For example, a tight chain of events, myths, and economic and status factors is at the bottom of the current health delivery disturbances. It can be documented that the shortage of physicians could, if one were tenacious enough, be traced to an elitist, economically based stance on the part of several generations of their leaders. The shortage of nurses is in large part a myth. The use to which nurses allow themselves to be put is the problem.

The health care system is overburdened now with a multiplicity of new workers. Now another, the physician's assistant, appears—for whose eventual good and with what legal implications? There is also a need for physicians (who, in the final

---

*Lysaught, J.: An abstract for action, New York, 1970, McGraw-Hill Book Co., pp. 1-23.

analysis, are legally responsible for activities relating to health and illness, as they frequently point out) to engage in collaborative relationships with others. They have a long history of handing down administrative fiats. Perhaps the solution is to ensure that with all reasonable and safe speed their heavy legal responsibility be shared with other licensed health workers. This action might make a vast difference in the way patients receive care in the future.

The rules that we talk about and know are not problematic. Those which cause difficulty and which can be classed as covert metarules are the ones that cause occupational identity crises, strains in work roles, and covert and unproductive operations, or games. As with individuals in their life-spans, professions often find themselves in identity crises, playing games of dubious worth and giving lip service to one set of rules for conduct and living out another every day. At least one truth is as certain at this moment as when it was expressed years ago:

You (the nurses of the present generation) will find yourself inevitably concerned with the educational problems of the day, with the social and civic movements of the time, with legislative efforts to sustain these, and will of necessity come to take your share in them; for nursing is bound up with every one of them.*

*From Nutting, M. A. In Lesnik, M., and Anderson, B.: Nursing practice and the law, ed. 2, Philadelphia, 1962, J. B. Lippincott Co.

References

1. Burnstein, E.: Interdependence in groups. In Mills, J., editor: Experimental social psychology, London, 1968, The Macmillan Co., p. 357.
2. Goffman, E.: Behavior in public places, New York, 1963, The Free Press, p. 4.
3. Rapoport, A.: Fights, games and debates, Ann Arbor, 1961, University of Michigan Press, pp. viii, ix, xiii.
4. Silber, J. R.: The pollution of time, Bostonia 45:9, Sept., 1971.

Bibliography

Laing, R. D.: The politics of the family and other essays, New York, 1969, Pantheon Books, Inc.
Lysaught, J.: An abstract for action, New York, 1970, McGraw-Hill Book Co.
Wheelis, A.: The quest for identity. In Ohmer, M., editor: Behavior disorders, New York, 1965, J. B. Lippincott Co.

6

Remarks on the physiological and psychological factors influencing addiction*

Elizabeth M. Maloney

A discussion that encompasses both the physiological and psychological aspects of addiction must necessarily be limited at the outset to certain aspects of the problem. Implicit in the title, for example, is the assumption that the various addictions have much in common. This assumption may well be fallacious, and, indeed, many people are beginning to think that it is. The existence of an addictive personality is becoming more and more open to question. For example, Blaine states the following:

We do know that there are vast differences among individual alcoholics and these differences depend on a wide array of factors, such as social and cultural backgrounds, intelligence and education, the stage to which drinking behavior has progressed and so on.†

He goes on to list a series of personality traits that he views as characteristic but makes the point that culture and social environment are extremely significant. It is my belief that they are more important than any listing of traits that, in the final analysis, are found everywhere in human life. Second, these trait listings have closed off entire areas of therapeutic endeavor. Postulating other ways of looking at the problem may offer alternate avenues of approach. The most successful relief of addiction to date has been through organizations that are largely constituted of nonprofessional persons. Careful study of their operations casts tentative doubt on some professional views. It is no secret that some ex-addicts feel that they are better equipped to deal with the problem than, say, psychiatrists have been to date.

For example, professional workers often mention *dependence* as one trait, or personality characteristic, that is considered to be prominent in the "addictive personality." The pertinent question that is never asked is how much dependence is abroad in the general population and what forms does it take? The latter half of the question is the most significant.[6] Then a more incisive question needs to be considered: how does it violate a social norm? For instance, it is socially acceptable for a woman to allow her husband to make all decisions, to dole out money for personal purchases, and to decide on such details as menus and rising and retiring times. It is not acceptable to lie about the house stoned on pot or alcohol all day. Yet the one may be finally as destructive as the other; both are bondage in terms of what we wistfully call the good life. Both can be viewed as excessively dependent behaviors. Which, then, exemplifies the dependent personality that the professionals postulate? Professional treatment involves labeling, and labels are deceptive in many ways.

Almost the same type of question could be raised about the many faces of addiction to various drugs. Those of us who grew to maturity on the exploits of Fu Manchu knew unequivocally who the drug fiends

*This presentation was originally prepared for an interdisciplinary conference sponsored by The Institute for Professional Nurses on Alcoholism and Drug Abuse, May 15, 1972, New Orleans. Permission for publication has been granted, and substantial changes have been made.
†From Blaine, H.: The personality of the addict. In Chafetz, M., editor: Frontiers of alcoholism, New York, 1970, Science House, Inc., p. 16.

were. In a doss house on a foggy night in the Limehouse section of London were rooms reeking with opium. Dimly seen figures reclined on grubby bunks, puffing their way to narcotized nirvana. Thus it was possible to separate the "fiends" from the rest of us. It is not so easy now. The man next to your office may be in serious trouble with barbiturates and amphetamines and the lady to your right suffering from alcoholism; the boy who lives next door may be managing his heroin addiction with methadone or not be managing at all. None of these individuals will be categorized as "dependent" or victims of "oral fixation" or anything else unless they reach professional hands. That they are unproductive, miserable human beings is undeniable, and, if that state is illness, then a large proportion of the population is sick. Therefore the eventual fate of the person involved depends on who is defining things, under what circumstances, and on what basis. Since each of us has only one life, that fate is vital.

At this point two arguments that will explicitly or implicitly underlie the rest of this presentation should be advanced. Both are open to controversy among persons interested in addiction, and both question whether some of the beliefs held about the addictive process are valid, partially valid, or, in some instances, not valid at all. First is this proposition: the physiological, or withdrawal, symptoms are the most dramatic and the best known to professionals in medicine and nursing but are of lesser import than has hitherto been considered to be the case. They serve as a theatrical focal point and, in fact, obscure the long-term problem. This does *not* posit denial of the severe physical and mental anguish that occurs in addiction. It does not overlook the deaths that have occurred from delirium tremens or the overdose in drug addiction. It does mean that the majority of addicts can be helped in about five days with good medical and nursing management, although some in the field believe that eight or ten days are preferable. Seale,[9] whose paper is probably typical of treatment protocols in alcoholism, is one of the latter. A summary of his views follows. With some variations they would probably

coincide with many others in the field. (Specific regimens exist in other areas of addiction as well.)

1. He speaks first of the immediate need to institute a physical and mental appraisal of the patient, noting that acute intoxication may produce a patient with head injuries, contusions, concussions, convulsions, fractures, and delirium tremens.

2. Next he refers to the great help that tranquilizers have afforded, since without further clouding consciousness they reduce agitation. He asserts that chlordiazepoxide (Librium), diazepam (Valium), and hydroxyzine pamoate (Vistaril) exert an anticonvulsive effect and that diphenylhydantoin (Dilantin) three times daily may prevent withdrawal or convulsive seizures. For the more acute "shakes" chlorpromazine hydrochloride (Thorazine) and promazine (Sparine) are helpful. Paraldehyde may be used if tranquilizers are not successful in controlling delirium tremens. Diagnosis of alcohol-related conditions is made at this time (e.g., gastritis).

There are many variations on this general approach, but one of the important points made by Seale is the attitude of the nursing staff as a treatment factor. However, opinions vary in the field of alcoholism as to whether nurses are necessary. These positions range all the way from total acceptance of the nurse as a valuable team member to total denial of such a worker's value. Seale puts it this way:

We have been fortunate in having the same nurses for a number of years. Many former patients have attributed the success of their stay and rehabilitation to the nursing personnel.*

On one end of the spectrum is that testimonial and at the other, the intention to have only the minimal legal coverage. Discernible reasons for both extremes seem to lie in the usual human factors and patterns—a hope that less expensive personnel will serve, personal perceptions or experiences that lead to the conclusion that other

---

*From Seale, F. E.: Treatment of the alcoholic in a clinical setting. In Texas summer studies on alcohol, Austin, Texas, July 13-18, 1969, University of Texas Press, p. 4.

workers can better be prepared on the job, and, probably the seldom discussed fact that nurses today are more knowledgeable and more vocal. To the less secure, this is a condition that is problematic but that can be managed by training paraprofessionals to a treatment attitude specific to a given rehabilitative unit. Of course, it may come as a shock to some nurses, but there are physicians who categorize everyone but themselves as paraprofessionals. It may come as a shock to some mental health technicians that nurses characterize them as paraprofessionals—and so goes the labeling and classifying game, which would be glorious fun if it did not affect the fate of the client, or patient, so much. As Roman[7] has pointed out, the "disease label has disease consequences," and so it does. Attaching labels to people is usually preceded by a steryotyping or a professional "hierarchical stance"[8] that is heavily attitudinal in nature and predictable in its operational effects. For example, the label *patient* in the psychiatric world, so quickly and so loosely applied at times, has disastrous consequences for some individuals not just during hospitalization but also, as Goffman[3] has remarked, for the rest of their lives.

The second assumption related to this presentation would take this form: the most urgent problems in consideration of the addictions are attitudinal and social. They are most closely related to two key concepts, deviance and stigma,[3] with the subabstraction of "passing" seen as related to the stigmatized of the world and the consequences of being stigmatized.

First, a seminal work[4] in the field of psychiatry will be cited as indicative of the direction that follows.

In a discussion of the "oppression of a label" Halleck cites the growing number of psychiatrists (such as Szasz, Leifer, and Menninger) who have identified the damage that labeling can do and the power of those who label in our society.

When an individual is given a medical label, society is encouraged to believe that his behavior cannot be controlled; a non-medical label, on the other hand, leads society to assume that an individual can control his behavior. Thus, a heavy drinker may be thought of as imprudent or ob-

noxious; however, once we call him an alcoholic, we assume that he cannot control his drinking.*

Indeed, according to all the standards we know and all the data we possess, he cannot control his drinking. Halleck continues as follows:

In the area of drugs, a man who uses alcohol or other drugs to excess may be overwhelmed with all sorts of personal and social difficulties and still maintain a respectable role in society. However, once he is labeled an alcoholic or an addict, he is cast into an entirely different social role; he is viewed as a person who is diseased. Some people will pity him, but a sizeable number will fear or scorn him.*

Eric Berne has said that "The vast literature on alcoholism is, with few exceptions, an apology for not being able to do much about it." He also noted that the word *alcoholic* is only about a hundred years old and makes an important point for those who would help the alcoholic in a professional sense. He said about the word *alcoholic* that "It is one of those words ending in 'ic' used by clinicians to mean a non-person, like 'schizophrenic' and 'psychotic'."†

At this point I would like to offer a tentative conclusion, one that is in accord with all the available literature but may deserve more prominence than it now apparently gets. This conclusion concerns aggression and one of its close correlates, power.[6] The covertly aggressive pattern (often hidden under an agreeable facade) and an equally unacknowledged drive for power might be considered central problems in the future as is the almost classic "dependent-orally fixated" combine now. As a beginning psychiatric nurse I was chief supervisor of the admission building in a large public hospital. One of my duties was to preside over the admission of patients. Among the recurring clients were alcoholically addicted men and women. Additionally, as a middle-management administrator, I encountered problems em-

---

*From Halleck, S. L.: The politics of therapy, New York, 1971, Science House, Inc., pp. 102 and 104.
†From Berne, E. In Steiner, C.: Games alcoholics play, New York, 1971, Grove Press, Inc., p. ix. Reprinted by permission of Grove Press, Inc. Copyright 1971 by Claude Steiner.

anating from this group, such as illicit but highly functional stills uncovered in locked ward kitchens and underground routes for the importation of fluid supplies. This focused my attention on the group; thus I was struck, as many have been before me, by three characteristics of this population. First, that after the shakes and incipient or actual delirium tremens were warded off, these persons were clearly marching to a different drummer than were the diverse psychotics in the unit. In short, after a few days they did not belong there. Second, none of the personnel was clear about where they did belong. Third, collectively they were an affable group, ever ready to work about the ward and to help confused or elderly patients and generally sociable. This characteristic remained in my mind many years after I had gone on to other things; some rumination then suggested that aggression and its useful, or productive, expression might well be the central dynamic and therapeutic factor in alcoholism, if not in drug abuse or other addiction as well. Let us revive the old simplistic psychiatric truism: frustration leads to aggression; aggression in turn can be expressed outwardly or turned inward against the self. Certainly the long-term ingestion of substances such as chemicals in quantities sufficient temporarily to obliterate reality is an extreme act of hostility toward the self. Also documented of late, although not so prominently, is the hostility so evident in what addiction does to those persons in the vicinity of the user. The whole picture, when this later facet is added, becomes one of rather massive aggression—retaliation and power over others.

Earlier in the chapter, one of the biggest problems regarding addiction was mentioned, that is, the attitudinal and societal factors that are so closely tied to addicts, ex-addicts, and families of addicts. Addicts are deviates in the sociological sense; deviates are stigmatized by their departure from the norm. As ex-addicts, they have essentially three choices: (1) to "pass" as normal or as never having been addicted, (2) to proclaim their addiction and identify with other ex-addicts, or (3) selectively to filter information to a small trusted group and

pass in the rest of their contacts in the business and social world.

I have already mentioned the destructiveness of labels as applied to any human being. To label is to stereotype and dehumanize; once dehumanization occurs, it is easy to rationalize anything that is done to the nonhuman other—even killing him. Szasz[10] has for the past decade been a burr under the saddle of the psychiatric establishment, stating among other things that "It is widely believed [that persons afflicted with mental illness] are psychologically and socially inferior to those not so afflicted [and must be cared for] even if that care requires interventions imposed on them against their will or incarceration in a mental hospital." One does not need to document that addicts are sociologically tenants of the same house. Becker,[1] in an excellent volume on deviance, has said that sociologists no longer confine themselves to "delinquents and drug addicts" but are widening their focus to include not only the who, why, and where of deviance but also the process of interaction between those who veer sharply from the norm and those who live in the normal world, if a normal world, in fact, exists.

To go back to the ways that declared deviants cope with their problem once they become ex-addicts, let us consider the decision to "pass." Goffman,[3] as has been pointed out earlier, makes clear that the constant price paid for "passing" is eternal vigilance against exposure, with all the ramifications inherent in discovery. On the other hand, it is generally well recognized that everyone has at least one skeleton in the closet. A recurrent joke makes this point lucidly. One man makes a public announcement, "Fly, all is discovered!" whereupon 95% of the town's population precipitately leaves.

The second choice, to proclaim addiction and join a group of ex-addicts, has found expression in a recognized social movement. In a publication called *Odd Man In,* Sagarin has characterized this phenomenon as follows:

The growth of an important social movement of open, voluntary and formal organizations . . . among people whom society has characterized as deviant people who are subject to scorn, discrimination, gossip, sometimes pity, and sometimes punishment, because they carry a stigma.*

Among the organizations he treats in his document are Alcoholics Anonymous, Gamblers Anonymous, The Mattachine Society, Synanon, and The Little People of America (dwarfs), to name a few. This source provides a description and critique of the various societies, or organizations, that attract the stigmatized of the American culture.

As to professional attitudes toward the addicted deviate among the patient population, Chafetz has the following comment about one group of addicts:

> What about alcohol excess! What is there about it that makes us self-righteous and punitive, moralistic, and inhumane? Even today the attitude towards alcoholic persons is different from that towards other ill individuals.†

The comment was made about what might be called the general (lay) public, but it is in keeping with the feelings of many workers in the so-called mental health field. This is one of the reasons why so many persons find work in the field of addiction so unrewarding, but there are also other reasons.

My impression, formulated over time, is that the physiological aspects of the addictive process, although important, have assumed too much significance vis-à-vis the total problem. The attitudinal and social aspects are far more urgent for the long term, and too often the theoretical framework or the professional educational process that teaches the conceptual basis for medical or nursing action fails in some part. The relevant sociological insights that might be useful are glossed over. For example, the deviant in society serves a not altogether healthy purpose in that, if one can put down the other person, one can put oneself up. Polarity rules judgmental classification: wicked-good, sinner-saint. On the other hand, society must maintain equilibrium and some order of morality, as it has been defined at a given point in history, so that an element of double binding

enters also to complicate matters. It is similar to the descriptions of neurotic interactions so ably developed by Horney many years ago. These essentially nonproductive operations are described by the common saying that it takes two to tango. Let us further examine the concept that the addict is frequently caught in a double- and sometimes triple-binding communication. On the one hand, society says, "You deviate, depart from your wicked ways, repent, and return to us," and, on the other hand, says in effect, "You are not like us; doubtless you will do it again" (e.g., become mentally ill, shoot up, or return to jail). There is some truth to this because recidivism is frequent. To use the neurotic parallel, a situation exists in which one person cons the other into commitment and then says blandly, "You misunderstood me all along." As Sagarin comments, "Any mutual adjustment and mutual approval between two individuals can be fundamentally embarrassed if one of the partners accepts in full the offer that the other appears to make."* "Come close–go away" is bad enough, but to add "I never said either in the first place" approaches the summit of distancing operations. Of course, anyone familiar with the more exquisite waltz of the neurotic game knows the pattern. The sado-masochistic elements of it become immediately clear to the observer and eventually to the engrossed players themselves. Although generalizations are sometimes of dubious worth, society apparently needs its scapegoats.

SUMMARY

To debate the efficacy of the so-called medical model as the major therapeutic approach to addictions is outside the scope of this discussion. I have stated elsewhere my belief that this structure is riddled with fallacies when it comes to the care of the mentally ill, in part because of the territorial and power needs of professionals. Be that as it may, addiction, too, is being treated according to that model, and it may be the best solution that this decade has to

*From Sagarin, E.: Odd man in, Chicago, copyright 1969 with permission of the publisher Quadrangle/ The New York Times Book Co.
†From Chafetz, M.: The prevention of alcoholism, Int. J. Psychiatry 13:331, 1972.

*From Sagarin, E.: Odd man in, Chicago, copyright 1969, with permission of the publisher, Quadrangle/ The New York Times Book Co., p. 123.

offer. Certainly there seems to be little willingness to look at new conceptual ways of dealing with the problem. So essentially we are still discussing what all of us call sickness, or loss of mental health, and it seems appropriate to close these remarks in that vein.

Everyone lives surrounded by rules, and, although acceptance or rejection of these codes does not mean disaster or success in terms of mental health, many of us have to abide by them as gracefully as possible even though not believing in all of them wholeheartedly. Those who cannot believe or act at all are "ill" or "deviate." The one we channel to "treatment" and the other to assorted institutions; sometimes we direct the same individual alternately to hospital and jail.

Mental health is an ambiguous and even autistic term, especially since the psychiatric labeling system in the hands of the vengeful can, with almost no effort, be used to classify any behavior as "sick." Flagrant paranoids can stalk the streets, but, as long as they do not utter their suspicions, they are not considered ill.

The entire psychiatric establishment needs reexamination in terms of its immense and submerged potential for power because many of its practitioners—physicians, nurses, social workers, and psychologists alike—are in danger of becoming the arbiters of morals and ethics in this country. The alleged use of the psychiatric institution for political punishment is already recorded in the world press. The mental hospital is, among other things, an institution of social control. As Cumming[2] points out, "All complex modern societies have a proliferation of agents and agencies charged with the social control of individuals"—physicians, social workers, policemen, etc. Addicts are the subjects of these agents' concern.

The mental health of the second-class citizen is always somewhat vulnerable. Probably the healthiest response would be an accumulation of sufficient power to challenge the established status holders to compel the respect due other human beings and particularly to ensure better health care for the sick.

Mental health is capable of many definitions. My own selection is one developed by Heath[5] in 1964, which resulted from a study of a group of Princeton students. He called his prototype of health "The Reasonable Adventurer," characterizing this person (as do similar lists of mental health attributes) as having "intellectuality, close friendships, independence in value judgments, tolerance of ambiguity, breadth of interests and a sense of humor." All these and more are characteristics possessed by many addicts, in common with much of the human race. While addicted, they are unable or much less free to use them.

The central thesis of this chapter has probably resulted in the substitution of one set of concepts for another in looking at the addictive process. As McClelland and his colleagues put it so well, "The essence of the problem lies in one's conception of the nature of psychological theories or explanation."* They further emphasize: *"The conventional model of a scientific theory dictates that it should lead to a crucial operational test which will confirm or reject it"** (italics mine). Nurses who are anchored with patients and their pathology for so many hours of the therapeutic day above all need a conceptual framework that can be put into practice. Finding ways of socially channeling needs for power and aggression might be more useful to addicts in the long run than some current theories and activities. Certainly it is worthy of further trial.

*From McClelland, D., Davis, W., Kalin, R., and Wanner, E.: The drinking man, New York, 1972, The Free Press, p. 332.

References

1. Becker, H. S.: The other side, New York, 1964, The Free Press, pp. 2-3.
2. Cumming, E.: Systems of social regulation, New York, 1968, Atherton Press, p. 6.
3. Goffman, E.: Stigma (notes on the management of spoiled identity), Englewood Cliffs, N. J., 1963, Prentice-Hall, Inc.
4. Halleck, S. L.: The politics of therapy, New York, 1971, Science House, Inc.
5. Heath, R.: The reasonable adventurer, Pittsburgh, 1964, The University of Pittsburgh Press.
6. McClelland, D., Davis, W., Kalin, R., and Wanner, E.: The drinking man, New York, 1972, The Free Press, pp. 1-98, 332-336.
7. Roman, P., and Trice, H. M.: The sick role;

labelling theory and the deviant drinker, Int. J. Soc. Psychiatry **14:**247, Autumn, 1968.

8. Schnall, S.: Personal communication, 1970.
9. Seale, F. E.: Treatment of the alcoholic in a clinical setting. In Texas summer studies on alcohol, Austin, Texas, July 13-18, 1969, University of Texas Press.
10. Szasz, T.: The manufacture of madness (a comparative study of the inquisition and the mental health movement), New York, 1971, Harper & Row, Publishers, Inc., p. xv.

Bibliography

Bateson, G.: Steps to an ecology of mind, New York, 1972, Ballantine Books.

Becker, E.: The revolution in psychiatry, New York, 1964, The Free Press of Glencoe, Inc.

Berne, E.: In Steiner, C.: Games alcoholics play, New York, 1971, Grove Press, Inc.

Blaine, H.: The personality of the addict. In Chavitz, M.: Frontiers of alcoholism, New York, 1970, Science House, Inc.

Chafetz, M.: The prevention of alcoholism, Int. J. Psychiatry **13:**331, 1972.

Maloney, E.: How to play the territorial game, Perspect. Psychiatr. Care **10:**31, 1972.

Sagarin, E.: Odd man in (societies of deviants in America), Chicago, 1969, Quadrangle/The New York Times Book Co.

7

Understanding and altering family relationship patterns

Joan M. King

Psychiatric nurses have become increasingly involved in family therapy, a relatively recent approach to psychiatric and mental health problems. This treatment modality focuses both on the identified patient and on his primary unit of socialization. Warkentin[6] views family therapy as assisting family members to develop a more satisfying life style that will encourage growth and reduce vulnerability to emotional injury.

The conceptualization and practice of family therapy has developed far beyond the original clinical observations that were the impetus for research and theory building. Initially, child psychiatrists[4] working with youngsters in individual therapy noted that therapeutic advancement was frequently impeded or undermined by family members. In an effort to overcome this dilemma therapists met with one of the child's parents to encourage increased cooperation. However, these meetings became therapeutic sessions for the parent, and, as parental conflicts were resolved, related conflicts in the child also improved without specific therapeutic intervention.

These observations can now be understood through viewing the family as an interdependent unit rather than as a collection of loosely related individuals.

CONCEPTUALIZATION OF THE FAMILY

Modern social systems theory applied to the family provides one means of understanding the dynamic interrelationships within this group. Buckley[2] defines a system as a complex of units related in a causal network such that each component is related in a more or less stable way to other components over any particular time span.

Campbell[3] has identified six criteria for determining a social system: boundaries, proximity of members or units, similarity of members or units, communication network, common goals or values, and resistance to change. Application of these criteria to the family not only establishes the family as a system but also furthers understanding of its inherent complexity.

A family exhibits boundaries: some belong and others do not. The elements of this system may be defined as individual members or as specific subgroups such as parents or children. Although we tend to consider families as being composed of two generations, this is not necessarily the case. In some instances families are trigenerational or include nonrelatives. A system and its boundaries may be defined in many ways, but some attention should be directed toward the impact of individuals generally excluded from a narrow definition of family unit. An "outsider" may be an integral part of daily family life, and, if so, he is involved in the system. Such individuals may contribute extensively to family tasks and needs. They may influence goals and the nature of the communication networks. This situation is frequently seen in one-parent families. A friend, neighbor, or housekeeper may assume some of the functions of the absent parent, thus becoming an influential force in the family.

Proximity of members is certainly a characteristic of family life. Even a member separated from the family unit may maintain proximity through emotional investment, communication, and maintenance of functions such as financial support or

53

advice giving. It is this physical, emotional, and psychological proximity that contributes to the influence of each member on the others.

Similarity of family members may be viewed at many levels. They are identified as similar through a common name and address. Marital partners may demonstrate considerable sameness through common agreements about the level of emotional intensity, closeness, and degree of honesty deemed mutually comfortable. These agreements, generally altered only in periods of crisis, provide one element for family commonality. Similarity also may be achieved through the process of children's identifying with parents. Expectations contribute to likeness. Similarity among family members is a frequent expectation in our society. This expectation can lead to the actual development of like behaviors and traits through what is frequently referred to as *labeling,* or the *self-fulfilling prophecy.*

Communication, both verbal and nonverbal, is the means by which relationships between component parts are maintained or altered. An open system is one in which information interchange is both internal and external to the system. The family that provides for the changing growth needs of its members and that is cognizant of changing social views illustrates an open system of interchange of information. This openness is an essential element in providing continuity, variability, and change. In essence, reception of new external data facilitates adaptation and learning and also maintains some degree of congruence between the family, its members, and society. Fresh internal messages provide awareness of changes within and between components of the system. Reduced adaptability is a consequence of a closed system, since new information is less available. Routinized activity and repetitive interchanges may indicate the existence of a closed system.

Each family develops communication patterns that are designed to convey necessary information and to maintain conflict within levels of comfort, or tolerance. Through the communication network members accommodate divergent goals, and roles, or behavioral prescriptions, are developed, maintained, and altered. Since family roles are intermeshed, the roles and their performance affect other family members as well. A flow of new information permits role flexibility to meet changing needs within the family. When these data are limited or lacking, roles that are maladaptive or irrelevant to present needs may be developed and perpetuated. This pattern limits the growth and adaptability of all family members.

Tension is a characteristic of any system. Relationships between component parts and the relation of the system to the external environment is not static. Rather a state of dynamic equilibrium exists to a greater or lesser extent. A stable system possesses a governing process that sets the limits of tolerated variability. In a family the system defines the extent of permissible divergence or change, and this allowance for deviation is the measure of tension for the family system. This definition is expressed in common values, goals and what is frequently referred to as "family rules." Whether explicit or implicit, these limits permit a range of alternative interactions as well as delineation of the unacceptable. In addition, individual members respond to another's exceeding the behavioral limits with attempts to return the erring individual to the acceptable range of behavior. Essentially each member attempts to set the range of activity for the others. These attempts may not be equally effective because some members hold greater influence due to role, status, or power. However, both direct and indirect efforts are made by all members at various times. This process of control, which provides some constraints with some freedom of choice, maintains a viable system with sufficient flexibility for common goal-directed behavior and individuation. The specific constraints and choices are not unalterable; they may be redefined through negotiation in an open system.

All social systems evidence some degree of resistance to external intrusion, and families are not an exception. Even an open system is not open indiscriminately. Families are concerned about the degree of control they exercise over their own destiny. They object, sometimes vigorously, to external influences that are in opposition to strongly held beliefs and goals. Youngsters may be forbidden to play with children deemed undesirable, or certain individuals may be unwelcome in a family home because of the anticipated influence on family members. Families resist intrusion.

Three of these systems theory concepts are particularly relevant to family therapy: resistance to intrusion, the interrelationship of units, and the communication network.

A family may seek therapy because one or more of its members is experiencing difficulty and pain. Although initiation of therapy implies a need for change, a resistance to change exists concurrently. The therapist's efforts may be viewed as an intrusion, and family mobilization to nullify this influence is a frequent occurrence. Family nullification efforts may be seen in attempts to include the therapist in the family system and thus control his impact. Cancelling or terminating treatment is another means of resisting intrusion.

A second significant concept for family therapy is that of the interrelationship of units. Considerable evidence suggests that symptoms are a product of the family system. An individual's behavior may not be congruent with social standards or personally adaptive, but it is congruent with and adaptive to the family system. This conception requires that the symptom-bearing individual not be considered the patient. Rather, what is "sick" is the pattern of relationships among family members that produces a need for symptomatology. For example, the pain and conflict of parents who argue constantly can be reduced by focusing mutual concern, attention, and effort on a delinquent child whose behavior has involved the family with school, police, and juvenile officers. Should this occur there may be some implicit encouragement to continue behavior that reduces a greater pain in the family. Such a system is dysfunctional because flexibility is insufficient to provide for the psychological, sociological, and intellectual growth needs of all its members.[5]

If a family is to endure and meet the needs of each individual, some accommodation must be made to all members and to any change in a single member or subgroup. What is new may be viewed as an intrusion that threatens the system itself or its components. In these instances efforts may be directed toward returning to prior relationships and behavior, since a change in any member necessitates some alteration in other members. This process may be seen in the members' intense negotiations with the changed individual to assume his old role, or another family member may assume the recently discarded function. In the latter instance, role maintenance permits members to continue existing patterns of family integration. In other families change may be accommodated with minimal stress. Growth or improved adaptation of any single member holds the possibility of eventual increased flexibility for the total system or its various members or both.

The third concept relates to the nature of the communication network. New information and messages that are not congruent with current functioning permit greater flexibility and adaptation. Helping families become aware of and examine the consequences of verbal and nonverbal messages between members provides new information that permits and requires altered relationships and behavior. This process is not undertaken with ease in a closed system. Again there is resistance to change; the therapist's messages may not be heard, may not be understood, or may evoke considerable discomfort and fear. Yet processing information, both internal and external to the system, is an essential component of therapy.

Systems theory alone is insufficient for understanding and altering family patterns that produce symptomatology. Theory related to the specific phenomena evidenced in the family is needed. In the family that will be discussed, a symbiotic relationship prevailed. Symbiosis emphasizes not only psychological aspects but also elements of systems theory.

FAMILY SYMBIOTIC RELATIONSHIPS

A symbiotic relationship as used in this chapter is one in which a vague intermingling of egos exists. It is characterized by ambivalence and a lack of identity and self-esteem and is not growth producing for either person. The normal symbiotic period of infancy is not the relationship under discussion.

Bowen[1] has identified the relationships presented in families in which a symbiotic attachment exists between parent and child. This pattern entails the collusion of all family members, although it is limited to a triad: mother, father, and child. Thus attention must be directed toward the marital pair and each parent's relationship with that child.

Parents in this situation exhibit a distant relationship, which Bowen has termed an *emotional divorce*. Both parents are equally immature. However, this may not be immediately observable. One parent denies his immaturity and assumes an over-adequate position; the second parent stresses his inadequacy without necessarily accepting himself as inadequate. In this manner the marital pair are integrated in an uncomfortable overadequate-underadequate role relationship.

The birth of a child superficially eases some of the difficulties inherent in the parents' relationship through a refocusing of attention and concern. The family gains a third member whose helplessness allows the mothering individual securely to assume the overadequate position. The mother-child relationship is an intense one in which each individual primarily invests in the other. This investment is maintained rather than gradually reduced, as occurs in the normal symbiotic relationship between mother and infant.

The child serves a distinct need for the mother, who projects aspects of her own immaturity to the child and then becomes overly concerned about the child in the areas of her projected immaturity. The mother's attention then can be directed toward the child's perceived inadequacies rather than toward her own. This pattern reduces the mother's anxiety in two ways: first, through projection and, second, through the ongoing interaction process. It has been observed that, as the mother becomes anxious, the child increasingly demonstrates in his behavior those elements that the mother views as inadequacies. This pattern permits the mother to reduce her own increasing anxiety by focusing attention on the child. She may worry about and attempt to correct the child's behavior.

In line with this pattern the mother concurrently imposes two incongruent demands on the child. The first, that of remaining helpless and unable, is generally communicated nonverbally. The second message involves an expectation for the child to develop into a mature, able individual. The latter is generally conveyed verbally and represents a conscious goal for the child's strivings.

Although this pattern has been discussed in terms of the mother's activities, it is not a one-sided occurrence. The child accepts and acts in accord with the mother's projections. The father also accepts the mother's view of the child. He permits the maintenance of the intense symbiotic pattern and consequently has only an ancillary relationship with the child.

These elements are reflected in the relationships of the specific family that will be discussed. The symbiotic pattern between mother and daughter is not so encompassing as that described by Bowen but was sufficiently prominent to deter growth of all family members, particularly mother and child.

Clinical data

Mrs. Leon, an orphan, came from a home broken by desertion and the death of her mother in a psychiatric hospital. She described herself prior to her marriage as being wild and unmanageable and having already had an abortion. Shortly after her marriage at 17 years of age, she discovered her 18-year-old husband was addicted to heroin and to his mother.

The pattern of this eleven-year marriage was that Mrs. Leon worked to support the family and assumed all responsibility for it. Mr. Leon could not be depended on to make or act on decisions. Also he frequently disappeared for weeks at a time. When they were together, Mrs. Leon attempted to get her husband to stop using drugs and to "act like a husband and father." They had been separated two years when therapy was sought for Lila, the older child.

Ten-year-old Lila had been referred to the agency because she was inattentive, disruptive, and unmanageable in school. Mrs. Leon was fearful that Lila would "drive me crazy" because she constantly was worried about her daughter. Lila was unmanageable at home, and Mrs. Leon feared she would become pregnant and involved in gang-related problems when she became an adolescent. She attempted to control Lila's behavior by keeping her in the house when she was not in school. While in the house, Lila taunted her brother and mother so extensively that Mrs. Leon "screamed" at her constantly but without effect.

Mrs. Leon repeatedly emphasized to the therapist that only she could have any effect on Lila's behavior. She viewed Lila's present problems as her fault because she had left her with a baby-sitter for eight years while she worked. Now Mrs. Leon wanted to return to work but believed that she could not because Lila's behavior was so uncontrollable that she could not be entrusted to a sitter.

Mrs. Leon expressed no concern about 9-year-old John, the only other child. She said that he did not have Lila's abilities but presented no problem to her or to the school.

During the initial family interview, Mrs. Leon, John, and Lila were present. Neither child would look at the therapist or respond when addressed. This behavior continued throughout the interview and brought screaming demands from the mother that Lila respond and explanations that John was shy. However, whenever the mother and therapist attempted to talk, turmoil ensued. Either Lila or John would kick, pinch, or spit at the other. A shouting battle between the children would follow, and Mrs. Leon would scream at Lila to "stop picking on John." She seemed not to notice that John frequently started the battles and was as involved as Lila. When the children ignored her commands, she turned back to the therapist and continued what she had been saying. Communication was impossible with the two children crying, screaming, running, and jumping.

The therapist attempted to get the mother to set limits; when she did not, the therapist forcefully told the children to sit in their chairs and be quiet while she and their mother talked. The children obeyed briefly. Mrs. Leon obviously did not like the therapist's setting limits for the children. She repeatedly requested that "You tell me what to do," or said, "I need someone to tell me what to do so I can do it right, and then Lila will be alright." However, her attempts to control the children when asked to do so were ineffectual. She assured the therapist that she had tried everything, and nothing worked with Lila; she seemed to be implying that this would fail, too.

The parental relationship, as described by Mrs. Leon, reflects the overadequate-underadequate pattern. It also reflects efforts to confirm her competence through repeated unsuccessful attempts to rescue her husband from addiction. Mrs. Leon apparently turned to Lila for those gratifications that were not forthcoming in the marriage and for assurance of her adequacy. However, the potential intensity of the mother-child relationship was diluted by reality factors.

Mrs. Leon achieved a feeling of some adequacy though supporting and managing the family and through focusing attention, energy, and worry on the physical and legal concerns related to her husband's addiction. The necessity for a baby-sitter also provided the children with input from external sources and reduced the degree of maternal control over the children through her absence.

The mother-daughter relationship was an ambivalent one that appeared to be predominantly negative. In matters of control, or dominance, neither would budge; any compromise with an existing position could be achieved only through the other's accomplishing impossible tasks. This pattern was illustrated in an argument about Lila's visiting a neighbor child. Mother stated that she would let Lila play outside only after she could prove that she was trustworthy outside. On the other hand, their relationship demonstrated more positive aspects of mutual caring, support, and concern. Lila enjoyed household tasks, and her mother fostered and responded positively to Lila's voluntary efforts in cooking, cleaning, and ironing.

Intervention

The following goals were established for therapy: to reduce the intensity of the symbiotic relationship, to facilitate Mrs. Leon's understanding of her relationships with others, and to institute effective limit setting. Each of these broad goals will be discussed separately, although in practice this rather false separation did not occur. Efforts were directed toward several goals simultaneously, and gains in one area were also reflected in other areas.

The major task in therapy was to reduce the intense mother-daughter emotional involvement. The common strategy of increasing the parents' involvement with each other could not be used, since this was a one-parent family.

Information about the mother's relationships with others outside the family was sought, to determine resources available for support and perhaps increased involvement. Mrs. Leon was found to be virtually isolated. She had maintained but a tentative relationship with her only relative because she feared embarrassment if her sister discovered that she was married to an addict. Furthermore, she lived in a neighborhood where few adults spoke English. The language barrier and life style of neighbors limited potential relationships.

The therapist elected to form an alliance with Mrs. Leon, since her resistance to intrusion seemed likely to block treatment efforts unless she believed herself to have retained some control and unless she obtained rewards at the beginning of therapy. Also this alliance would permit the therapist to offer needed support and guidance while encouraging Mrs. Leon to develop relationships with others. Consequently the therapy sessions were divided; half the time was spent with the total family, whereas the other half was devoted to Mrs. Leon alone.

This strategy was effective in lessening resistance by gradually altering Mrs. Leon's initial perception of the therapist. At first she viewed the therapist as someone who would tell her that she was at fault and give directions related to how she should change. As time passed, she spoke of her surprise in finding support in the relationship. This support appeared to act as an incentive to give consideration to some of the therapist's comments.

The pain and frustration that Mrs. Leon was experiencing in her relationship with Lila was used to help her achieve some distance in that relationship. Initially Mrs. Leon perceived all comments related to lessening the intensity of her and Lila's emotional involvement and the length of time spent together as an indication that the therapist viewed her as a bad mother. She defended her view that anything less would encourage Lila to become a "bad girl." However, she recognized that her screaming insistence that Lila change her behavior was ineffective. Also she was open to the suggestion that part of her over-response was caused by the frustration that she experienced because she had no present adult gratifications.

Mrs. Leon would not consider returning to work but, with considerable support and encouragement, began attending classes to obtain her high school diploma while the children were in school. This arrangement was a compromise that permitted outside interests as well as close contact with Lila. Through this activity she met others who eventually became friends. The combined effect of focusing attention on her studies, achieving in school, and developing friendships permitted Mrs. Leon to lessen the emotional involvement with her daughter. Lila was allowed greater freedom outside the home and began to relate to others more positively in the school, neighborhood, and home.

This change was not accomplished smoothly. Both mother and child have an investment in maintaining the symbiotic relationship, and both experience the tug of this pattern when some distancing occurs. Mrs. Leon seemed to need preparation for the inevitable attempts to reestablish the prior closeness. The goal was to assist Mrs. Leon to withstand Lila's behavioral pleas and remain in school. Mrs. Leon was asked to discuss with the therapist her anticipations of Lila's behavior and means of responding in these situations. In a similar manner her own possible discouragement with school was discussed.

Throughout the time that Mrs. Leon attended school she required encouragement, but she had a particularly difficult time during the first several months. Lila skipped school and instigated several fights in the neighborhood; her mother remained in school only with considerable effort.

As Mrs. Leon developed friendships with classmates, she began leaving the children with a sitter. Initially she spoke of her fear and guilt for enjoying these brief outings. In time this was reduced through emphasizing that she needed and deserved adult companionship and recreation. Through a friend Mrs. Leon met a man with whom she became infatuated. Although this investment functioned to separate her further from Lila, it soon became apparent that the relationship was inherently problematic: the man was an alcoholic.

This new relationship provided a natural avenue to explore Mrs. Leon's relationship with her husband and some of her own needs and patterns of relating to others. She began to recognize similarities in her relationships with her husband, daughter, and boyfriend. Gradually she became aware of her participation in the painful realities of her marriage. She could no longer view herself as a victim of a "bad" marriage and her husband's addiction or as a rescuer of the weak and helpless. She began to express a desire for a more mature relationship and subsequently stopped seeing her boyfriend.

Mrs. Leon's greater understanding of her needs and participation in painful life experiences provided a new vantage point from which to view her fears that Lila's life would be a repetition of her own. She was able to modify her idea that she alone could prevent the feared reoccurrence. Discussion emphasized the need for self-understanding and internal rather than external control. She tentatively began to give both children greater responsibility for their behavior and to act in the more consultative capacity of helping them to anticipate the consequences of their actions.

The third goal of therapy, as originally stated, was to help Mrs. Leon set realistic expectations and limits for herself and the children. Neither she nor the children expected compliance with limits, and consequently family life was chaotic. Initially Mrs. Leon was unable to recognize that her empty threats and inconsistent expectations promoted the children's unruly behavior. The therapist worked with Mrs. Leon to identify specific expectations for the children and means of enforcing these desired behaviors. It was agreed that Mrs. Leon would be responsible for carrying out these limits and that the therapist would assist only when necessary. In family sessions Mrs. Leon conveyed these expectations to the children but needed frequent reminding to function as a limit setter. The children also needed to have their attention focused on their mother's directions and her new parental role. This was accomplished through simple observations and questions, such as "Did you hear what your mother said?"

Mrs. Leon was more successful in controlling the children's behavior in the sessions than she was at home. She complained of their misbehavior frequently; it was difficult for her to maintain consistency. The idea that the children should be held responsible for their own behavior was even more difficult to accept. She viewed this as an abdication of parental responsibility and anticipated that Lila would become a juvenile delinquent as a result. Limit setting remained haphazard at home until satisfactions derived from relationships with friends increased Mrs. Leon's need to depend on the children's internal controls.

As the children's behavior improved and she obtained pleasure from adult interests away from home, Mrs. Leon began to consider returning to work. This idea was strongly supported because holding a job would function as an ongoing guard against returning to the prior emotional intensity between mother and daughter. It also held the possibility of greater freedom and continued growth for all members of the family. Mrs. Leon was hesitant about leaving the children after school without a sitter, but the children maintained that they were too old for a sitter. The total family responded enthusiastically to the suggestion of involving the children in the local YMCA activity program after school. This plan provided some adult supervision while offering the children greater exposure to other adults and to peers. The family made plans to divide specific household tasks to assist Mrs. Leon when she returned to work.

The total family response to plans related to Mrs. Leon's return to work indicates family growth in more mature behavior and relationships. In terms of systems theory distinct changes were evidenced in the communication network. The system became open to and used new information, with consequent changes in goals, values, and the nature of relationships among family members. These changes were resisted by individual members; therapeutic strategies were developed to reduce resistance and facilitate movement toward the goals of family therapy.

SUMMARY

The application of systems theory to the family provides one means of comprehending the complex interrelationships demonstrated in family life. This conception, coupled with theory specifically related to family pathology, provides the family therapist with a means of approaching inhibiting family patterns that produce symptomatology in one member.

References

1. Bowen, M.: A family concept of schizophrenia. In Jackson, D. D., editor: Etiology of schizophrenia, New York, 1960, Basic Books, Inc.
2. Buckley, W.: Social and modern systems theory, Englewood Cliffs, N. J., 1967, Prentice-Hall, Inc.
3. Campbell, D.: Common fate, similarity, and other indices of the status of aggregates of persons as social entities, Behav. Sci. 3:17, 1958.
4. Gyarfas, K.: Personal communication, 1966.
5. Satir, V.: Symptomatology: a family production. In Howells, J., editor: The theory and practice of family psychiatry, New York, 1971, Brunner/Mazel, Inc.
6. Warkentin, J.: Marriage—the cornerstone of the family system. In Pollak, O., and Friedman, A., editors: Family dynamics and female sexual delinquency, Palo Alto, Calif., 1969, Science and Behavior Books, Inc.

8

A family case study

Jean Shannon

To a special magic box, a sunflower in a strawberry patch,
a struggling sea gull, and the Rock of Gibraltar.

He would often and sometimes constantly ramble on about being of alien seed, a victim of the Cosa Nostra, or the founder of a movement for a Los Angeles free state. He would speak of the help he had given his brother to become Emperor of China and of his plans to refuse a mission to the presidency, since he feared assassination. He was seemingly oblivious of the comments or directions of others as he aimlessly spoke of being controlled by aliens who had the secret for perpetual life or of his illegitimate birth to a woman who lived down the street. His thought and speech patterns could be labeled delusional, illogical, disorderly, sterotyped, difficult to understand, and obviously not in the service of reality testing. He evidenced ambivalence in his emotions toward others, indifference to matters of normal importance, and inappropriate laughter and anger and generally appeared preoccupied or "off in his own world." His behavior may be termed a bit crazy, mad, or abnormal, or for the sake of formality he may be labeled as schizophrenic.

A diagnosis is made based on behavioral cues emitted by the patient, but what is known of his experience? Laing[6] defines a person in a twofold way: in terms of his experience, as a center of orientation of the objective universe, and in terms of his behavior, as the originator of actions. The divorce, or split, between experience and behavior that Laing describes in reference to the "normal" alienated masses may be seen not only as it relates to the perpetuation of sanity within an insane world but also as it relates to the perpetuation of

"craziness" in those who may be truly sane.

Traditional approaches to psychopathology, incorporating such terms as *illogical, irrational,* or *nonsensical* as referents to behavior, evidence this split, since they limit their own experience of the patient to his behavior or "inner world" rather than to his total experiential being. Delusions about the Cosa Nostra and psychotic behavior such as withdrawal are seen as distortions of and inappropriate responses to the outside world. Behavior is seemingly unrelated to experience.

Incorporating the assumptions that behavior is a function of experience and that observation and action occur in a social field of reciprocal influence and interaction, new approaches to mental illness attempt to bridge the gap between behavior and experience by pursuing a better understanding of the patient's overall life concepts. Such approaches are often termed *transactional,* or *interactional,* and have a framework that may be thought of as a process made up of the interrelated behaviors of two or more persons or groups, in which each step of the rational progression arises logically out of the preceding steps.[9] This process of interaction may be thought of as an open system possessing the characteristics of open systems, such as wholeness, nonsummativity, feedback, and homeostasis. The key element in the interactional approach is communication, which is viewed as the vehicle of the overt manifestations of relationship.[10] Examination of the communication patterns and relational system of the patient is carried out to facilitate the therapist's experiencing of the patient as one who not only acts on but also experiences, interprets, and reacts to an outer world.

Perhaps the most important relational system available for study and treatment is the family. Hence family therapy has evolved as a major treatment modality within the interactional approach. The following case study is about a family, one of whose members was previously described. This patient has evidenced recurrent psychotic behavior for the past six years and has weathered numerous hospitalizations and treatment approaches. Family therapy was initiated with the goal of attaining a deeper understanding of the patient's experience and behavior within his interactional world, as a means of studying the dynamics of the family system and their relation to the schizophrenic process, as a promising treatment approach for a family-bound patient, and as a means of providing me with my initial experience as a family therapist. The following study of this type of therapy will include a description of the family, an analysis of system dynamics in terms of related theory, a description of the therapeutic process, and a discussion of the learning experience. It is hoped that the reader may reach a deeper understanding and knowledge of the patient's experience and that the delusional and psychotic behaviors of the patient will assume new meaning—for the Cosa Nostra may be alive and well in terms of the patient's experience within an interactional reality, and our own "crazy" perpetuation of the gap between experience and behavior may be what keeps the patient "crazy" and the therapist "sane."

DESCRIPTION OF THE FAMILY

The E. family consists of the two parents, Alfred and Elaine, and three children, George, 26, Ralph, 23, and Linda, 20 years of age. Alfred is a stocky Italian, whose middle age shows in his gray hair and expanding waistline. He likes to eat, and his countenance generally reflects contentment. He often has the warmth and appeal of a big teddy bear but can also show his teeth and his stubbornness. For this he is frequently referred to as the "blockhead." He likes to laugh and frequently has a joke to tell. He is the playful daddy to his daughter, a peer to son George, the loyal protector of his "crippled" son Ralph, and the con-

sistent adversary of his wife in their symmetrically escalating game of one-upmanship. He is described by himself and his family as a "sucker," who goes out of his way for those who would never reciprocate, and by George as a "turtle" who plods along through life giving free rides to those who would hop on his back. He is the operator and part owner of a small independent poultry business and claims to struggle to meet the requirements of middle-class suburban life.

Elaine is friendly and outgoing and wears her smile like a badge. She is lean, a bit wrinkled, and often nervous. Her pointed face is often drawn with fatigue. She keeps a clean house, cares much for her children, loves to have company, drinks coffee all day, and smokes too much. Most of her waking hours are spent thinking about or caring for her son Ralph, and her outside activity is limited. She is not so submissive as her husband might wish and can easily match wits with him in their numerous arguments. She is often in opposition to her son George, fighting his efforts to dominate her. She delicately blends the elements of peer loyalty and companionship with motherly concern and protection in her relationship with her daughter, and she is the worried, anxious, loving, guilty, and heartbroken mother of her son Ralph, always searching for a solution to his problems.

George is the dynamic achiever of the family, always succeeding and never failing, always right and never wrong. Although short in stature, he is perhaps the "biggest" member of the family. He is the spokesman, the "prosecuting attorney," the "big brother," and often the surrogate father. He is quick to find fault with others and delights in presenting his eloquent, lengthy, and footnoted put-downs. He often appears obsessed with his own ideas, seemingly unable to tolerate differences in others. Yet with all his egotism, domination, and intolerance, he is seeking to know himself and to relate better with other persons.

Ralph is the oversized, baby-faced, fair-haired failure of the family. His prolonged adolescence never seems to end, as the child in his eyes says, "Mother me," and his psychotic outbursts say, "Let me go." He often appears to be the house "pet"—well cared for, well fed, and having no responsibility, always on a leash or tied to a pole in the backyard. He is bright and witty; his "out talk" is often intricate and rather ingenious. He is the sick and often embarrassing brother to George, who resents his lack of initiative and effort to improve himself. He is the cohort and supporter of his sister in her efforts to achieve independence, and he is the submissive son and often subtle protector of his father. To his mother he is a demanding child insisting that he be treated like a man.

Linda is the sparkling, attractive "sweetheart queen," the family's gift to a social world. She is ever smiling, ever teasing, and ever playfully seductive, but she often has to struggle to maintain her "sweet," delightful role while fighting for her independence. She is always willing to help a friend and looks to nursing or teaching as her means of making a professional contribution to society. To her brother George her efforts to maintain a free and uncompulsive spirit are regarded as irresponsible, and he is often irritated by her chronic lateness and her lack of achievement motivation. To her proud parents she is the loving and caring daughter—a joy to have with them. As Alfred repeatedly states, "The only thing wrong with Linda is that she wasn't born a twin." To Ralph she is someone to cling to when his friends have all left him.

Alfred and Elaine married in their mid-twenties. Elaine found Alfred to be a manly, rugged, stable, charming, and self-assured gentleman, who showed her many good times. Alfred found Elaine to be a charming girl who had her "right foot forward," was fun to be with, and made efforts to please him. Each asserts that he missed seeing the "bull-headed stubbornness" of the other. The first years of their marriage are described as "stormy," since their mutual intolerance of each other's differences caused many arguments.

An early dispute, which has continued throughout their marriage, was concerned with place of residence. Elaine wanted a suburban home situated near her mother. Alfred wanted a home near the business, which meant living next door to his family. For more than eighteen years they lived in Phoenix, close to the business. Other chronic and long-standing arguments stemmed from their differing approaches to child rearing. George was a pale, sickly baby with chronic gastrointestinal upsets; therefore they often argued about the best approach to feeding him. Their different methods of dealing with Ralph have also been a source of constant and continuing conflict throughout the marriage.

Ralph was born within a few years of George and because of congenital strabismus underwent three eye operations within the first four years of his life. Alfred still accuses Elaine of overprotecting and "babying" Ralph from the time of his birth, and Elaine accuses Alfred of not giving enough love or attention to him. Two years after Ralph's birth, Linda was born. She rarely caused friction between her parents and seems to have had a happy childhood. As the children grew up, they had little contact with any other neighborhood children, perhaps due to a difference in ethnicity. They spent most of their playtime in the backyard with their cousins who lived next door. Linda describes the group in this way: she was the only girl and because of this often got her way; George was "Mr. Intelligent" and able to achieve by outwitting others; the cousins were "Mr. Football" and "Mr. Big Star," able to hold their own or "show off" in competition; and Ralph was a cross-eyed, gentle, and sensitive sissy, who refused to fight back and who always tried not to show his hurt. Alfred thought that Ralph showed signs of abnormality at the age of 5, since he would often twist the arms and legs off Linda's dolls or "daydream and wander" while in grade school. Several times he encouraged his wife to take Ralph to a psychologist, but she would "blow up" and deny any abnormality. It was not until Ralph's adolescence that Elaine, too, began to question the normality of his behavior.

During his freshman year of high school Ralph became progressively more withdrawn, had chronic physical ailments such as colds, and eventually came down with mononucleosis. Despite his ailments he was able to spend enough time in school to complete the year. However, his life at school was no better than his physical status. His chronic daydreaming irritated one of his teachers to the point of spanking him in front of the class—a tremendous embarrassment for a young adolescent. Ralph insisted on switching schools and, finding his insistence somewhat extreme, his parents took him to consult a psychiatrist. This physician pronounced him a normal adolescent, and Ralph entered another high school as a sophomore. Later in the year he relapsed with mononucleosis from fatigue. During the summer prior to his junior year, his mother's wish finally was realized, and the family left Phoenix and moved to the suburbs. This move meant further change and another adjustment to a new high school. Early in the first term Ralph contracted a severe intestinal flu; on recovery he accused his father and sister of poisoning him. Adamantly maintaining this paranoid ideation, he was hospitalized for the first time, and after a brief period of rest and medication, he "pulled out of it." During the second term, while trying to make up the subjects he had missed, he developed a "nervous twitch" in his neck and eventually began accusing others again of poisoning him. He was rehospitalized for a two-week period but on discharge had not recovered so fully as before. He began to talk incessantly of politics and of his run for governor. By midsummer his "paranoid" and "grandiose" behavior had greatly increased; he began breaking and throwing things and refused his medication. Once again he was admitted to the hospital and during his five-week stay was given heavy shock treatments. He recovered enough to complete his senior year of high school without much difficulty, and he remembers this as one of his happiest years. He became more involved in activities at school and developed a strong social tie with a group of boys in his class. He then went on to junior college and completed a semester. However, he became highly nervous in the spring, and by fall his behavior had progressed to overt psychosis. At this time Ralph claimed that others were "seeking revenge" on him, and he disavowed membership in his family by insisting that he was the illegitimate son of a woman who lived down the street. Concurrent with his adoption of a new mother was the adoption of her son, Steve, as his brother. He believed that Steve had given him the love and companionship that he had always needed and thought that they might have had a homosexual relationship. He also claimed to have been abandoned by his father in California and to have organized a movement for a "Los Angeles free state." He was admitted to the state hospital, where he remained for a period of three months. After discharge he was treated in the day hospital or as an outpatient in the community mental health center. During this period he made some often unsuccessful attempts at resuming his studies and did some part-time work in his father's business. Within a year of his discharge the progression to psychosis began again. His delusional talk increased, and he became restless. Unable to sleep at night, he would come into his mother's room and insist on staying, or he would bang on her door or call to her during the night. One day he lost control and hit his mother while insisting that he was the son of Jackie Kennedy and that his mother was a fraud. Since Ralph refused to be hospitalized, Alfred felt compelled to get a petition, and the police took him to the hospital. During his hospitalization he was apparently unable to remain in contact with reality long enough to pursue a "normal" conversation. In addition to the various delusional ideations already mentioned, he spoke of being controlled by aliens and of being a "computerized human fighting a computer war." When visited by his mother, he acted in an infantile manner, stroking her neck and repeatedly calling her "mommie." After a month of hospitalization and some improvement he was transferred to the day hospital for care. Some of the elements of the behavior that he recurrently exhibited while in the day hospital were described at the beginning of this chapter. During this period the E. family was referred for family therapy and began involvement in this process in the early part of October, 1971.

Unfortunately, the activities and behavior of other members of the family during Ralph's adolescent years are not well known. Alfred claims that Elaine changed dramatically from her usual overprotective position to one that was demanding and disciplinary. He believed that this change was an important causal factor in Ralph's recurrent "blowups" and often criticized his wife for being "so hard on the boy." Elaine asserts that Alfred remained relatively uninvolved with Ralph and was lenient with him. Although each parent was critical of the other, as Ralph became "sicker" they tried to avoid arguing in his presence. During this period George was living away from home, spending four years in the seminary and then attending college. Linda was pursuing the normal activities of a young, popular adolescent girl and often took Ralph under her wing by sharing her friends and activities with him. Alfred was working hard and was overburdened by the bills for Ralph's care. Elaine spent most of her time worrying about or attempting to care for Ralph and exploring the various theories and treatments of schizophrenia.

Ralph's illness was upsetting to the family, and they evidenced great concern for his welfare. Despite this, their concepts of and approaches to the problem varied. George believed that Ralph had hypoglycemia (since he himself had this disease) and advocated dietary adjustment as one approach to treatment. He thought that Ralph's behavior was also the product of his various life experiences. He advocated a learning theory approach to his brother's behavior and consistently made attempts not to reinforce, sometimes to the point of punishment, his brother's "sick" behavior. He was often critical of his parent's "leniency," claiming that they positively reinforced the irresponsible, pressureless, and sick life of his brother. Linda, not so adamant as George, believed that a lack of overt reinforcement should be coupled with understanding and kindness. Alfred thought that the boy was simply sick and probably always would be. He tried to be accepting, understanding, and protective of his "crippled" child. Elaine, spending more time with and feeling most responsible for Ralph, consistently found herself in a double-bind situation. Sensing his feelings of inadequacy and loneliness, she responded to his childlike behavior with "mothering," realizing at the same time that her protection perpetuated his inadequacy and did not fulfill his need for growth and independence. If she did not provide the mothering, he often became sicker; yet, if she did provide it, he never got "better." Because of this double bind it was impossible for her to decide on a consistent approach. She suffered distress in facing her inconsistency and also criticism from other members of the family. Understandably she often appeared overtly anxious.

The differing opinions on and approaches to Ralph's illness caused debate and criticism within the family. However, their unified concern made them amenable to working together and facilitated their involvement in the family therapy process.

ANALYSIS OF THE FAMILY SYSTEM IN TERMS OF RELATED THEORY

A core concept of family psychotherapy is that the mental illness of one member is a symptom, or aspect, of a greater, interlocking family pathology. Schizophrenic symptoms in the patient, such as thought and affective distortions, are related to the context of similar distortions operating subclinically in the family. The various theories of family psychopathology differ from each other in a number of ways—from their terminology to their assumptions about schizophrenia, in their focus, and in the degree of their concern with social roles of personality dynamics. Varying orientations to the subject generally stem from psychoanalytic, role, and communication theories and are not necessarily contradictory. An attempt will be made to relate the important aspects of relevant theory as they relate to the dynamics evidenced in this particular family.

Utilizing primarily psychoanalytic theory as his framework of analysis, Kramer[5] describes family epigenesis in terms of a *family relationship system*. He views the psychopathology of the child as evolving from the pathology in the marital relationship. He considers the attraction of the two spouses as being based on their mutual seeking in each other of some solution to their own neurotic problems. The traits that one is attracted by in the other are actually character defenses against the other's own deeper and similar immaturity. A mutual projection system is developed in which each spouse objects to, complains about, or feels uncomfortable with various characteristics of the other person, which serve as handy targets for projections of undesirable elements of the self. The mutual projection system may evidence itself in several common types of marriages such as the conflictual marriage, the overadequate-underadequate marriage, and the "united front" marriage. However, the pathology of these marriages does not necessarily affect their stability. The projection system meets the need of the couple to handle their own inadequacies and by its very nature as a system is self-perpetuating.

With the addition of a child to the family, there is not only a shift in the relationship system but also the possibility that one or both parents may see the child as another opportunity to resolve their neurotic problems. Due to the normal mother-child symbiosis, it is the mother who becomes most involved with the child, and by focusing her attention on his deficiencies, she becomes less aware of her own inadequacies. By coping with the inadequacies of another she is caused to feel more adequate. The father becomes more comfortable with his wife as her projections are displaced from himself onto the child. Consequently, he, too, reinforces the wife's preoccupation with the child's deficiencies, and eventually the persistence of symptoms in the child comes to serve the equilibrium of the family system. The child becomes motivated to be deficient or to have symptoms because this type of behavior serves to lessen the anxiety of the parents. The family system becomes stable and self-perpetuating, based on the reciprocal projection of the members. Some evidence of the dynamics involved in Kramer's theory may be seen in the E. family.

First of all, the numerous conflicts of the couple may be seen as based in their own mutual projection system. Incapable of facing their own inadequacies in dealing with their son's psychosis, they criticize one another's approach. Second, evidences of the beginning and perpetuation of the three-way projection system whereby the symptoms of the child serve to stabilize the marriage may be seen in Elaine's possible overprotection of Ralph in his childhood. Third, the self-perpetuating nature and stability of the system is evidenced by the continuance of the marriage despite a high degree of conflict and by the efforts of members of the system to resist change. Such resistance is demonstrated by Alfred in his acceptance and protection of his child's pathology; by Elaine in her recurrent overconcern and dependency-inducing behavior, despite her overt wish to discontinue this; and by Ralph in his recurrent attempts to elicit mothering behavior from others, despite his overt wish for independence.

In a vein similar to that of Kramer, Bowen[3] describes the immaturity and projection of the parents and an early attachment to the mother as important factors in the development of the pathology. He describes the mother-child relationship as active and intent, hallmarked by demands of the mother for the child to remain helpless and at the same time to become a gifted and mature person. The mother's overconcern and complaints about the patient can be regarded as externalizations of the mother's own inadequacies. He also sees projection occurring on the level of physical illness, whereby the soma of one person reciprocates with the psyche of another, and the child may become physically ill if the mother is feeling overly anxious. Bowen uses the concept of *emotional divorce* to describe the married life of the parents. The term encompasses a wide range of behavior but in general indicates a lack of sharing personal feelings and of mutual tolerance. He asserts that the mother views the child's attachment to her as due to the father's lack of interest. He also states that the father cannot have a primary relationship with the patient until he can become emotionally involved with his wife.

Discussing the choice of the scapegoat in a multichild family, Bowen claims that the birth of a physically deficient or deformed child might come closer to fulfillment of the emotional need of the mother. He believes that the main threat to the mother-child symbiosis is the growth process of the child, especially in adolescence, and views the psychosis as an unsuccessful attempt by the adolescent to adapt his severe psychological impairment to the demands of adult functioning and independence. In light of Bowen's formulation, the E. family may be seen to evidence the following pathologic characteristics: projection and mutual intolerance in the parents, indicating emotional divorce; an overactive and intense mother-child relationship; numerous physical ailments of the patient that may indicate an empathic representation of his mother's anxieties; the blaming of Ralph's attachment to Elaine on Alfred's indifference; the choice of a physically deformed child (Ralph with strabismus) as a scapegoat; and the development of the psychosis in adolescence, indicating the threatening nature of the growth and independence of the child.

In their clinical work Whitaker and Malone,[12] describe patterns in the schizophrenic family similar to those described by Bowen. They frequently find evidences of a dominant mother–inadequate father relationship and an attempt by the parents to gratify needs through their children rather than through each other. This is observable in the overinvolvement of Alfred and Elaine in their children's activities rather than each other's.

Lidz[7] utilizes extensions and applications of psychoanalytic and role concepts in his analysis of the family. He claims that a critical etiological feature in development of schizophrenia is the blurring of age and generation boundaries within the family. The consequence is that identity development within the child is distorted and inadequate. He describes a lack of role reciprocity in the family that is associated with distortions in role-appropriate behaviors for the various age-sex groups within

the system. Consequently, distinctions between the generations are not realized, the normal parental coalition is not maintained, and the children become involved in parental conflicts with the parents competing for the child's alliance. Blurring of age-sex boundaries and distortions in role-appropriate behavior are evidenced in the E. family by George's apparent assumption of the father role in his dealings with both his parents and siblings and by Alfred's assumption of the mother role after Elaine's change in behavior during Ralph's adolescence. Lidz also describes the threatened outbreak of both murderous and incestuous wishes during adolescence and sees these as playing an important part in the schizophrenic breakdown. Ralph's continual pursuit of his mother both day and night prior to his hospitalization may be seen as possible evidence of such incestuous wishes. Lidz utilizes the terms *marital schism* and *marital skew* to characterize the disturbed parental relationship. In both of these processes, the partners fail to meet each other's deep dynamic needs, which paves the way for the induction of the child by either parent into a pathological alliance. Marital schism, whereby the family stays together despite overt disagreement, best describes the relationship in the E. family.

Wynne and Singer[13] hypothesize that the disorders in schizophrenia derive from disordered patterns of interaction within the family. They describe four main features of the family of the schizophrenic as follows: first and foremost, patterns of handling attention and meaning are fragmented, amorphous, poorly integrated, and disjunctive; second, styles of relating are erratic, inappropriate, and highlighted by fluctuations between distance and closeness; third, there are underlying feelings of pervasive meaninglessness and emptiness in the family; and, finally, the overall structure of the family is characterized by maneuvers that serve to deny or reinterpret the reality of anxiety-provoking feelings and of the underlying meaninglessness of the relationship. Some of these elements are apparent in the transactions of the E. family. Amorphous and fragmented patterns of handling attention and meaning

are exemplified by the tendency of a discussion to shift in the object of attention
during the family sessions. Inappropriate
distance is also demonstrated by various
members of the family, especially Alfred,
when deep-seated and anxiety-provoking
feelings are evidenced by one of the other
family members. Also there are maneuvers
that serve to deny or reinterpret the reality of anxiety-provoking emotions. George's
expression of feelings of inadequacy and
fear of failure and Elaine's expressions of
feelings of exclusion are approached intellectually by other members and responded
to with comments such as, "You shouldn't
feel that way."

Another important theory and one that
has gained wide support from such researchers and therapists as Bateson, Jackson, Haley, and Satir is communication
theory. The general theory is often identified with the idea of the *double bind,* and
within the theory communication is viewed
as equivalent to human behavior, rather
than as only one aspect among others. The
theory postulates that the schizophrenic
must live in a world where the sequences
of events are such that his unconventional
communicational patterns will be in some
sense appropriate.[1] The unconventional
and distorted communication of the patient becomes more understandable when
seen in light of his interactional experience and exposure to the double-bind transaction. The *double bind* is defined as a
special type of learning situation from
which the growing child cannot escape, a
situation in which he is the victim of incongruent messages that require him to
deny important aspects of himself or his
experience.[8] Watzlawick[10] defines the ingredients of the double bind as follows: (1)
two or more persons are involved in an intense relationship that has a great degree
of physical or psychological survival value
or both for one, several, or all; (2) a message is given that is so structured that it
asserts something, it asserts something
about its own assertion, and these two assertions are mutually exclusive; and (3)
the recipient of the message is prevented
from stepping outside the framework of
this message, either by commenting about
it or by withdrawing: he cannot react to

it, but neither can he react to it appropriately, since the message itself is paradoxical. Defining the connection of the double
bind with schizophrenia, Watzlawick adds
the following two criteria: (1) when double
binding is of long duration, it will turn
into a habitual and autonomous expectation regarding the nature of human relationships and the world at large, an expectation that does not require further reinforcement and (2) the paradoxical behavior imposed by double binding is in turn
of a double-binding nature, which leads to
a self-perpetuating pattern of communication. The behavior of the overtly disturbed
communicant if examined in isolation sat-
isfies the clinical criteria of schizophrenia.
The double-binding communication presents a "damned if you do and damned if
you don't" situation for the child who is
trapped by the incongruent demand and
forbidden to draw attention to his predic-
ament. The incongruence of the assertions
in the communication may take the form of
affect and context discrepancies or may be
involved in a dichotomy between verbal
and nonverbal expression.

Bateson and his associates[1] describe the
family in which the double-binding mechanism operates as follows: A mother who is
made anxious and hostile by the threat of
too much closeness with her child responds
to her hostility by asuming a too loving
attitude toward the child. In an effort to
control her anxieties she manipulates communications to produce a degree of emotional proximity that she can tolerate. The
child becomes aware that her attitude hides
a basic hostility, but, if he is to receive
whatever love he can get, he must not permit himself to communicate this knowledge
to her. "The child is punished for discriminating accurately what she is expressing
and he is punished for discriminating inac-
curately—he is caught in a 'double bind'."
The father may be outraged by the mother's
behavior, but he remains passive because of
the peculiar or strained relationship he has
with his wife.

Faced with the untenable absurdity of
the situation, the child may respond by
consistently searching for clues and meaning to the messages and behavior of others
in the most unlikely and unrelated phe-

nomena, or he may respond to the illogic by complying with any and all injunctions with complete literalness and abstain from any independent thinking. Such behavior would perpetuate the inability to distinguish between the trivial and the important, the plausible and the implausible. A third possible reaction would be to withdraw from human involvement. These three forms of behavior as reactions to the double bind are suggestive of the clinical pictures of schizophrenia.[10]

Weakland[11] describes the double-bind situation as it occurs in three-way interaction. By grouping the two parents into an apparent unity a perception of "oneness" and its implications of single or consistent messages may occur when, in fact, the two parents are communicating separately to the child. The use of the pronoun *we* prior to a demand by one parent in conjunction with the perception by the child of covert disagreement between the parents makes for a contradictory message. Also marriages dominated by conflict and emphasis on differences and separateness that continue to remain intact and stable are contradictions in themselves. On the level of action the couple communicates relatedness and dependence of some kind; yet at the same time they are denying it.

Evidences of double-binding communication are apparent within the E. family. Elaine is able to describe her own inconsistent, contradictory, and double-binding messages to Ralph, and his resultant bind may be termed classic. In essence, her various behaviors and messages say, "Be a good little boy, and grow up." By obeying this command and growing up Ralph would have to disobey it by not being a little boy. He is faced with a paradox, is totally unable to respond appropriately to the demand, and yet must react. In his attempts to avoid his mother's inevitable disappointment or punishment, he tries to eradicate his commitment to respond by withdrawing from viable contact with his environment or by attempting to invalidate or make obscure his own responses. Since he has been forced to face the repeated double-binding message throughout his life, especially in adolescence, the double bind turns into an autonomous expectation re-

garding the nature of human relationships and the world at large. Consequently, his inappropriate responses are carried over to other relationships and contacts outside the family. Following is an example of his obscure and seemingly irrational responses during a therapy session:

> Elaine (to Ralph): Why do you talk those subjects at home and when company comes but not here?
> Ralph: What? That Amos is in the Cosa Nostra and active? I know for sure he is. What's wrong with it? Subjects aren't irrational.
> Therapist: What's the question? Is this what you wanted, Elaine?
> Alfred: He's coming up with what you wanted.
> Elaine: He has not answered my question. Why not talk "subjects" here?
> Ralph: Not the place for it. You don't go and tell people that your uncle's in the Cosa Nostra and active in the machine because there is an FBI, and, if they were to prove it, they would arrest him.
> Therapist: This is not the place to bring up material because you might get these people in trouble?
> Ralph: That's right. They'd use the radio station as a front.
> Elaine: What we say here is confidential.
> Ralph: That's my irrational talk, but it's not really irrational because it's the truth.

This excerpt exemplifies not only the patient's inappropriate and obscure style of relating but also the rationality of such responses in terms of his experience within a recurrent double-bind situation. Experiencing his family as the "Cosa Nostra machine" and fearing that he might reveal their activities to the FBI (the therapists), precipitating his family's "arrest," he avoids his position as the "front" and tries to keep from "signaling."

The reciprocal nature of the double bind is also evidenced within the family. Not only is Elaine giving Ralph a dual message, but his frequent response to that message is also double binding in nature. He responds by saying, "Treat me like a child and satisfy all my needs, including my need to grow and be like a man." By treating him like a child she cannot fulfill his need to be a man and vice versa. Consequently, she too is in a bind and cannot respond appropriately or break the cycle of reciprocal double binding without ceasing to give the double-binding message herself. To stop would eventually free the patient and stimulate his growth but would initially cause upset, disturbance, and confusion within the system.

Further confusing messages emerge from the parents as they remain unified despite overt divergence. This contributes to Ralph's perplexity in response to Elaine's message to him: "Be a man," for, if he were a man as are his father and his brother, rather than making her happy, he would produce nothing but conflict.

In summary, the various theories of family psychopathology, regardless of approach or emphasis, highlight the interactional nature of the patient's pathology. The differing approaches broaden our understanding not only of family dynamics and the development of pathology but also of the patient's behavior and experience within a transactional system.

THE PROCESS OF THERAPY

The ideal yet practical goal of family therapy is a more meaningful relationship for the parents and separation with consequent meaningful marriage and parenthood for the children.[2] In addition to the individuation of family members, other goals of family treatment include the removal of symptoms and consequences of a mutually destructive mode of living, the provision of workable models for identification, the removal of obstacles that stand in the way of the family's relational growth, the achievement of freedom for raising and resolving controversial issues, and the improvement of the family's dynamic exchanges with the larger community.[2] Also Jackson[4] states that the use of family psychotherapy increases the chances of breaking the schizophrenic's communication "code," since the therapist is present to trace the process by which communication moves to a pathological level.

With such goals in mind and a rationale emanating from the various theories focusing on the transactional or system dynamics of pathology, the family therapy process was initiated with the E. family. Initially, all family members were interviewed individually. This procedure was carried out to get some idea of each family member's individual life style and of his perceptions and evaluation of family problems and the patient's illness. After the collection of this data the parents were interviewed together to get some notion of their receptivity to family therapy and for preliminary evaluation of their marital relationship and mutual reactions to family life and pathology. The entire family was then brought together for an assessment session. This session was dominated by confronting behavior on the part of George, who was open in his expression of negative feelings and reactions toward his brother's "crazy" behavior, and by seemingly conscious and deliberately obstructive behavior on the part of Ralph. Alfred and Elaine appeared content to let their children "run the show" and made little effort to exert control. Linda remained less active than either of her brothers and made occasional attempts to straddle the fence between them. Ralph appeared to be the center of two subsystems, one involving his parents and the other, his siblings.

After this session the obvious interaction patterns, apparent family problems, and other pertinent information about the family were evaluated and assessed and a treatment approach initiated. Involved in the assessment process were the two co-therapists and others involved in the learning experience. A decision was made to initiate therapy with the parental unit, to follow up the patient's case individually, and eventually to incorporate the patient and possibly others into the therapy with the couple. This approach was advocated for the following reasons: (1) Alfred was highly resistant to involving his disturbed son in a situation in which the normal confrontations and behaviors of others might upset him; (2) the complexities and difficulties involved in controlling the entire system would have been burdensome and perhaps overwhelming to a novice therapist; (3) assuming the existence of (due to the numerous theoretical formulations) and having been partially exposed to some degree of pathology in the marital relationship, therapeutic work with the couple would presumably benefit not only the parents but also the entire family system. The couple was agreeable to this plan if it would be of help to their son.

After preliminary assessment the therapeutic work with the E. family may be divided into two phases. Phase 1 involved eleven one-hour weekly sessions with the couple and the cotherapists and approximately the same number of weekly one-hour sessions with the patient and one of the therapists. Phase 2 (still ongoing) involved ten one-hour weekly sessions with the entire family. An attempt will now be made to highlight some of the important dynamics and process evidenced throughout the two phases.

During the first two sessions with the couple, much of the discussion centered around Ralph, he apparently being the focus of activity and attention. The couple argued about their differing approaches to Ralph, each advocating and substantiating his own approach while condemning the approach of the other. Each complained that the other one never listened, and neither one appeared to try to listen. Elaine tended to avoid answering direct questions or confrontations posed by her husband and evidenced tangential and circuitous patterns of communication. Alfred appeared so convinced of his own "rightness" and so resistant to change that he was oblivious to what his wife had to say. In response to this the therapists attempted to clarify the nature of the disagreements, refocus from the content to the relational aspects of the conflict, investigate the couple's means of coming to agreement, and maintain a focus by preventing rambling and avoidance maneuvers.

During the next two sessions the couple was able to discuss aspects of their own relationship and issues not directly related to Ralph. Both spoke of their resentments toward the other. Elaine claimed to resent her husband's expectations, and Alfred asserted his resentment of Elaine's lack of compliance with his wishes. Many past issues were brought up, and the couple argued about events occurring twenty-five years ago as if they had happened the day before. Each continually attempted to reject or invalidate the opinion of the other. Generally there was less rambling, but

communication remained defensive and confusing at times. The couple's relationship appeared to be a symmetrically escalating game of one-upmanship. Possibly because of feelings of inadequacy and insecurity the partners clung to their positions or behaviors and were unable to tolerate the divergence of the other. Each seemed constantly to project his own inadequacies onto the other, causing the other partner to sink and keeping himself afloat. In dealing with these feelings of inadequacy, efforts were made by the therapists throughout therapy to be ego supportive to each partner. Attempts were also made to clarify the content and meaning of communication. During this "fiery" period, Alfred showed some resistance to dealing with the marital problems by suggesting that some of the other children be incorporated into the session. This suggestion was resisted by the therapists, since there was an obvious need to work on the problems of the couple. At the day hospital during this intial period of family therapy, Ralph showed some improvement. Able to relate better to others, he began planning his future but consistently resisted discussing his family.

After a two-week break the topic of discussion reverted to Ralph and the problems he was now having with George regarding choice of school. George preferred that Ralph not attend the school in which he was teaching. Alfred found George's feelings and their expression harsh and inappropriate, and he wanted to bring him into the session so that the therapists could "straighten him out." The suggestion was made that both George and Ralph come in to work on this problem. A discussion of Alfred's "overprotective" feelings followed, since he remained resistant to bringing Ralph into the session. Elaine appeared to favor bringing in both sons. To get a better picture of their decision-making process, the decision was left up to them at the end of the session. During the next session one of the therapists was gone and the couple arrived alone and twenty minutes late. Evidently Alfred had persuaded Elaine that it would be better for only George to attend; however, he could not come. The session was slow moving and boring, and attempts by the therapists to focus on the satisfying aspects of the couple's relationship were met with expressions of fatigue and seeming lack of interest. These numerous resistive maneuvers may have been due to a continued desire to escape discussion of their marriage and to the first absence of one of the original therapists. The couple's lateness, caused by Elaine, may also have been a covert expression of her disapproval of their "joint" decision to bring in George alone.

During the following three sessions, broken up and followed by cancellations on the part of the couple, their relationship was again the topic focused on. This was a productive period of therapy for the couple and involved discussion of their difficulties in expressing positive feelings, the progression of their relationship throughout the history of the marriage, resentments about being excluded from each other's activities, fears and accusations of infidelity, and their mode of expression of positive feelings. Despite the overtly destructive nature of their many arguments, it was discovered that positive feelings do exist between the couple and are expressed in subtle, although possibly inadequate, ways. During this period the therapists attempted to differentiate intellectualizations from feelings, to clarify discrepancies between messages sent and messages received, to elucidate the relational meaning of content issues, and to maintain and stimulate the focus on the couple's relationship. Relational issues become more apparent, such as the battle for power, dominance, and the one-up position, the existence and expression of positive feelings were found to exist, communication became clearer, and each partner seemed to listen more to the other. The decision was made to incorporate the children into the therapy during this progression because of the continued concern of the couple, the recent discharge of Ralph from the day hospital, and the belief of the therapists that the couple had made progress and had a workable understanding of problems. At this point Ralph was showing further improvement, and his communication and relational patterns were

clearer. However, because of his improvement his medication (fluphenazine [Prolixin]) was changed from intramuscular to oral administration, and he became negligent about taking it. During the following weeks he became agitated and reverted to his "out talk."

The remaining two sessions with the couple were dominated by discussion of the causes of schizophrenic behavior, the relation of this behavior to conflict in the marriage and the double-binding messages of the parents, the power and control issue within the marriage, discrepancies between verbal and nonverbal behavior in their communication, Elaine's feelings of inadequacy in dealing with her son, and their feelings about their therapy and the upcoming involvement of others. One of the therapists was absent and was again represented by a substitute during the first of these sessions, but this seemed to have less of an effect on the interaction. Generally the sessions were characterized by greater input and interpretation on the part of the therapists.

Phase 2 began and continues to be a dynamic series of sessions with the entire family. After a structured discussion of their expectations of family therapy, George immediately presented himself as the spokesman for and dominator of the group. He continually bombarded Elaine with accusations and complaints about her approach to Ralph's diet. Several "coalitions" and "marriages" within the family became apparent. George appeared to be in coalition with his father and a surrogate husband to his mother as he dynamically extended the conflict between them. Linda maintained a shaky coalition with her mother and appeared seductive to both George and her father. Ralph acted as the rescuer, often distracting the conflict with unrelated inputs and appearing uninvolved in the struggle for power that was obvious among the others. The therapists generally felt that they had been invaded, experienced greater anxiety, and felt pressured to exert some control in the situation. Plans were made to attempt greater control and to provide more structure to the following sessions. These plans included efforts to prevent "runaway" arguments by dealing with the clarification and interpretations of individual message transactions, to call on others for comments to prevent total domination by one, and to encourage attempts at listening and empathizing with others. During the week after this session Ralph became physically ill and appeared depressed and preoccupied. Although sufficiently recovered to attend, he missed the next family therapy session.

The second family session was dominated by a discussion of Ralph's absence, his position in the family, and the subtle reinforcement that all the family members give to his exclusion. During an individual session with Ralph that week he described himself as "uptight"—wanting to be "the trigger man to blow up the world." He spoke of being an archangel and agreed with the therapists' interpretation that he acted as a modified savior for his troubled family. After receiving the encouragement of the therapist and some family members, he consistently attended the family sessions. At this point, individual therapy with the patient was terminated to facilitate the emphasis on family rather than individual pathology and to prevent a division of therapeutic work and goals and an impractical protective alliance between patient and therapist.

The third session, attended by all, involved a structured discussion of the positive aspects of each member. This exercise was introduced by the therapists not only to provide greater structure and to facilitate control of the session but also to break the pattern of unending arguments and put-downs. George appeared to have the greatest difficulty with the expression of positive feeling and often qualified his positive remarks with negative ones. Despite the structure George still tried to dominate.

During the fourth session several procedural changes were initiated. Visiting consultants and traditional observers were present in the room to observe and make input into the session, and the tables were removed so that the family and therapists could sit in a circle. This session was highly intense, dramatic, and productive and involved the revelation and discussion of deep-seated feelings. Role expectations of the parents and extended family were discussed by the children, and their resultant feelings of pressure and inadequacy were brought to light. The expectations of George to succeed and of Ralph to fail were emphasized, and George's feelings and fears of failure were revealed for perhaps the first time in his life. The therapists generally felt overwhelmed by the numerous changes and by the intensity and pace of the session. This session was followed by a one-week break because of vacation.

The remaining sessions of therapy to date have been productive and mainly involved work on problems and relationships within various subsystems or between individual members. The termination of individual therapy and resultant feelings about it were dealt with, and the struggle for power and intolerance of differences within Linda's and George's relationship were thrashed out. Also brought to light were Ralph's perceptions of his mother's expectation of him to be "crazy" forever, his resentment of the price he pays for being crazy, his ambivalent feelings about his dependent role, and his protective feelings and behavior toward those who help to maintain the security of his present dependent status (e.g., Alfred). Also discussed were Elaine's feelings of confusion and inadequacy in dealing with the double-bind situation, Alfred's overprotective role, Linda's struggle for independence, the treatment of Ralph as a child by all family members, George's father surrogate position, and the expectations and desires involved in George's and Ralph's sibling relationship. Throughout the sessions the therapists were actively involved in clarifying and interpreting the issues, relationships, and communications and in attempting to elicit deep-seated feelings and meanings behind the various messages. During this period the family appeared committed to the process of family therapy and actively worked to explore and resolve problems. When faced with the option to resume therapy after a summer break rather than terminate it, they unanimously decided to continue.

Consequently, the process of therapy has

not ended but will continue. Realizing the necessity for change within their system and making efforts to effect it, the E. family has not only made considerable progress but also evidences a promising potential for the achievement of the goals of family therapy.

THE LEARNING EXPERIENCE

Perhaps most important of all my work with the E. family has meaningfully revealed to me the transactional qualities of experience. Man is not an isolate whose experience and behavior are solely determined either by inner or by outer forces. He experiences himself by experiencing the outer world and vice versa. All behavior stems from experience within a relational world, since man himself exists only in relation to that which is outside himself.

Assuming a lack of proof to explain the cause of schizophrenic behavior in terms of physiological abnormality, such behavior must then be seen to arise from an experiential-relational context. The inappropriate, irrational, and nonsensical behaviors of the schizophrenic become appropriate, rational, and sensible when viewed in terms of their relational tie to an absurd outer world. Distorted and "meaningless" communication becomes realistic and meaningful.

When I first became involved with the E. family, Ralph's behavior appeared psychotic and unrelated to anything. The family therapy experience enabled me to gain a better understanding of his experience within a system whose dynamics and communication patterns, especially in terms of the double bind, relate well to the schizophrenic's experience and resultant behavior.

Needless to say I learned much about system dynamics operating in the family unit, including the self-perpetuating nature of pathological dynamics despite efforts toward change.

In relation to my role as a cotherapist I discovered that I tended to react to the authority and ability of the other therapist (my teacher) by assuming the role of junior adult or child, vacillating between independent and dependent functioning. During her absences from therapy I would assume an adult role. Because of my perceptions of the authority of the cotherapist, I often felt like a sibling in relation to the members of the family. Also the family appeared to treat me like a sibling and to look to my cotherapist for authority.

In relation to my roles as individual and family therapist, I found myself to be comfortable when able to keep them separate but had difficulty handling the switch when individual therapy with Ralph was terminated. I had difficulty in defining my relationship and in responding to him when in the family sessions. I often felt confused—not knowing what to do with myself. I was so afraid of evidencing bias or of showing overconcern for him that I became too reserved.

Through the experience I also came to learn of my ability to block efforts at understanding or acting as therapist to those I personally dislike. This occurred throughout the beginning of therapy with the entire family, since I consistently complained about or condemned George's "obnoxious" behavior rather than attempting to understand it in terms of his experience within a transactional reality or in terms of my own projections. I have also found this learning to be helpful in regard to my relationships with and reactions to other people in general and have discovered my own ability to overcome intolerance of others.

Last, I have come to realize more than ever before the value of experiential learning. I could never have grasped the meaning of experience without experiencing. No one could have made me realize the nature and effects of the transactional family system. My involvement within the system itself, my experience of it, my feelings about it, and my actual work with it not only facilitated my learning about the nature of mental illness but also gave me a meaningful experience. By discovering the meaning of experience, my experience attained meaning.

References

1. Bateson, G., Jackson, D. D., Haley, J., and Weakland, J.: Toward a theory of schizophrenia, Behav. Sci. 1:251, 1956.
2. Boszormenyi-Nagy, I.: Intensive family therapy as process. In Boszormenyi-Nagy, I., and

Framo, J. L., editors: Intensive family therapy, New York, 1965, Harper & Row, Publishers, p. 133.

3. Bowen, M.: A family concept of schizophrenia. In Jackson, D., editor: The etiology of schizophrenia, New York, 1960, Basic Books, Inc.

4. Jackson, D. D.: The monad, the dyad, and the family therapy of schizophrenics. In Burton, A., editor: Psychotherapy of the psychosis, New York, 1961, Basic Books, Inc.

5. Kramer, D. H.: The theoretical position; diagnostic and therapeutic implications, Proceedings of workshop on family therapy, Oak Park, Ill., 1968, The Family Institute of Chicago.

6. Laing, R. D.: The politics of experience, New York, 1967, Pantheon Books, Inc., p. 23.

7. Lidz, T., Cornelison, A., Fleck, S., and Terry, D.: The intrafamilial environment of schizophrenic patients. II. Marital schism and marital skew, Am. J. Psychiatry 114:241, 1957-1958.

8. Mishler, E. G., and Waxler, N. E.: Family interaction processes and schizophrenia; a review of current theories, Int. J. Psychiatry 2: 375, 1966.

9. Schvaneveldt, J. D.: The interactional framework in the study of the family. In Nye, F. I., and Berardo, F. M., editors: Emerging conceptual frameworks in family analysis, New York, 1966, The Macmillan Co., Publishers.

10. Watzlawick, P., et al.: Pragmatics of human communication, New York, 1967, W. W. Norton & Co., Inc., Publishers.

11. Weakland, J. H.: The "double-bind" hypothesis of schizophrenia and three-party interaction. In Jackson, D., editor: The etiology of schizophrenia, New York, 1960, Basic Books, Inc.

12. Whitaker, C. A., editor: Psychotherapy of chronic schizophrenic patients, Boston, 1958, Little, Brown & Co.

13. Wynne, L., and Singer, M.: Thinking disorders and family transactions, paper presented at the American Psychiatric Association, Los Angeles, May, 1964.

9

Group psychotherapy with chronic patients in a community setting

Helen K. Grace

One of the major problems confronting mental health caregivers relates to the chronic patient. Although intensive efforts have been made to move the mentally ill out of custodial settings and into the community, the recidivism rate for chronic patients remains extremely high.

Mental health workers are immersed in record-keeping activities associated with admitting and discharging patients repeatedly. In analyzing the work of staff in agencies one finds that much of their time is spent in associated "intake" proceedings with little remaining for treatment activities. Once patients are discharged from state hospitals, they are referred to community clinics, but rarely do they appear for an appointment. Staff speaks disparagingly of the hopelessness of working with chronic patients. Predictions are made as to when particular ones will reappear on an emergency basis in need of hospitalization. The public health nurse in the community observes these individuals regressing but feels unprepared to offer assistance.

From the patient's perspective, discharge from a state hospital assigns him to a lonely and hostile world. Family members constantly look for signs that he is becoming "disturbed." Even the most legitimate expression of anger arouses fear in those around him. If the former mental patient seeks employment, he faces the dilemma of deciding whether to tell the employer his history and risk being turned down or not to report his history and face the possibility that his employer will find out; in the latter case he lives in constant fear of disclosure. In many instances the mental outpatient becomes immobilized. He has been told by hospital staff to go to the mental health clinic for follow-up care. Little consideration is given as to whether the client knows how to take public transportation to the clinic, whether he has adequate money for the carfare, or if he knows how to use the telephone, should he have access to one, to call the clinic for an appointment. Attendance at a mental health clinic poses additional problems; it reaffirms to the community and to the family that this individual has "mental problems" and therefore must be "watched."

Given this complexity of forces, how can one assist the chronic patient in readjusting to the community setting and thus prevent repeated hospitalizations? This chapter reports a two-year group psychotherapy endeavor with a core group of eight chronic schizophrenic patients in a community clinic setting. All eight patients had either been hospitalized for extensive periods and had been recently discharged from a state hospital or had had multiple hospitalizations in recent years. At the end of the two-year period none of this group had been rehospitalized. This chapter will (1) review literature relevant to group psychotherapy with chronic schizophrenic black patients, (2) describe the setting and the group members, (3) identify group themes and delineate the underlying process, and (4) draw implications from this experience pertinent to follow-up care for chronic schizophrenic patients in the community.

REVIEW OF THE LITERATURE

Withdrawal and isolation from meaningful and supportive social relationships characterizes the schizophrenic patient. Will describes this process as follows.

Through a series of anxious contacts with his fellows he has become increasingly unsure of himself, isolated and lonely. Relatedness to and communication with one's kind are essential to human survival, and some aspects of schizophrenic behavior may be looked upon, not only as evidence of disorganization and desocialization, but as complicated obscure communicative endeavors designed to preserve some semblance of social living.*

The goal of group psychotherapy based on this formulation of the problem becomes that of providing an experience in which the individual may develop skills in relating to others and in learning new and more effective patterns of communication.

The psychodynamics of schizophrenic behavior present a particular set of problems in establishing a therapeutic relationship. Much of the literature relating to schizophrenic behavior speaks repeatedly of the intense dependency needs as a problem in therapy. As Searles states the problem, the schizophrenic seeks another person to assume complete responsibility for satisfying all his needs, both physiological and psychological, although the other person is to seek nothing from him. The therapist from the patient's view is omnipotent and the sole source of help.[3] The therapist faces a dilemma: on the one hand, the patient must experience some gratification of his dependency needs if he is to trust himself to the relationship[5,6]; on the other hand, the therapist must not play the omnipotent role, which only makes the patient feel increasingly powerless and helpless. A part of the work in group psychotherapy becomes that of developing a means of relating to the intense dependency needs of the group.

Further characteristics of the chronic schizophrenic patient "consist essentially in an impairment of both *integration* and *differentiation*."[4] The group experience should be structured to facilitate this process. The individual needs to experience himself as a person of worth in his own right; the group affords a setting in which he can begin to see himself as one who is different from others. Additionally, a group composed of members who have shared similar experiences affords a safe place in which each may achieve a new perspective on his past. Review of the past provides the individual with an opportunity to gain new understanding as to the meaning of his behavior at a time of great upset. Traumatic experiences need no longer be dissociated but may be talked about in a safe environment; thus the most degrading experiences can be integrated into the totality of each one's being.

The problem of building positive self-identifications within group members becomes complicated when the patients are black and the therapist is white. The black patient has been socialized to view the white man as all powerful and himself as powerless and dependent. Grier and Cobbs explain the black situation as follows:

It is necessary for a black man in America to develop a profound distrust of his white fellow citizens and of the nation. He must be on guard to protect himself against physical hurt. He must cushion himself against cheating, slander, humiliation, and outright mistreatment by the official representatives of society. . . . For his own survival, then, he must develop a *cultural paranoia* in which every white man is a potential enemy unless proved otherwise and every social system is set against him unless he personally finds out differently.*

With this set of treatment problems, how may participation in group therapy be of value to black chronic schizophrenic patients?

First, the use of the group treatment modality diffuses the transference and thus provides an opportunity for finding appropriate ways of meeting the dependency needs of the schizophrenic.

A group of chronic schizophrenic patients tends to form what Bion characterizes as a dependency group. In such a group the members tend to behave immaturely and attempt to cause the leader to assume responsibility for them. The task for the therapist in such a group is to move each of the group members toward greater independence.

It is hoped that the group will advance

---

*From Will, O.: The schizophrenic reaction and the interpersonal field. In Appleby, L., Scher, J., and Cumming, J., editors: Chronic schizophrenia, New York, 1960, The Free Press of Glencoe.

*From Chapter 8, in Black Rage, by William H. Grier and Price M. Cobbs, copyright 1968 by authors.

from a dependency unit to one in which individuation occurs. Schutz delineates four stages of group development: (1) the *narcissistic* phase, in which members do not relate to one another, (2) the *inclusion* phase, in which they are primarily concerned with acceptance or nonacceptance, (3) the *power* phase, in which the struggle to separate from the therapist begins, and (4) the *intimacy* phase, characterized by cooperation and peer feeling.[2]

During the individuation, or power phase, group members begin to challenge the leader. In groups composed of schizophrenic members pairing frequently occurs as a means of coping with the guilt associated with opposing the leader.[1] The leader in her interaction with the group must be comfortable in allowing the patients to challenge her. In groups of schizophrenic patients it is particularly important that the leader allow pairing to occur among members if they are to cope adequately with their feelings of anger, on the one hand, and the associated guilt, on the other.

In groups of black patients it becomes even more difficult for them to move to a point where individuation may occur. Individuation may occur only in an atmosphere in which basic trust has been established within the gathering. According to Grier and Cobbs, the following is necessary:

The essential ingredient is the capacity of the therapist to love his patient—to say to him that there is a second chance to organize his inner life, to say that you have a listener and companion who wants you to make it. If you must weep, I'll wipe your tears. If you must hit someone, hit me, I can take it. I will in fact, do *anything* to help you be what you can be—my love for you is of such an order.*

To summarize, group therapy with black chronic schizophrenic patients must be focused on (1) first finding a satisfactory balance in meeting patient dependency needs, (2) moving from a dependency type of group to one in which individuation may occur, and (3) throughout the course of therapy allowing the black patients to ventilate their rage at the white therapist without becoming defensive or, on the other hand, overly guilty. The therapist must be committed to bearing the brunt of the rage from the past indignities experienced by the patient on the basis of being black and "mentally ill."

DESCRIPTION OF THE SETTING AND OF THE GROUP MEMBERS

I became involved with this group as a faculty member of the graduate program in psychiatric-mental health nursing at the University of Illinois. We as faculty had made the decision that we, as well as students, would become more heavily involved in providing mental health services in a community context rather than in isolated clinical experiences, as has been common in the past history of the graduate program. This change in our program was based on a belief that locating ourselves within the community context would allow us to follow the patients throughout the mental health system, as they availed themselves of services.

A particular interest of mine, stemming from experience in working within the state mental health system, centered around the problem of maintaining chronic schizophrenic patients in the community without the necessity of their returning to the hospital. With this in mind I, along with one of the graduate students, developed a psychotherapy group within one of the Board of Health mental health clinics. The group was recruited from intake conferences in which all patients discharged from the state hospitals servicing the area were automatically referred for "aftercare" services. All group members were contacted by telephone and interviewed by the graduate student before they entered the group. This group was co-led for the first year of its existence. During the second year, I led the group, since the student had completed our program.

The core* patient group was composed of the following eight members.

*From Chapter 8, in Black Rage, by William H. Grier and Price M. Cobbs, copyright 1968 by authors.

*Core members are defined as those who most consistently attended throughout the course of the group's history, in contrast to other members who entered and left the group in shorter periods of time.

MRS. A: 30-year-old divorced mother of two children. History of hospitalization for past ten years. Hospitalized in six different state hospitals; diagnosed in all as chronic schizophrenic. Separated from husband. Children residing with paternal grandparents in a distant state. Currently lives alone in a rooming house situation.

MRS. B: 33-year-old, twice-married woman. No children. Just discharged after second hospitalization when she was described as hallucinating and delusional. Now having severe difficulties with her husband.

MRS. C: 56-year-old separated mother of eight grown children. Hospitalized for most of past twenty years. Currently living with youngest daughter and three children in housing project.

MRS. D: 47-year-old, married, mother of two sons. Eleven prior hospitalizations during the past fifteen years. Currently maintaining home for husband and adolescent son.

MRS. E: 58-year-old mother of a 40-year-old retarded schizophrenic son, who also became a group member. Eight previous admissions in past ten years.

MR. F: 40-year-old son of Mrs. E, who has been hospitalized and in schools most of his life. Last hospitalization was for five years.

MR. G: 28-year-old unmarried man, living with mother. Two previous hospitalizations. Last hospitalization was for one year.

MR. H: 62-year-old married man. Numerous hospitalizations over past twenty years. Separated from his wife because she doesn't like it when he listens to the "voices."

This core group of eight members maintained themselves in the community for the entire two-year period. Another member, although he did not remain in the group for the entire period and required rehospitalization, was influential in determining the direction in which the group moved.

MR. I: 28-year-old single male, living with mother. Sister also hospitalized at same hospital.

All members shared a history of repeated hospitalization; they were poor and black and had been extruded from the community.

PHASES OF GROUP DEVELOPMENT
Narcissistic phase

During the first phase of the group development each individual addressed comments directly to the group leaders. It was as if each member had his story to tell but was little involved with other group members. At this stage each member evaluated the leaders' responses to him as an individual. Main themes in the first session revolved around circumstances surrounding hospitalization.

MR. I: I had had a vision that someone was going to die. . . . My mother put me in the state hospital because of this.

MRS. A: When I got sick, I couldn't eat. Daddy took me to the hospital. I was sick with pneumonia. They kept me in the part of the hospital for sick people.

At this stage many of the group members remained silent. Although first contributions of group members centered around denial of any need for psychiatric hospitalization, they then tentatively tested out the leaders' responses to reports of more disturbed behavior.

MRS. A: I had another vision before coming to the hospital where I saw President Kennedy coming through a light switch.

MR. I: You needed a man, that's what it was. My trouble is that I don't get enough sex . . . but all women want is money. I'd have to get a job to support one.

In this early phase of development, with a group composed of schizophrenic members, the group productions were extremely fragmented. The leaders in turn felt frustrated and helpless to try to bring any coherence into the meetings. It was difficult to get the group working together as a whole, rather than as a set of separate individuals.

Dependency phase

The first theme that began to unify the group was the racial issue. Through discussion of a racial theme, the group members were able to begin to develop a basic trust relationship with the coleaders. The student coleader of the group was a light black woman, whereas I was the only white person in the group. In the first session the racial topic was introduced, but the group members were not ready to pursue this.

MR. I: I'm sick because I'm a black man. (He went on to discuss how the system had made him ill.)

GROUP LEADER: Do you feel like a second-class citizen in this group?

At the first introduction of this theme, the group leaders attempted to establish a climate in which discussion of this sensitive area would be possible. Identifying the underlying meaning of the communication and relating it to the feeling tone within the group in an attempt to reduce anxiety, was the method used.

In the second session, the racial theme was reintroduced.

MRS. A: In the middle of the session shows the group members pictures of her children.

MR. I: I didn't know that you were that old. Your children are such beautiful chocolate color. I wish I were that color. (Mr. I was a very light black man.) I'm growing a mustache, and I wish it would really be black.

MRS. A: You're a shitty yellow.

MR. I: I didn't know you felt this way about me. . . . Some people think there is an advantage to being dark.

MRS. D: I think it's your personality rather than your color that counts.

From this the group fled into a discussion of religion.

MR. I: The Bible is the greatest story on earth. God was a white man.

MRS. A: I wished I could have lived back in those days.

MR. I: I wished I could have been a disciple.

Later in the session they returned to the racial topic.

MRS. A: Do you think people are jealous of skin color?

MR. I: I am of Indian ancestry. My people on both sides have been discriminated against.

MR. J: There is prejudice all over the place. Black people are prejudiced against black people.

MR. I: A light-skinned Negro is nowhere. When he's a child he's too light for black people and not light enough to be a white person.

After this meeting participants began to pair up outside the group for shopping trips and to engage in other activities together.

Discussions of God were frequent. This theme was an expression of their intense dependency needs. For a time they quarreled over whether God was white or black. They reached a compromise in which God had a combination of the features of both coleaders. Clearly they had expectations that we would perform miracles and be all loving and all giving to them. Confronted by the extreme dependency needs of the group, we considered it important to respond in some way to these demands without playing the omnipotent role that they wished us to assume. A goal established for the group was to build up a supportive network in which the participants would begin to rely on one another for support outside the group sessions. We decided that one way to approach this problem was for us to provide role models through visiting each member's home. The goal was to use this experience to make them comfortable in having other members to their houses and establishing social relationships. Each individual was visited, and these visits then were discussed within the group meetings. At these sessions coffee was regularly provided and usually some type of cookie, cake, or pastry. As the group developed, members assumed responsibility for providing treats for the others. The group moved into a phase in which they openly shared their feelings.

MRS. A: (Speaking of unhappy experiences with her father and stepmother) "You know, when my father gets older, he is going to need me, and I am going to turn my back on him."

OTHERS: Replied that they could understand her feelings.

MR. I AND MRS. K: Talked of how their families watch them for signs of illness.

MR. I: It's good to have this group to come to where we are understood and accepted.

As the group developed this feeling of closeness to one another, they expressed a desire to go on outings together. The first one was to the Black History Museum. The following week, discussion focused around this visit.

Mr. G, Mrs. A, and Mrs. C related to Mrs. D, a member who had not accompanied them, the details of the trip and discussed the displays that most impressed them: a replica of a mutilated slave (Mrs. C), African sculpture (Mr. G), a picture of Martin Luther King, Jr. (Mrs. A), and the murals painted on the basement walls depicting the history of black people in America. From this Mrs. C proceeded to discuss cotton picking in the south—how much was picked and the number of bales. An analogy was made between this description and the conditions of slavery depicted in the mural.

The discussion introduced a topic disturbing to the group. Whenever the group became frightened, they turned to a religious theme as a means of coping with the anxiety. Mrs. C at a prior meeting had stated that she wanted to talk about "my kingdom." At this point she stated that she wished to talk about this.

MRS. C: Emphasized that it was not "your" or "the" kingdom, but "my kingdom" that she wished to talk about and asked the group to consider the Bible verse "Seek ye first the kingdom of God and his righteousness, and all these things shall be added unto you."

GROUP: Looked at "my world" as the present one filled with hate and killing.

MRS. A: "We all have to die."

MRS. D: You know, they say that God knows just how much you can bear, but I don't know. . . . Some people have more than their share of trouble.

The session ended when Mrs. A and Mrs. C asked if the time had come to close and stated their need for medication. Throughout the course of the group's history, the members had difficulty in expressing anger either within the group or outside it.

Each time a disturbing theme developed, they reached out to one another for support. As the group relationship developed, they became comfortable in reviewing disturbing experiences of the past in the "safe" environment of the group. Discussion of hallucinations, experiences in state hospitals, and difficult experiences with family members were shared. The leaders attempted to help group participants define the experiences that had precipitated acute psychotic episodes and encouraged them to talk about the factors precipitating upsets within the context of the group. At the beginning of each weekly session, the members reviewed events that had occurred since their last meeting. Troubles with a teen-age son, divorce proceedings instituted by a separated husband, difficulties with welfare payments, and medical and dental problems all became topics to be shared in the group. Instead of looking solely to the leaders, as they had at the beginning of the series of sessions, group members relied on one another for help in their problem-solving endeavors.

Individuation, or power, phase

The group made little movement into the individuation phase of development. The power maneuvers that were made were covert, except for one instance in which Mr. I openly challenged me as leader of the group. Mr. I's attendance at meetings had become increasingly irregular. He refused to take medications because, he said, "They destroy my nature." He had picked up a girl who moved into his home to live with him and, on reporting this to the group, expressed anger at his mother for not accepting this arrangement. The group afforded him little support, and he felt increasingly isolated. After an absence of several weeks, Mr. I came into a group session one morning and sat extremely close to me. He began a tirade likening me to Eve in the garden. "It is always women who betray men." In the midst of the conversation he called me "nigger," saying that I was just like all the rest of the black people. Although disturbed, he was expressing underlying feelings common to the group. This could have been a positive experience for both Mr. I and the group. However, the staff in the agency heard the interaction. (This center had only partial partitions separating rooms, and all staff could hear what was going on in the other areas.) In reviewing the situation later, black professional staff became upset at the idea of a patient's calling a "white doctor," "nigger." They called the police, who appeared at the center; Mr. I ran away and never returned to the group. Group members certainly could not be free in expressing their anger if they had to expect such an outcome.

Separation phase

Throughout the last year of work with the group, my primary focus was on making them less dependent on me as the leader and more self-directed. Frequently I would leave the room to get their medications, encouraging them to continue the discussions. Although they always stated that they could not get along without a leader, the minute I would leave the room their laughter and talk belied this statement. During the last year, when I had to be absent from the group, they were encouraged to meet by themselves. Plans for termination were made six months in advance of the last meeting date. At that time, the group was given the opportunity of deciding its future. It could continue to meet in the center or in members' homes, join other groups, or terminate altogether. The members decided not to meet as a group, as they said, "because it wouldn't be the same without you." After they stopped meeting as a group, however, they were comfortable in visiting one another at home, frequently telephoned each other, and did many things together in pairs or in larger groups.

They continued, on an informal basis, a tradition of having picnics, developed within the last year of the group's history. Members took great pride in bringing the food: some brought cold meat and bread for sandwiches, others brought cake, potato chips, and pop, and still others would fry chicken or make some other contribution to the gathering. The final activity of this group was a picnic on the lakefront. Each individual was dressed in his best clothing, and each came with his contribution. The message came through loud and clear: "We are somebody."

At the termination of group sessions, all the members were integrated within the community. Mrs. A had developed a stable relationship with a boyfriend; Mrs. C was a valued caretaker of her grandchildren at home while her daughter worked; Mrs. E was maintaining a home for her son; Mr. F had been placed in a job-training program; Mr. G had gone through a job-training program and was awaiting placement; and Mr. H was reunited with his wife and caring for her after an accident in which she had broken her leg. Only Mr. I had returned to the state hospital.

SUMMARY AND IMPLICATIONS

Work with this group demonstrates the possibility of maintaining chronic schizophrenic patients in the community for a prolonged period with minimal professional input. The goal of making this group self-directed and independent could have been achieved to a greater degree had there been a meeting place within the community other than in the mental health center. The chronic schizophrenic patient needs to experience the stability that comes in meeting with other individuals experiencing similar problems. He needs to have a safe place to speak of his fears, anxieties, and problems. But this type of experience could be structured outside the boundaries of an official mental health agency. In the black community utilization of the churches as meeting places would be one possibility. Community workers could be responsible for maintenance of the groups with outside consultation from mental health professionals. Whether chronic patients with prolonged histories of psychiatric hospitalizations would ever be able to function in a job situation is questionable, but they could find meaningful places within their family constellations. The grandmother who baby-sits so that a daughter can go to work is performing a valuable function and should be supported in this.

The goal of group psychotherapy with chronic schizophrenic patients should be that of helping each individual develop a more positive image of himself as a person of worth. Accomplishment of this end can best be achieved through a recognition of the intense dependency needs and the difficulties of differentiation experienced by this group and then use of the group process to facilitate working through these difficulties.

References

1. Fried, E.: Individuation through group psychotherapy. In Sager, C., and Kaplan, H. S., editors: Process in group and family therapy, New York, 1972, Brunner/Mazel, Inc.
2. Schutz, W. C.: FIRO, New York, 1958, Rinehart & Co., Inc.
3. Searles, H.: Dependency processes in the psychotherapy of schizophrenics. In Searles, H.: Collected papers on schizophrenia and related subjects, New York, 1965, International Universities Press, Inc.
4. Searles, H.: Integration and differentiation in schizophrenia; an overall view. In Searles, H.: Collected papers on schizophrenia and related

subjects, New York, 1965, International Universities Press, Inc.
5. Sechehaye, M. A.: Symbolic realization, New York, 1951, International Universities Press, Inc.
6. Whitaker, C. A., and Malone, T. P.: The roots of psychotherapy, New York, 1953, Blakiston.

Bibliography

Grier, W., and Cobbs, P.: Black rage, New York, 1968, Basic Books, Inc., Publishers.

Rioch, M. J.: The work of Wilfred Bion on groups. In Sager, C., and Kaplan, H. S., editors: Process in group and family therapy, New York, 1972, Brunner/Mazel, Inc.
Will, O.: The schizophrenic reaction and the interpersonal field. In Appleby, L., Scher, J., and Cumming, J., editors: Chronic schizophrenia, New York, 1960, The Free Press of Glencoe.

Section II

Pediatric nursing

with an introduction by
Marion H. Rose

The chapters that follow deal with a variety of topics related to pediatric nursing. However, two unifying themes cut across the diversity of topics. One of the themes is that to truly help children nurses must work with them in the context of their total family situation. This theme is particularly strong in the first four chapters of this section. Riddle's and Struempler's chapters poignantly reveal the detrimental effect of lack of family unity and strength on the care of the child and on the lives of significant family members, particularly the mother. Shea and Harris discuss how personnel and the organization of care within a hospital can assist families during the crises of illness and hospitalization.

The second theme concerns the need to critically study individual children as a basis for learning how to work with children both in and out of the hospital. Gallagher and Rose both present material on one child that illustrates how each coped with the experience of hospitalization. Robischon in her excellent chapter does not deal directly with either of these two themes; however, her study does point up the importance of the development of children in investigating the etiology of the practice of pica.

As in previous volumes, it continues to be my hope that the chapters that follow will contribute to the improvement of the care of children and their families.

10

Caring for children and their families

Irene Riddle

The concept of family-centered care in the nursing of children is generally endorsed by nurses, but the extent to which this concept is demonstrated varies substantially in nursing practice. There is a tendency on the part of nurses to equate the concept with policies such as unrestricted visiting hours for parents in a children's hospital or an active teaching program for parents in an ambulatory pediatric care setting. Such policies in themselves do not necessarily confirm the provision of family-centered care; confirmation can only be found within the process of nursing itself.

Nurses who demonstrate the concept of family-centered care in the process of nursing each child are those who are sensitive to the point of view of the child. They perceive that his parents are of crucial importance to him; they recognize that his health problem is a family problem and that his health needs are a family concern. They search to find the specific meaning of the child's health problem to him and to his family.[5] They seek to determine the nature and extent of assistance needed by the child and family to master their health problem and to meet the future with increased competence and confidence.

A commitment to caring for families within the framework of pediatric nursing practice extends the scope of responsibilities of the nurse.[13] The commitment calls for a systematic method of assessing the nursing needs of each child and the particular family unit of which he is a member. It is this phase of the nursing process that ensures individualized care. Assessment data also provides the most reliable rationale for the use of professional resources.

Recent literature contains valuable guidelines for nursing assessment that focus on the child. Erickson[9] points out the importance of obtaining information about each child's life situation and experiences from his mother, as well as obtaining information directly from the child through observation and interaction. Thompson[17] discusses growth and development as a basis for assessing each child. Barton[1] describes the use of play as an assessment tool and points out that play affords a means of gaining information about children that may not be obtained in any other way.

This chapter will focus on the family unit and will suggest some guidelines for nursing assessment. The value of the suggestions will be determined by their usefulness to nurses who are committed to implementing the concept of family-centered care in the nursing of children.

THE FAMILY AS THE FOCUS OF CARE

Every family is a dynamic entity; change over time is a universal characteristic of families as well as individuals. At any given point in time a family can be considered in terms of the individuals who make up the unit and in terms of the systems that characterize the total unit.

The nuclear family unit represents the model structural pattern of the family in our society. Parsons[15] cites two basic functions of the nuclear family: the primary socialization of children and the stabilization of adult personalities. These functions imply a process of development through family life for both children and parents.

Individual development within the family

The psychosocial development of each individual throughout the life cycle has

85

been described by Erikson[10] in terms of a sequence of eight phase-specific developmental tasks. In usual circumstances the first three of these tasks are accomplished within the nuclear family unit; subsequent tasks involve a broader social context and other social institutions. Successful accomplishment of one task increases potential for success with the next task. Successful accomplishment of each task also results in the establishment of a certain basic quality of strength, which Erikson[11] terms *virtue* to imply both inherent strength and active quality. Erikson identifies hope, will, purpose, competence, and fidelity as the basic strengths or virtues derived from childhood and adolescence and love, care, and wisdom as the central virtues of adulthood.

Individuals who approach parenthood within a loving relationship after having firmly established the basic strengths of childhood and adolescence are perfectly suited for the responsibility. But reality is seldom perfect, and certain personal strength may be insecure, perhaps still rudimentary, as individuals become parents. For those who possess basic hope, parenthood offers opportunity for further development of all human strengths. The primary quality of hope, which stems from the first phase of an individual's life experience, is the fundamental strength. Without sufficient hope no human endeavor is worthy of effort, and the hopeless parent will find parenthood hopeless. Those who lack sufficient hope must be identified so that they can be assisted in establishing a firm basis of this essential quality. Only then can parenthood become a growth-promoting process for the parent and for the newly born.

In describing parenthood as a developmental phase, Benedek[4] reminds us that every woman brings all her past experience to the task of becoming a mother and ever man brings all his past experience to the task of becoming a father. This single statement, which appears disarmingly simple, indicates the dynamic complex that exists when two individuals, each with a unique life history, unite in the common endeavor of creating a family. Insecure personal strengths can be compounded or compensated in the union. One individual's limited strength of purpose, weakness of will, doubtful competence, or tenuous fidelity can mature over time when fostered by a corresponding quality of strength in another. Even a limited capacity to care can be expanded through another's loving, trusting expectation that responsibility for caring will be fulfilled. Erikson defines care as the "widening concern for what has been generated by love, necessity, or accident," and states further that care "overcomes ambivalence adhering to irreversible obligation."*

The basic strengths established in childhood and adolescence are refined and synthesized into the qualities termed *motherliness* and *fatherliness* in adults. A commitment to parenthood facilitates the maturation of these qualities into the highly specific functional expressions of mothering and fathering. Benedek makes a clear distinction between the biologic fact of motherhood and fatherhood and the interactional processes of mothering[3] and fathering.[2] It is the basic distinction between creating a new life and sustaining that life.

Infancy, childhood, and youth comprise a prolonged period of vulnerability, but the specific nature of the vulnerability changes with each phase of development. Therefore parents are faced with changing responsibilities in fostering each child's growth over time. Developmental tasks are shared by parents and children, as are many problems that arise in the course of time. Tasks and problems are stress evoking; with accomplishment of each task and resolution of each problem, children and parents both realize new adaptations and new levels of strength. In this way the process of family life is a developmental process for each family member.

The family as a unit

At any given point in time, a family can be described in terms of systems that characterize the total unit. These systems reflect patterns of functioning within the ongoing process of family life.

---

*From Erikson, E. H.: Insight and responsibility, New York, 1964, W. W. Norton, Inc., p. 131.

Each family member contributes a specific configuration of real and potential strengths and vulnerabilities to the unit. The success of any family in maintaining a quality of life that ensures the development of individual members does not depend on any single characteristic of any one particular member. The crucial factor is the composite strength or total resources that the family realizes as a unit. Four family unit systems are of special significance as indicators of composite strength: the communication system, the economic support system, the emotional support system, and the system of seeking and using help.

Communication system. Communication pertains to the exchange of meaning between and among family members through a common system of verbal and nonverbal symbols. An open communication system encompasses all family members and facilitates the free exchange of meaningful expressions. An open system also implies flexibility in patterns of communication among members based on use of appropriate communicative symbols.

Economic support system. Economic support is essential for the maintenance of the family unit. Economic resources are required to meet the basic needs of family members; a dependable system of economic support provides the family with a sense of security for the future as well as the present.

Emotional support system. Emotional support is also essential for the maintenance of the family unit. Emotional resources are required to sustain individual members during periods of vulnerability; a dependable system of emotional support provides each member with assurance that support will be available when needed.

The system of seeking and using help. Maintenance of the family unit requires the use of resources outside the nuclear boundary. In addition, problems arise within each family from time to time that call for the use of specialized resources. The family's ability to seek help when a problem cannot be resolved implies recognition of the need for help and knowledge of possible resources. The family's ability to use help implies active effort and collaboration in working toward a resolution of their problem. The ability to use help also implies that it is available when needed.

These four systems, although interrelated, are not necessarily interdependent. Each system can be viewed as a functional variable. A family unit may reflect a dependable economic support system with a severely restricted communication system. The interests and energies of both parents may be so deeply invested in the process of building up family economic resources that they have little interest or energy left for meaningful exchanges with their children. The restricted communication system may eventually split into two distinct, closed systems, one between parents and the other among the children. Another family unit may reflect an open communication system, but emotional resources of each member may be so meager that only needs can be communicated. Still another family unit may reflect adequate systems of communication and support, yet the family may be unable to seek help from outside its boundary when a certain problem arises. Family pride may inhibit action, perhaps because the family possesses a false sense of autonomy, perhaps because the nature of the problem connotes social disapproval. Inability to seek help with a problem may also be due to lack of knowledge of possible sources of help. The hardships engendered as problems that remain unresolved usually take their toll on the emotional resources of each family member and may eventually destroy family unity. These brief examples demonstrate that family unit systems, although interrelated, can reflect various combinations of characteristics at any particular point in time. Together they describe the manner in which a family functions as a unit, regardless of the family's structure, membership composition, or socioeconomic class.

ASSESSMENT OF FAMILIES WITH HEALTH PROBLEMS

The existence of a health problem in a child is a stress-evoking experience for him and for his family. The magnitude of the stress is partially determined by the nature of the problem and the therapeutic regimen the child is required to undergo. A family's ability to master the stress that a health problem evokes is a function of the composite strength the family realizes at the time the problem occurs and the nature and extent of assistance each member realizes in mobilizing strengths to deal with the problem. The aim of family-centered nursing care is to ensure that all family members are provided with the assistance they need to deal with a health problem successfully.

In the reality of professional service, nurses often find that they are limited in terms of the number of family members with whom they come in contact. This limitation in no way attenuates the importance of the concept of family-centered care. Nurses can provide indirect supportive care to family members they may never encounter through working effectively with those they do.

A systematic assessment of each child and individual members of his family is complemented by gaining a perspective on the entire family as a unit. This perspective ensures that the needs of all family members will be taken into account in the caring process. The information the nurse acquires over time through direct observation and interaction can be analyzed to ascertain distinguishing characteristics of the family's structure, communication system, economic support system, emotional support system, and system of seeking and using help. These characteristics can then be used in determining the nature and extent of assistance the family needs in dealing with their health problem.

The structure of the family unit

The nuclear family structure, in which parents and their children constitute an independent unit, represents a well-circumscribed theoretical model. Realistically, this structure is subject to considerable modification. In preparing this chapter, I compiled data on the family structure of a random sample of fifty hospitalized children. These data will be presented because they emphasize the importance of an individualized consideration of the family structure of each child as a basis for family-centered care.

The fifty children in the sample ranged in age from 3 days to 12 years, and all were patients in a pediatric hospital of an urban medical center. The children had been hospitalized for treatment of diverse types of health problems. Some of the problems were acute, others were chronic. Some required a short hospital stay, others required a long-term stay. Genetic disorders, congenital defects, accidental injuries, and newly acquired illnesses with both favorable and unfavorable prognoses were all represented in the sample. Some of the children had been hospitalized on an emergency basis; others had been admitted on a scheduled, elective basis.

Thirty-six children, or 72% of the total sample, were members of two-parent families who maintained independent households. Six of these children had experienced the loss of one of their natural parents from the family unit through divorce and the acquisition of a new parent through remarriage. Five of the thirty-six children were experiencing prolonged separation from their fathers, either because of military service or prison confinement. One of the children, a baby girl, was in the care of foster parents until she could be adopted into a permanent family. Nineteen of the thirty-six independent two-parent family units maintained close ties with extended family members (great-grandparents, grandparents, aunts, or uncles of the children) and perceived their relatives as helpful. The remaining seventeen two-parent families either did not have any ties with extended family members or did not perceive the members as helpful. Within this group of families, relatives were often perceived as being too needful to be a source of help.

Fourteen children (28% of the total sample) were members of one-parent families at the time of the study. One of these children, a 10-year-old boy, had been reared in an institutional setting since the death of his mother when he was 6 years old. He and his brother were weekday residents of a boys' home and spent the weekends with their father. There were no relatives available to assist this family unit. Another child in this group, an 8-year-old girl, had lost her parents when she was young. She was a member of an independent family unit consisting of her paternal grandmother and 10-year-old brother. The child's grandmother did not perceive any relatives as helpful because of their own needs. The remaining twelve children belonged to single-mother families; divorce was a factor in eight of these families. Seven of the single mothers maintained independent households; two of these mothers perceived relatives as helpful. Five of the single mothers and their children resided with and were economically dependent on extended family members (grandparents of the children).

Nineteen mothers in the sample maintained either full-time or part-time employment outside the home. Daytime child care was provided by the father in one instance, by an extended family member in seven instances, and by a nonrelative caretaker in eleven instances. The fifty family units contained a total of 136 children. The number of children per unit ranged from one to eight, and a new baby was expected in four families at the time of the study.

These data provide a representative description of the focus of family-centered care: children and their families, each circumscribed by a particular structure and each confronted with a particular health problem.

Systems of the family unit

An estimate of the composite strength of each family confronted with a health problem can be derived from the characteristics that distinguish the systems of the family as a unit. These characteristics thus afford a useful means of identifying the nursing needs of individual family members.

In considering family unit systems, the nurse engages in a mental method of processing or categorizing information as it is acquired in the caring process.

Communication system. The nurse can discern whether the family's communication system is open or restricted on the basis of information gained through interacting with family members and observing interaction among members. If the system is restricted, certain members are probably being denied opportunity to express their feelings about a health problem and are most likely being denied needed emotional support. Support depends on an open communication channel. When necessary, nursing intervention can be planned to facilitate communication among family members and to offer emotional support to needful members.

Information about family communication systems is contained in the following excerpts from two nursing situations. The situations involved the infant sons of two young couples. Each couple had one other child of toddler age. Mr. and Mrs. A's baby, Davy, and Mr. and Mrs. B's baby, Jimmy, were both in the hospital for surgical correction of pyloric stenosis.

In talking with the nurse, Mrs. A said, "I knew something was wrong when Davy kept throwing up, but he took his feedings so well each time—I kept thinking he'd keep the next one down. Finally I tried to get in touch with my pediatrician, but he was gone for the weekend. I was so worried, but I decided to wait and try feeding Davy real slow. I kept burping him about every ounce; he'd do O.K. one time and throw up everything the next—really hard. When I got my pediatrician on the phone Monday, he said I should get Davy right to the hospital and he'd meet me here." . . . "I knew it was serious, but I didn't have any idea he'd have to have an operation." Mrs. A's eyes filled up with tears; she twisted a crumpled tissue in her hands as she said, "Poor little tyke. I sure hope he does O.K." . . . Later in the conversation, the nurse asked, "How do you think your husband feels about Davy's problem?" Mrs. A replied, "Dave? He never feels anything—at least he never acts like he does. He spends so much time at the station rebuilding old cars—him and his buddies. That's where he works. He spends so much time there he might as well live there! He's at home now though; he stayed home to take care of Mary. He's real good with her; they get along swell together. He's gonna bring her with him this evening. I can go stay with her in the lobby while he comes up to see Davy."

This brief excerpt reflects the valuable information a nurse can gain about a family through listening attentively to one member. The nurse noted that Mrs. A used the first person singular pronoun in her explanation of Davy's problem. This prompted the nurse to explore Mrs. A's perception of her husband's feelings. From the pattern of restricted communication that characterized the A family, the nurse identified the need of both parents for opportunities to express their feelings and Mrs. A's special need for consistent emotional support. Through meeting these needs, the nurse hoped to facilitate communication between Mr. and Mrs. A.

A different system of communication characterized the B family. In talking with the nurse, Mrs. B said, "It didn't take us long to realize that something was very wrong. At first we thought it was just a minor upset. Jimmy would keep some of his feedings down; others he'd keep down for a while and then lose completely. Then he started vomiting up every one. . . . I thought maybe he had a milk allergy, but my husband said he couldn't have because nobody in our family—on either side—has ever had any kind of allergy trouble. Finally we decided to get in touch with our doctor. . . . I was pretty upset at first when we found out that Jimmy would have to have an operation. My husband says that it's probably easier for babies than anybody else—he thinks he won't feel all that soreness and stiffness—that he'll get well real fast and we can take him home." Later in the conversation, Mrs. B talked about her daughter and said, "I'm so glad my mother was able to come to be with Janie. My husband had to go to work today to make arrangements to be off tomorrow. He'll be here as soon as he gets off work."

An open system of communication within the B family was reflected in Mrs. B's verbalizations. The nurse recognized that the process of care directed toward Jimmy and Mrs. B would be extended to all family members through Mrs. B.

Economic support system. The nurse can discern whether the family's economic support system is dependable or undependable and then determine the impact of the health problem on the family's economic resources. Parents who are faced with serious financial worries because of a child's hospitalization may be unable to offer the child the emotional support he needs to cope with his experience. When necessary, the prompt initiation of a referral can reduce a family's distress over inadequate economic resources. The following summary of a nursing situation describes a family whose economic support system was severely threatened by a health problem.

Bobby G, 7 years old, was admitted to the hospital with multiple injuries after having been struck by an automobile. In talking with his mother, the nurse learned that Bobby's family consisted of his mother, an 8-year-old sister, and a 14-year-old sister. Mrs. G was employed at a restaurant; her income supported the family. She worked an early shift so that she could be home before her children returned from school. Her 14-year-old daughter was responsible for getting herself and the younger children off to school each morning. Mrs. G indicated that the family had been managing adequately with these arrangements. When Bobby was admitted to the hospital, Mrs. G wanted to stay with him during the day. She appreciated her son's need for her, but she had recently changed jobs and was worried that she would not be paid if she did not work. She demonstrated her anxiety in talking of all the time-payment bills she faced each month and the fact that she had no medical insurance. The nurse contacted the social worker as soon as she learned of Mrs. G's situation. Collaboration among health care professionals is essential in meeting the complex needs of families. With the assistance of the social worker and the nurse, Mrs. G was able to resolve her immediate financial concerns and support Bobby in dealing with his hospitalization. Mrs. G spent each day with her son until he indicated that he could manage all right if his Mom returned to work and just visited in the late afternoons.

Emotional support system. Through observation and interaction in the caring process, the nurse can discern whether the family's emotional support system is dependable or undependable. As was noted earlier, the ability of family members to support each other depends on open communication channels. An open system of communication does not ensure emotional support, however. A health problem may deplete a family's emotional resources to the extent that members cannot support each other. The impact of a health problem on the emotional resources of a family is significantly determined by the nature of the problem, the economic implications of the problem, and the nature and number of other problems confronting the family simultaneously. Nursing intervention can be planned to extend emotional support to all needful family members. The following excerpts from two nursing situations demonstrate the development of different plans of care based on assessment of the emotional support systems of the families.

Mr. and Mrs. M admitted their 4-year-old son Timmy to the hospital for a tonsillectomy. He was a little shy with the nurse at first but responded to her interest in his suitcase by opening it and showing each item he had brought to the hospital. Throughout the admission procedures, Timmy's behavior indicated that he had been carefully prepared for his hospital experience.

In talking with Mr. and Mrs. M, the nurse learned that they had a clear understanding of Timmy's surgery. Mrs. M said, "We hate to put him through this—he's never been in a hospital before—but we can't have him go through another winter like the last; he was sick more than he was well. He just loves nursery school, but he had to miss so many days." Then Mr. and Mrs. M talked about the explanations they had given Timmy. Their conversation reflected their trustful expectations concerning the quality of care their son would receive in the hospital. The nurse asked how Timmy had responded to learning that he would have a very sore throat after his operation. Mrs. M replied, "Well, he's had lots of sore throats before due to infections, but I don't think anybody ever really understands how something will feel before actually feeling it. Timmy's usually pretty crabby when he's sick—I guess we all are. Tomorrow he'll probably hate the whole world when he wakes up from the anesthetic." Then Mr. and Mrs. M and the nurse talked about

measures that would promote Timmy's comfort after his tonsillectomy.

In conversation with Mrs. and Mrs. M the nurse also learned that Timmy had a 2-year-old brother named Mike who was being cared for at home by his grandmother. Mr. M explained that he wanted to be home in time to put Mike to bed. He smiled as he said, "Grandma will be needing some help by that time. Mike's a real handful—on the go every minute." Mrs. M said that she had decided to stay with Timmy through the night because he had never been away from home overnight before. She felt he would rest better and thus get along better after his operation.

The dependable emotional support system that characterized the M family was quickly recognized by the nurse. A plan of nursing care was then developed to facilitate parental care. With the assistance of the nurse, Mr. and Mrs. M supported their son throughout his hospital experience. A different plan of care was called for in the following situation.

Mr. and Mrs. J brought their 4-year-old son Danny to the hospital for a tonsillectomy. During the admission procedures Danny and his parents manifested anxious tension. Danny began to cry when the nurse approached him; his mother tried to coax him to respond; his father showed increasing impatience with Danny and with Mrs. J. The nurse spent some time talking with Danny; gradually his crying subsided, and he consented to being weighed. The nurse decided to postpone additional physical assessment and invited Danny and his parents to the playroom. Mr. J stayed with Danny, and Mrs. J talked with the nurse.

In conversation with Mrs. J the nurse learned that Danny knew he was coming to the hospital to get his tonsils taken out. Details regarding his hospital stay had not been explained. Mrs. J appeared apprehensive when the nurse suggested that Danny would benefit from knowing what to expect. She replied, "He gets upset so easily; he's a very emotional child. I decided it was best not to tell him he was going to have an operation, but my husband told him anyway. John thinks I'm making too much over this whole thing, but he's really just as concerned as I am." The nurse reassured Mrs. J and offered to talk with Danny about his stay in the hospital. Mrs. J agreed with some hesitancy.

A short time later the nurse had opportunity to talk with Mr. J while Mrs. J stayed with Danny in the playroom. Mr. J told the nurse that his wife was very nervous and apologized for her behavior. He said, "She insists on staying with Danny tonight; I keep telling her he'd do fine on his own and she'd rest better at home, but she won't change her mind." The nurse also learned from Mr. J that he had to work the next day but would spend the evening with his wife and son. There were no other children in the family.

The nurse quickly recognized that the J family's emotional support system was not adequate to deal with the health problem that confronted them. Mr. and Mrs. J perceived Danny's hospital experience from different points of view, and the discontinuity was placing severe demands on their emotional resources. Neither parent was able to provide Danny with the support he needed to deal with the experience. A plan of nursing care was developed to extend emotional support to Mr. and Mrs. J while providing Danny with direct, consistent assistance in dealing with his hospital experience. As the nurse worked with Mrs. J, she was gradually able to mobilize latent resources and provide Danny with the maternal support he needed.

The system of seeking and using help. Within the nuclear family, the system of seeking and using help is primarily a parental responsibility. A child's health problem must be recognized as a problem by his parents for them to seek professional health care. Then the child's health care must be perceived as helpful by his parents for them to collaborate with care.

In considering the family's system of seeking and using help, the nurse endeavors to find answers to the following questions: How has the family managed problems in the past? How do the parents perceive their child's health problem and health care needs? What are their health care expectations? How are the needs of other children in the family being met? Are relatives, neighbors, or friends available to assist the family? Are they perceived as helpful by the parents? What other problems are confronting the family and how are they being managed? Do any unrecognized health problems exist within the family? From information acquired over time, the nurse can discern whether the family's system of seeking and using help is effective or limited. If the system is limited, the nurse must identify the most suitable strategy for assisting the family toward a more effective system.

Margie F, 5½ years old, was admitted to the hospital because of obesity.[16] She was to undergo a comprehensive evaluation at the request of her mother. Margie's chubby appearance was in marked contrast to her mother's slim stateliness.

The nurse who assumed responsibility for Margie's care in the hospital learned that Mrs. F had been divorced shortly after Margie's birth. Mrs. F had two other children who were in their teens and a good friend named Mr. B who was a frequent visitor in the F home. Margie referred to Mr. B as her daddy, and Mrs. F explained that he was the only real father Margie had ever known.

In the process of caring for Margie, the nurse observed that Mrs. F made frequent references to Margie about her weight and size. Clothing was often cited as too snug; many foods were identified as too fattening. Mrs. F seemed compelled to keep Margie reminded of her obesity. Mr. B did not visit Margie in the hospital, but Mrs. F stated that he did not consider Margie's weight problem to be a problem.

The nurse also learned that Margie had undergone two other evaluations in two different hospitals and had been under the care of four different physicians prior to her present physician. From this history and observations and interaction in the caring process, it became clear to the nurse that Mrs. F kept seeking additional help for Margie's health problem because she was unable to use the help offered her.

Margie's physician, an endocrinologist, could not detect any physiological basis for her obesity and initiated a psychiatric referral. Mr. F contacted the psychiatrist one time while Margie was in the hospital but did not follow through on scheduling an appointment after Margie's discharge. Mrs. F wanted a rapid, dramatic resolution for her daughter's health problem; she could not accept the professional judgment that the resolution was within her own realm.

The nurse who worked with Margie and her mother during their hospital stay recognized that help, in the nature of a trusting relationship, would have to be made consistently and continuously available to Mrs. F for her to use it eventually. The understanding and acceptance that the nurse extended to Mrs. F and her daughter developed into a trusting relationship over time. The nurse's care continued long after Margie was discharged from the hospital. The nurse made help available through telephone contacts and home and clinic visits. Gradually the nurse was able to detect changes in Mrs. F's behavior that indicated that she was beginning to use help.

This nursing situation describes only one of many possible limitations that can exist in a family's system of seeking and using help. Each situation requires an individualized approach to the family and the development of an individualized plan of care.

In working with each family, the nurse can discern the characteristics that distinguish the family's communication system, economic support system, emotional support system, and system of seeking and using help. These characteristics reflect the family's composite strength in dealing with their health problem and afford a useful means of identifying the nursing needs of individual family members.

SUMMARY

Implementation of the concept of family-centered care calls for a systematic method of assessing the nursing needs of each child and his family. A consideration of the family as a unit ensures that the needs of all family members will be taken into account. From information gained in the caring process, the nurse can ascertain distinguishing characteristics of the family's structure, communication system, economic support

system, emotional support system, and system of seeking and using help. These characteristics can then be used to determine the nature and extent of assistance the family needs in dealing with their health problem.

The nurse who is committed to implementing the concept of family-centered care in the nursing of children is committed to providing each child and his family with the assistance they need to master their health problem and meet the future with increased competence and confidence.

References

1. Barton, P. H.: Nursing assessment and intervention through play. In Bergersen, B. S., Anderson, E. H., Duffey, M., Lohr, M., and Rose, M. H., editors: Current concepts in clinical nursing, vol. 2, St. Louis, 1969, The C. V. Mosby Co., pp. 203-217.
2. Benedek, T.: Fatherhood and providing. In Anthony, E. J., and Benedek, T., editors: Parenthood, its psychology and psychopathology, Boston, 1970, Little, Brown & Co., pp. 167-183.
3. Benedek, T.: Motherhood and nurturing. In Anthony, E. J., and Benedek, T., editors: Parenthood, its psychology and psychopathology, Boston, 1970, Little, Brown & Co., pp. 153-165.
4. Benedek, T.: The family as a psychologic field. In Anthony, E. J., and Benedek, T., editors: Parenthood, its psychology and psychopathology, Boston, 1970, Little, Brown & Co., pp. 109-136.
5. Blake, F. G.: The child, his parents and the nurse, Philadelphia, 1954, J. B. Lippincott Co.
6. Debuskey, M., editor: The chronically ill child and his family, Springfield, Ill., 1970, Charles C Thomas, Publisher.
7. Duvall, E. M.: Family development, Philadelphia, 1971, J. B. Lippincott Co.
8. Elliott, K., editor: The family and its future, London, 1970, J. & A. Churchill, Ltd.
9. Erickson, F.: Nursing care based on nursing assessment. In Bergersen, B. S., Anderson, E. H., Duffey, M., Lohr, M., and Rose, M. H., editors: Current concepts in clinical nursing, vol. 2, St. Louis, 1969, The C. V. Mosby Co., pp. 171-177.
10. Erikson, E. H.: Identity and the life cycle, psychological issues, vol. 1, monograph 1, New York, 1959, International Universities Press, Inc.
11. Erikson, E. H.: Insight and responsibility, New York, 1964, W. W. Norton, Inc., pp. 111-157.
12. Eyres, P. J.: The role of the nurse in family-centered nursing care, Nurs. Clin. North Am. 7:27, 1972.
13. Fagin, C., editor: Family-centered nursing in community psychiatry, Philadelphia, 1970, F. A. Davis Co.

14. Parad, H. J., editor: Crisis intervention: selected readings, New York, 1965, Family Service Association of America.
15. Parsons, T., and Bales, R. F.: Family, socialization and interaction process, New York, 1955, The Free Press, pp. 16-17.
16. Shearer, P. S.: Juvenile obesity: a nursing approach, Master's project, 1971, Department of Nursing, Saint Louis University.
17. Thompson, J.: Human growth and development: a basis for nursing assessment. In Steele, S., editor: Nursing care of the child with long-term illness, New York, 1971, Appleton-Century-Crofts, pp. 1-26.

11

A mother of a child with facial and other visible anomalies

Lorraine Struempler

A mother who gives birth to an anomalous child has feelings of defeat, guilt, and shame because she sees the child as an extension of herself. She feels that to produce this child she, too, must be imperfect.[6,7] This feeling of imperfection is reinforced by the reactions of all who see a child who looks different.

Lis[4] and Allen[1] emphasize that correction of the defects through surgical procedures and other therapy is an aid to make the child more acceptable. However, there are limitations in what can be done to correct the anomalous individual. Corrective measures leave their scars and create tensions in the mother and other family members so that this adds to the disappointment and anger.

In this chapter the struggles of a mother handling her feelings about a defective child will be portrayed. The investigation was carried out over an eight-month period of time. During this time I saw the mother and child during the child's three hospitalizations and two clinic visits. In addition, I visited the home on eight occasions and talked with the mother (Mrs. B) many times on the telephone.

Mrs. B had three children from her first marriage. They were 7, 11, and 12 years of age at the time of her second marriage, about three years after she obtained a divorce from her first husband. Mrs. B became pregnant a few months after her second marriage and gave birth prematurely to twin girls, both of whom died within twenty-four hours after birth. She became pregnant again two months after the death of the twins. This pregnancy ended with delivery of a girl, Linda, who had gross physical anomalies.

Linda's anomalies included clefts, or incomplete union, of both lower eyelids; bilateral cleft lip and palate; constricting bands on the right foot and leg, which pulled her foot into an external clubbed foot position; arrested growth of the second and great toe, with webbing of the second and great toe stubs of the same foot; and arrested growth of the first, second, and third fingers of the left hand, with webbing of the first and second fingers. Linda was hospitalized twice before I met her and Mrs. B. These hospitalizations, when Linda was 3 and 5 months of age, were for beginning correction of the lip and leg deformities.

HOSPITALIZATION AT 9 MONTHS OF AGE

I met Mrs. B and Linda when Linda was hospitalized at 9 months of age for surgical repair of her right lower eyelid. A segment of skin from behind her ear was grafted to the cleft of her right lower eyelid. The upper eyelid was sutured to the lower for traction.

While we were waiting for Linda to recover from anesthesia after her surgery, Mrs. B told me about events surrounding Linda's birth. She recalled the sadness, mourning, and bereavement she suffered for two days after being informed that her child had a big hole in her face. It took these two days for her to muster up enough courage to ask to see the child. When the baby was brought to her, she recalled trying to remove the blankets from the baby's face four times before she accomplished it. After she looked at the baby's face, the nurse began to point out the other deformities of Linda's hands and feet. Mrs. B related, "I didn't know about them before."

95

Mrs. B's hope for a perfect child was expressed when she said, "I lost twins eleven months before Linda was born. They were perfect, but they only weighed a little over one pound each." She voiced her feeling of inadequacy as a woman by saying, "When we had Linda, I thought I had lost my ability to have babies."

After seeing Linda's eye the second day after surgery, Mrs. B reacted with much control and was pleasant and cheerful to everyone in the hospital. However, she went home that night and cried and vented her anger and disappointment on the family by being "crabby" with the other children. She said, "I seem to have to go through this each time. It hits me for a day. I am just a beast."

Mrs. B attempted to treat Linda as a normal child and did attain enjoyment in playful activities with her. However, ambivalence in her feelings of love and hate were expressed at the time of discharge when her thoughts turned to having Linda at home and in the community. She attempted to be realistic and honest about Linda's appearance. Her inner feelings and her deliberate control of them were voiced when she said, "I used to play with her and say, 'make an ugly face.' I don't do that anymore; I say, 'make a funny face'." Taking Linda out in public was difficult. She said, "People would stop and stare and look." She tried to shut it out by saying, "Now I don't even see them."

After several surgical procedures her dreams of having a perfect child by means of plastic surgery began to dim. Mrs. B met a teacher at a school picnic who had a lip repair that did not look very good. Mrs. B said, "I think I have been under the wrong impression as to what could be done with plastic surgery. I thought they could do almost anything to make it look normal. . . .but I guess that is not right."

INTERIM BETWEEN HOSPITALIZATIONS

Mrs. B called me a month later after she had visited the physician and been informed that half the eye graft had not taken. She projected her anger and disappointment about this onto other aspects of Linda's behavior. It seemed that nothing

about Linda was right. Linda, now 10 months old, was on a food jag. She was not eating fruit or drinking milk; her primary interest was cereal. Mrs. B seemed to feel she was not being a good mother because Linda was not eating the proper diet. Mrs. B expressed other feelings about the demands made by Linda when she said, "I have run out of things to keep her busy." She voiced helplessness and frustration in her inability to control anything about Linda.

When Linda was about 12 months old, Mrs. B was notified of the date of Linda's next hospitalization. At this time Mrs. B expressed feelings of inadequacy and insecurity as a person and expressed fears of losing everything. She projected her angry feelings onto her husband and criticized his lack of concern about the mortgage and other debts. In this way some of her anger was diverted from Linda.

HOSPITALIZATION AT 12 MONTHS OF AGE

When Linda came in for surgery, Mrs. B expressed guilt, anger, death wishes, and fear of losing Linda. The events surrounding Linda's birth reappeared with more pain and ambivalence. As she said:

I was just thinking of how I felt about Linda a year ago. When I saw her the first time, I thought she just looked like a bunch of garbage. . . . Mom and my husband went to church right after she was born and prayed that God would take her so I wouldn't be burdened with her. . . . This time all kinds of things went through my mind, more than ever before. I even had visions of her in a coffin. . . . If it would have happened first, it wouldn't have been so bad, but it would be different now. . . . I have time to really enjoy her. I love her so much. She is all right mentally.

Mrs. B expressed fear of losing Linda. She seemed to project some of her anger about Linda onto her mother and husband because of their prayers the night Linda was born. At the same time a life without Linda would be intolerable and would be further punishment for the mother.

PROBLEMS OF DISCIPLINE AND TRAINING

Management of Linda on the day of discharge was focused on matters of discipline.

The problem of disciplining Linda was compounded by the mother's feelings of anger, overprotection, and pity. With almost any child conflicts arise between the mother and grandmother concerning management; this conflict is exaggerated even more when the child is handicapped. Mrs. B said, "Mom thinks I am too strict with Linda. I keep telling her if she had her twenty-four hours a day, she would see that some limits were set." Mrs. B expressed a need to separate her identity from Linda and have temporary release of her burden when she said, "I would like to get a job a couple of nights a week."

Mrs. B also needed to prove Linda's mental competence and her ability to learn. This was an area in which she could exert some control, in contrast to the anomalies that she could not control. On arriving home from the hospital, she said, "I can hardly wait to get started with her toilet training." She interpreted the hospital personnel's feelings about and focus on Linda's defects when she said, "I wish the nurses at the hospital could see her when she is home. . . . She is so much different." She then excused the personnel when she said, "Well, they can't let her run around like this, so how can they know what she is like."

ADJUSTING TO LINDA'S PHYSICAL APPEARANCE

Mrs. B's sensitivity about the feelings of strangers and their inability to see what is normal rather than abnormal about Linda was revealed in a conversation Mrs. B had with another mother in the orthopedic clinic. This mother said, "When I come here, I feel lucky." Mrs. B responded, "If it wasn't for Linda's appearance, she would be normal in every aspect. We love her now. When she was born, I didn't know whether to keep her or throw her in the garbage can." Mrs. B paused for some time as though reflecting on what she had said, and, as if to compensate and reestablish reality, she said, "Now I wouldn't have her any other way."

The following example illustrates Mrs. B's sensitivity to Linda's appearance. It also suggests that people may tend to see more defects in children with anomalies than are

really present. Mrs. B had a picture taken of Linda by a commercial photographer. She was pleased with the proofs and selected one for enlargement and tinting. However, she "blew up" at the photographer when she noted that in the finished photograph one eye was painted blue and the other brown. She said, "My baby may have a lot of things wrong with her, but her eyes are the same color!"

The staring reaction of other children and the anger, hostility, pity, and guilt expressed by other parents was evident in the following incident in the orthopedic clinic when Linda was 16 months of age. A girl of about 6 years of age stared at Linda, then pointed her finger at her, and asked her father in a loud voice, "What's wrong with her nose?" The girl's father gritted his teeth, made a swinging motion toward his daughter's face, but stopped short of slapping her, saying, "Shut up!" He then squatted on his knees to block his daughter's vision of Linda. His daughter shifted to the side and continued to stare at Linda. Mrs. B said, "I just hate it when parents want to slap their children for saying something. The children don't know. They need to have it explained to them."

PROBLEMS OF CARE, CONTROL, AND CONFLICTING FEELINGS

Surgery for the second-stage palate repair and additional reconstruction on her lip was scheduled for Linda when she was 17 months of age. At this time Mrs. B expressed feelings of increasing inadequacy, insecurity, anger, and depression that spread to all areas of her life and herself. She said, "I am not taking care of the house, I am bored . . . I think I am going through the menopause. I am just all bound up . . . I don't care about cooking. Linda has a diaper rash. She always gets it before she goes to the hospital. Then I have to work real hard to get it cleared up." Mrs. B projected her anger and lonely feeling onto her husband. "He is so thoughtless, that is all it is. I told him the only good thing he gave me was Linda. . . ." She enumerated her husband's many faults and said he needed to see a marriage counselor. Then she expressed her own feelings. "I am so depressed . . . I am grumpy. I fight with everyone."

Cohen[2] says that the desirable resolution is to lose the fantasy attached to the child, but behind the denial remains the dammed-up pain and anger, creating constant anxiety.

Mrs. B described herself on the evening before Linda's admission as follows:

> I was just terrible . . . . I thought I was going to have a nervous breakdown. I was just horrible. I was yelling at everyone. I was worse than I ever was. I feel real bad about it now. I feel guilty because I was so horrible. I can't make them understand how I feel! They don't know what it is like.

After surgery Mrs. B attempted to be realistic about Linda's appearance. She asked, "How do you think she really looks?" Without waiting for an answer she said, "Pretty awful, huh? I always thought so."

Mrs. B had conflicting feelings about disciplining Linda. She was also concerned about whether other people perceived her as a good mother. She said, "Linda was bad in the hospital yesterday. I said, 'give mommy a kiss?' She hit me instead. If she hadn't been in the hospital, I would have slapped her on the behind." She expressed restraint of punitive actions because of Linda's defects. "There was a nurse across the hall. If she had seen me do it, she would have said, 'did you see what that mother did to that poor child?'. . . . You are home now, Linda; you will have to learn."

The burden of Linda's care and the failure of hoped-for miraculous surgery added to the normal difficulty in handling a toddler. On Linda's second day home Mrs. B said, "Yesterday, I couldn't do a thing with her. She was so bad even I couldn't stand her! And that is pretty bad. I paddled her and was rather cross with her. She has been a lot better today." Anna Freud[3] found that a child demands a surplus of attention from the mother during hospitalization and after discharge. The child may also express aggression against the mother and show revenge.

Mrs. B's need to protect, control, and mother Linda was clouded by feelings of guilt, anger, and martyrdom as expressed in the following: "Linda wants to run around.

I am afraid to let her, as she is so unsteady on her feet. She might fall and bust that lip open." It was as though she must prove that she was a good mother. If something should happen to Linda, it would be the "bad mother" that was appearing and would show that she really didn't love the child.

The stress and strain of overprotecting Linda to compensate for her anger and guilt had an impact on Mrs. B's strength. One week after Linda's discharge from the hospital Mrs. B looked tired and exhausted. She had large circles under her eyes, and her hair was untidy and unkempt. She expressed anger toward her husband and about the burden of Linda. She said, "I have to watch her so close when I am here alone with her, I don't even go to the bathroom unless I take her with me. Children her age get into things so fast."

Mrs. B's stress and anxiety continued to mount. Tension and irritation spread throughout the household. To cope with her stress, Mrs. B kept the two older children home from school to care for Linda so that she could "get out." She had her hair done, went out to lunch, went shopping, and subsequently felt much better.

A lot of "mental working through" of her feelings about Linda is still necessary. It is doubtful if complete acceptance of Linda as she is will ever occur. At the time of this writing Linda is 5 years old and will be attending school next year. Mrs. B is working for a company selling pots and pans on a door-to-door basis. She enjoys her work, and it gives her an outlet and a feeling of accomplishment.

SUMMARY

A mother of a child with visible anomalies, especially of the face, is constantly confronted with the painful barbs of stares, rejection, and finger pointing. Surgical procedures carry with them dreamed-of hopes of perfecting a face, an arm, or a leg. Each hospitalization promotes recall of the grief surrounding the birth of the child. Painful memories and reworking through the angry hostile feelings on being given and giving birth to the defective child continue.

The stress of having and caring for Linda produced in Mrs. B pent-up guilt and anger. Mrs. B's hostile expressions were controlled in the hospital environment but found release at home in angry outburst toward family members. Her angry outbursts resulted in guilt feelings, further lowering of self-esteem, and then additional need to release her pent-up anger. The anger and inadequacy of her own feelings were expressed in the fear of losing everything, including house, home, family, and her sanity. It was as though she became locked in her own pain and loneliness. Rejection by hospital personnel and by her family added to her loneliness and anger.

Mrs. B's anger and guilt toward Linda after her hospitalization at 17 months of age resulted in overprotection and fostered overdependency. The burden of an active toddler, expressing normal negativism, kept Mrs. B constantly struggling to contain the "bad mother" in her.

Mrs. B recognized her need to establish her own identity apart from Linda. She wished to be rid of the child, but the fear of something happening to Linda provoked further guilt and resulted in a feeling of martyrdom. Loneliness and isolation in her own misery were expressed in boredom, lack of interest, and inability to socialize with others.

Adjustment became more difficult after each hospitalization. As the hope of having a "normal" child dimmed, anger hostility, death wishes, and guilt about her feelings expressed themselves in longer and more violent angry outbursts. These, in turn, added to her lowering of self-esteem and guilt.

Mrs. B's complete resolution of her grief and ultimate acceptance of Linda will perhaps never occur. New adjustments and repeated disappointments will continue for Mrs. B throughout Linda's life. A traumatic time for Linda and her mother will probably occur when Linda starts to school.

Nurses can aid the mother in coping by looking at the child rather than at the defects and by treating the mother with consideration and respect. Perhaps, as Murray[5] says, most parents seem able, ultimately, to forgive inadequate knowledge and service if their professional counselors have shown that they care that their clients are troubled and are earnestly trying to understand and help.

References

1. Allen, J., and Lelchuck, L.: A comprehensive care program for children with handicaps, Am. J. Dis. Child. 3:230, 1966.
2. Cohen, P.: The impact of the handicapped child on the family, Social Case Work 43:137, March, 1962.
3. Freud, A.: The role of bodily illness in the mental life of children, Psychoanal. Study Child 7:69, 1952.
4. Lis, E. F., Pruzansky, S., Koepp-Baker, H., and Kabes, H. R.: Cleft lip and cleft palate; perspectives in management, Pediatr. Clin. North Am. 3:995, 1956.
5. Murray, M.: Needs of parents of mentally retarded children, Am. J. Ment. Defic. 63:1078, 1959.
6. Solnit, A. J., and Stark, M. H.: Mourning and the birth of a defective child, Psychoanal. Study Child 16:530, 1961.
7. Tisza, V., and Gumpetz, E.: The parents' reaction to the birth and early care of children with cleft palate, Pediatrics 30:86, July, 1962.

12

Social problems surrounding the high-risk infant

Cheryl Hall Harris

There have been several recent articles on nursing techniques required for the care of high-risk neonates; however, few focus on the social dynamics that surround the critically ill newborn. Nurses are frequently required to understand the human behavior exhibited by parents and to respond appropriately to several types of emotional situations that arise in a neonatal intensive care unit (NICU). This article will discuss some of the social difficulties that confront parents and staff who are involved with high-risk newborns.

Although the thought that she might have an infant with physical problems may enter an expectant mother's mind, practically no one anticipates producing a newborn infant with a life-threatening illness. Virtually no couple plans, either emotionally or financially, to have an infant requiring immediate and extensive treatment or with possible long-term physical or mental disabilities; yet many such neonates are born. Of the more than 3.5 million pregnancies that reach 20 weeks of gestation per year in the United States, 50,000 neonates die within the first month. At least 100,000 neonates will be mentally retarded (with an I.Q. of 70 or less) due to complications of pregnancy or delivery, and 50,000 will have severe, but often correctable, congenital anomalies.[1]

Nurses who work in postpartum units, as well as those involved in the NICU, should recognize these circumstances and help parents cope with them. Most parents require a great amount of support and reassurance that is realistic to the situation. In addition, they need to understand their newborn's condition, treatment, and the equipment used for his care. In many centers a multidisciplinary approach to the parents of high-risk newborns has been found to be the best means of achieving these goals. The following section describes the approach utilized by the staff of the NICU in which I am involved.

MULTIDISCIPLINARY APPROACH

Several key personnel are necessary for a multidisciplinary approach, including the staff neonatologist, the neonatal social worker, the visiting nurses, the nutritionist, and the nurses who are involved in the direct physical care of the infants. Each person performs his own functions, but there are overlapping areas in which more than one team member is involved. A brief description of each member's functions is given here.

The staff neonatologist is primarily responsible for ensuring that the best possible physical care is given to each neonate within the NICU. In addition, the neonatologist participates in the neonatal follow-up clinic, is responsible for collecting data on treatment and subsequent development of the infants, is involved with parents, and coordinates the efforts of the rest of the team in providing comprehensive care to the neonates and their parents.

The neonatal social worker has many roles—discusses with parents their apprehensions about their critically ill newborn, seeks out available community resources, and interprets emotional problems of the family to the staff. Home visits are frequently made to assess the family structure and to delineate problems that were previously unknown. The neonatal social worker also follows up neonatal patients if they are readmitted to the hospital for such problems as failure to thrive or child abuse.

The visiting nurse makes a predischarge visit to the infant's home to assess whether adequate supplies for the newborn are available and whether the mother is looking forward to the infant's homecoming. The type of living conditions the infant will face on dismissal from the hospital is also assessed. After obtaining this information in a nonthreatening manner from the mother, the visiting nurse relays impressions to the hospital staff so that they are aware of home conditions before the infant is dismissed. After the infant's discharge the visiting nurse makes frequent visits for health instruction and counseling of the mother. The visiting nurse, by providing continuous long-term support, probably is the closest contact the mother has with a health professional. The visiting nurse knows what the mother is taught in the clinic regarding feeding, developmental expectations, and infant stimulation; therefore this information can be reinforced during visits.

The nutritionist provides information concerning infant nutritional requirements for both parents and staff. In addition, the nutritionist is available to instruct parents in feeding techniques and to describe community resources for obtaining infant foods that are free to indigent families.

The supervisor of infant care and the head nurse of the NICU are responsible for supervising the nursing care given the critically ill neonate. They also collect and relay information about parental visiting patterns and attitudes toward their infant.

Once a week, a meeting is held that is attended by the staff neonatologist, the neonatal social worker, the visiting nurse liaison supervisor, the head nurse of the NICU, and the supervisor of infant care. These health workers discuss all the patients who are currently undergoing treatment in the NICU, as well as those either seen in the neonatal clinic the preceding week or those who failed to keep their clinic appointments. The decision is made as to which patients require additional help and which no longer require the services of, for example, the visiting nurse.

These meetings serve to allow all members of the nursery to share available information about the infants and to alert everyone to any possible problems so that they can be corrected.

This, then, is how the team functions in the NICU in which I am involved. Throughout the remainder of the chapter, specific examples will be given, using case histories to illustrate the interrelated functions of this health team. As mentioned earlier, one of the important issues discussed during the weekly meetings is the visiting patterns of parents while their infant is in the NICU.

VISITING POLICIES FOR PARENTS

When a high-risk newborn is first identified, he is transferred as soon as it is feasible to the neonatal intensive care unit, where proper staff and equipment exist to give him the best possible care. This usually necessitates his being transferred to a hospital away from his mother, who will probably worry about his condition. The nurses and physicians who are involved with the neonate's care must communicate adequately with the infant's parents to keep them aware of his current condition.

As soon as she is physically able, the mother should be brought to see and touch her infant, as suggested in the study by Barnett and co-workers.[2] This group of investigators studied the effect of early maternal-infant separation on both partners during their subsequent relationship. Included in this article were reports of mothers who disclosed that they first felt "close" to their infants when they were allowed to touch, see, feed, or care for them. In this pilot study mothers were divided into two groups: Group I mothers were allowed into the nursery to touch and care for their newborns from the onset of their admissions, and Group II mothers were allowed to view their infants from behind a window but were not allowed into the nursery until the baby reached 2,100 grams and was placed in a discharge nursery. Both sets of mothers were interviewed during the infant's hospitalization and after his discharge. The mothers were rated on their commitment or attachment to the infant, their confidence in their mothering abilities, as well as their ability to establish an efficient method of caring for the infant.

Barnett's group hypothesized that mothers in the second group would be less emotionally attached to their infants than mothers in the first group and that they would deprive their infants of adequate stimulation when they became responsible for their care. Although these investigators believed their hypotheses were substantiated by their observations, they thought the sample was too small in this pilot study to draw definite conclusions; therefore they are continuing with further research. However, they did discover that (1) mothers can be introduced into an NICU without either disrupting the care given by the staff or clinically endangering the infant by exposing him to infectious organisms and (2) nurses' attitudes about allowing parents into the NICU changed from initial skepticism to enthusiastic support for the idea. The permanent medical staff and visiting pediatricians also approved and supported the plan once they had a chance to see its benefits.

Robson[12] describes the importance of eye-to-eye contact between a mother and her newborn child. This early and continuous contact is necessary to fulfill needs of both mother and baby. A mother is involved for several months in the complete care of her infant, which may be an unrewarding experience except for the eye-to-eye contact and social smiles of the infant. Several investigators have remarked at the pleasure that new mothers demonstrate when they decide their infant "sees" them. Since Rheingold discovered that ". . . not physical but visual contact is at the basis of human sociability. . .,"* it could be concluded that eye-to-eye contact in early infancy may relate to later psychological development of the infant.

These ideas serve to support the theory that mothers should be allowed into the neonatal intensive care unit, since eye-to-eye contact is virtually impossible from

across the room. The following case illustrates the difficulties that may be encountered if a mother does not come to see her baby, either by her own choice or because of hospital regulations.

A male infant (T.D.) was admitted to the NICU at the age of 6 weeks with extreme difficulty in breathing, secondary to a congenital laryngeal constriction. He was the secondborn twin of an unwed white mother of lower socioeconomic class. His male twin was normal and went home with his mother after the usual four days of hospitalization after delivery. The mother lived approximately eighty miles from the hospital in which the NICU is located.

T.D. continued to have difficulty, and eventually a tracheostomy was performed. Although his mother had been encouraged to visit from the time her infant was first admitted, she came only once. After T.D.'s tracheostomy was done, the social worker and nurses began stressing to the mother that she should come and learn to take care of her baby in preparation for his dismissal. The mother came, intending to visit for an entire weekend. However, after seeing him only once, she decided to place him in a foster home rather than to take him home herself. He was dismissed to a foster home located in the same town in which the mother lived. Although the foster mother encouraged T.D.'s natural mother to visit him, the natural mother has not done so. Several months have passed, and the situation remains unchanged.

The dynamics of this case are probably more involved than they appear on the surface, but there are several facets that can be examined. Perhaps of primary importance is the fact that this mother had a normal infant twin whom she took home to mother, so that it was natural that she concentrate her initial efforts on him. Since she did not visit her newborn in the NICU, she never developed normal maternal attachments to him.

Although transportation was a problem for this mother, our social worker was able to help make the necessary arrangements so that the mother could come to visit. When the mother did finally come, she seemed to feel no mothering attitudes toward her baby and rejected him with the excuse of his physical difficulties (i.e., his tracheostomy). The nursing staff did explain that many mothers have learned how to care for an infant with a tracheostomy and that T.D. would not be dismissed until his mother felt comfortable in taking care of him.

---

*From Rheingold, H. L.: The effect of environmental stimulation upon social and exploratory behaviour in the human infant, Determinants of Infant Behaviour 1:143, 1961.

Of equal interest was the nursing staff's reaction to this mother when it finally became obvious she had no intention of taking her infant home. The staff had become fond of T.D. and were angry with the mother for electing to place him in foster care. However, they were relieved to find the foster mother so loving and interested in learning to take care of the baby.

To further support the theory that parents should be allowed liberal visiting opportunities, Faranoff and co-workers[5] have recently published the results of their study, which shows a correlation between infrequent visiting patterns of parents and subsequent reports of their children being admitted to the hospital because of failure to thrive or abuse. The nursery used in the study (Case Western Reserve Babies and Children's Hospital) permits parents twenty-four–hour a day visiting and telephoning privileges.

The study sample included 149 infants who had been hospitalized for longer than fourteen days and were followed up in the newborn follow-up clinic or by their private physicians for six to twenty-three months. Of the 149 infants, there were thirty-six whose mothers visited or called less frequently than five times per two-week period, and among this group there were nine disorders of mothering. These nine children were either battered, abandoned, or diagnosed as failing to thrive with no organic cause for their failure to gain weight. No disorders of mothering occurred in the group of mothers who visited more frequently than five times per two-week period.

The study concluded that parents of high-risk newborns who do not come to visit their infants may not form normal attachments to them. Furthermore, this group recommends that (1) a record be made of all visits and telephone calls made to the intensive care nursery, (2) the records be reviewed weekly to determine visiting patterns, and (3) the cause of infrequent visits be investigated so that appropriate action may be taken.

UNWED MOTHERS

The preceding section concerned with visiting patterns implies that there are two parents who planned to have their baby and eagerly awaited his arrival. A different set of circumstances exists in cases involving unwed (and frequently teen-age) mothers. Such a mother is described in the next example.

This mother came from a low-income family and had the additional handicap of coming from a broken home, where she had received poor mothering, inadequate prenatal care, and poor nutrition and lived in substandard housing.

A.M. was born eight weeks prematurely to a 14-year-old unwed black mother. The infant had a few problems during his hospitalization, which were related to his prematurity, mild respiratory distress syndrome, and a slight heart defect (patent ductus arteriosus). He recovered well and was dismissed to his mother's care. His mother was apparently unable to provide normal mothering performance; she did not cuddle or talk to him or stimulate him appropriately. She fed him minimally, even though she had been instructed in proper feeding techniques. She did not keep her neonatal follow-up clinic appointments. Our social worker became involved with this young mother early to try to help her cope with her financial difficulties and to try to teach her mothering behaviors. The nursing staff provided the mother with information about the physical care of her infant and stressed the importance of holding and interacting with her infant. At the time of this writing the infant is faring well in his physical development, but emotionally and intellectually his outcome is uncertain.

Certain maternal behaviors are accepted as normal maternal-infant interaction such as holding and cuddling an infant, talking to him, and playing with him, as well as the direct physical care activities necessary for his physical well-being. Mothers who themselves may have been deprived of proper maternal stimulation do not seem able to respond adequately to their own infants.[3] Many times, teen-age mothers seem particularly unable to understand the necessity for interacting with their infants, although they may give appropriate physical care. These mothers appear to treat their infants as though they were dolls. Unfortunately, children of mothers who fail to perform proper mothering activities may at least be emotionally deprived and at worst become the victims of physical abuse or fail to thrive. Nurses involved in the care of infants should focus their attention on how mothers interact with their babies and then strive to improve undesirable situations.[13]

The dilemma is, of course, how can health personnel teach the nebulous concepts of "mothering?" The answer is complex and not fully understood, yet the importance of establishing this aspect of the mother-child relationship cannot be overemphasized. These mothers frequently have many emotional and physical stresses beyond those produced by becoming a mother. If the nurse can provide a warm, understanding, nonjudgmental atmosphere, the mother may be able to relax and learn how to love her baby. Nurses should point out the baby's developing skills, such as smiling and holding a rattle, in such a way that the mother can become aware of the behavior and be proud of her infant's accomplishments.[11] The mother should be taught *how* to stimulate her baby by talking to him, providing him with toys, etc. Another way to direct mothers in learning the emotional aspects of mothering is to stress the importance of holding an infant during his feeding and utilizing the "on face"[9] position to look at him. Mothers should be instructed never to prop a bottle because the infant may have physical difficulties with a propped bottle and also because this is a means of reemphasizing the emotional benefits of holding an infant during his feeding. The problems of teaching mothering are great, but the effort that is expended toward solving these problems is often well rewarded and can be considered a type of preventive medicine.

BLACK INFANTS AND WHITE STAFF

Problems can arise for both staff and parents when the infant is black and the staff that cares for him, including physicians, nurses, and social workers, is primarily white. Redmann[9] describes nurses' avoidance of parents of black children because they feel black adults are inferior or because they are afraid of them. White nurses may also have preconceived notions of how the black family may react to certain problems and may generalize their assumptions to include all black families. For example, the white nurse may expect black parents not to want their infant or not to be too concerned over his death. If parents do not come to visit their infant, perhaps due to transportation difficulties, the nurse may assume that they do not care about their infant rather than investigate the cause of their infrequent visits.

Most white hospital nurses do not know the living situations of black families; often these nurses tend to believe that the conditions are worse than they actually are. Redmann[9] suggests that educational sessions should be provided for nurses to teach them ". . . about the beliefs, value systems, and social practices of members of the black race living in the area."

Black parents may fear that the white staff is hurting their child unnecessarily. A black infant in the neonatal follow-up clinic required blood studies that called for 5 ml. of blood. The physician explained to the infant's mother that he intended to draw blood and she consented, although she apparently did not realize that he had to draw the blood from a peripheral vein as opposed to a finger stick. When he had completed the procedure, the mother voiced extreme agitation and anger that he had employed the method that he had used and stated that she felt this was an unnecessary procedure. Much counseling was required to calm this mother and to elicit her cooperation in the future.

In the next example the mother did not believe continued hospitalization was necessary for her infant's well-being.

A black male infant was admitted with congenital elliptocytosis, a blood disease that leads to anemia. He did develop a progressively severe anemia but was not clinically ill. The physicians wanted to keep him in the hospital for observation and to transfuse him if this should become necessary. The mother felt that his dismissal was being delayed unnecessarily and after pressure from the infant's father decided to sign the infant out of the hospital against medical advice. A skillful physician finally persuaded her to leave the infant in the hospital, since taking him home might lead to further illness and perhaps the infant's death. The staff thought the mother's hostility was based in her mistrust of the staff's intentions and her belief that they just wanted to keep her infant from her. After further counseling sessions with the mother, the social worker seemed to overcome these feelings of mistrust. The mother has since been very cooperative in bringing her child for follow-up care.

This case is an excellent example of how

the social worker performs an integral role in the multidisciplinary approach.

FINANCIAL PROBLEMS

Another difficulty that confronts the parents of high-risk infants is the great financial burdens. Most insurance policies do not cover the first days or weeks of a newborn's hospitalization. If an infant is sick, these are usually the most expensive days, and bills that run into thousands of dollars are not uncommon. Perhaps the most depressing financial circumstance for parents occurs when a baby survives long enough to sustain a large hospital bill and then expires, leaving the family with a financial obligation but no child. Some hospitals make provisions for this circumstance, but many do not.

Since most parents do not expect their baby to be sick, they do not make provisions for exorbitant hospital costs caused by a newborn's illness. A real crisis may result for young parents with no reserve funds. Nurses are often painfully aware of financial crises confronting parents such as the one described in the next case.

Twins were admitted to the NICU because of extreme prematurity. Each weighed approximately two and one-half pounds; the little girl was the sicker of the two, whereas her brother had a rather uneventful course. Their father owned his own television repair store, which provided adequately for his wife and three other children. When the twins were dismissed after approximately two months of hospitalization, the boy's hospital bill totaled $5,000, and his sister's was $7,000. The father attempted to pay the bills but finally declared bankruptcy when it became apparent to him that he would never be able to completely pay the bill and provide for his family too.

Third-party payments for neonatal care will probably become more widespread when neonatal care advances from the small investigational scale to general availability. I recommend that the public be made aware of the specific financial problems confronting parents of newborns, so that pressure can be brought on insurance companies to include this age group in their policy coverage. Perhaps federal assistance should be made available for parents with infants in this specific situation until adequate health care insurance becomes a reality. In addition, social workers can occa-

sionally find private funds to help parents in financial distress; therefore the social worker should be involved in any such case.

THE INFANT WITH CONGENITAL ANOMALIES

Parents of an infant with congenital anomalies often face overwhelming guilt over having produced a defective child. The mother frequently blames herself for something she may have omitted or committed during her pregnancy. Imagine her guilt if this infant was unwanted and unplanned or if the mother had attempted a self-induced abortion. The extended family may suggest that this infant is punishment for a "sin" the parents have committed. Inevitably, the question arises: Why did it have to happen to *our* baby?

This traumatic episode in the lives of the infant's family is difficult for staff members to comprehend or help the family overcome. Infants with anomalies may precipitate the breakdown of a family that may have had previous difficulties. Therefore these parents should receive careful support and counseling from all members of the nursery team, and perhaps a psychiatrist should be available as well.

Some anomalies are caused by genetic disturbances, and parents will require counseling. Ideally, genetic counseling should be done by someone who knows the parents well. This counseling consists of explaining the defect, its cause, and the chances of the couple producing another child with this same defect. The decision is left to the parents as to whether they will take the chance. In some anomalies no direct inheritance characteristics are known, and in these cases the parents will be informed of this by the person doing the genetic counseling.

THE DYING INFANT

Interaction with grieving parents should be carried out by a nurse with information about the grieving process and one who can help to support the bereaved parents. Nurses should realize that the grief response consists of several stages.[4] The first response on learning about a death is shock and disbelief. This response may last from a few moments to several days, but finally periods of despair and anguish take over as the reality of the loss becomes conscious. As the person moves into the stage of developing awareness of the loss, he may demonstrate somatic signs as described by Lindemann.[8]

Lindemann describes acute grief as a definite syndrome with somatic symptoms such as loss of appetite, a tight feeling in the throat, an empty feeling in the abdomen, a need to sigh, and tension or mental pain. This syndrome may appear immediately after the crisis or may be delayed or apparently absent. Lindemann[8] also notes that "Severe grief reactions seem to occur in mothers who have lost young children." Furthermore, he states that if proper emotional support and management is given to the grieving person, prolonged and serious alterations in the person's social adjustment may be prevented.

The next example describes a mother who was involved in anticipatory grief. She grieved initially over the threat of death and then showed few signs of grieving after her infant's death. Engel[4] states that in anticipatory grief there is more opportunity to work through the initial awareness; therefore the period of shock and disbelief is less prominent when death does occur.

M.M. was the first infant born to a middle-class, married, white mother. The infant was born with a severe congenital anomaly called *gastroschisis*. She was transferred to the NICU within a few hours after birth, where she underwent surgery to correct her defect. Her parents were told that she would probably die. During the next few weeks the surgeons continued to be pessimistic about the infant's chances for survival. The parents came to visit their daughter frequently, but neither of them wanted to touch her. The infant progressed nicely for two months, and as the time for her dismissal neared, her mother was encouraged to learn to take care of her. She was very reluctant to learn to change the small dressings that were required but was eager to learn other aspects of care. The baby was dismissed with a Dacron netting over her abdomen and returned to the surgery clinic regularly for further procedures. During one of her routine clinic visits the infant suffered a cardiac arrest and expired despite vigorous resuscitative efforts.

The mother showed immediate signs of shock and sorrow at the time, but during the long-term follow-up sessions with the physician and the social worker she did not appear to grieve and in-

deed seemed almost relieved at her infant's death. The physician who was involved in the case explained to the perplexed staff that since the mother had initially been given no hope that the infant would live, she essentially separated herself from the baby and grieved as though she had died during her hospitalization. Since she had already undergone her grieving and mourning process, she did not need to work through them again at the time the infant actually died.

Frequently, the parents cannot accept that there is anything wrong with their infant or that he will probably die. They may become belligerent toward the staff and reject the diagnosis, as occurred with the parents in the following case.

K.B. was the first child born to a couple who had each had children by previous marriages. This infant suffered from severe asphyxia at birth, and the physicians informed the parents that they feared that the infant would be severely brain damaged as a result of the insult at birth. The infant was unable to cry, suck, or swallow when he was first admitted to the NICU. The parents refused to believe that the infant would have difficulties, and they cited any improvement in his condition as proof that he would be normal. The baby generally improved and was able to be dismissed on oral feedings. Subsequently, his father told the staff that they had been incorrect in their diagnosis and that he was certain that his infant would be normal.

The infant required a great deal of care at home. When it became apparent that he could not be sustained with either nipple or gavage feedings, he was readmitted to have a gastrostomy performed. He had seizures almost continuously and was heavily medicated for this problem. Eventually, he contracted pneumonia secondary to his inability to swallow his saliva, and on his third admission to the hospital he died. The parents required extensive support from the social worker and other staff members to help them in their grieving process.

These parents required a great amount of understanding from the nursing staff during their infant's initial hospitalization. The staff was able to comprehend the reason for the parents' belligerence, since the father especially did not want to admit that his infant would have mental deficiencies. One must remember that severe mental retardation is an exceptionally difficult prognosis to accept. When the baby did die, his family was relieved on one hand and grief stricken on the other.

Parents often have feelings of ambivalence about a dying infant, as illustrated in the following case.

K.R. was admitted with a complicated tracheo-esophageal fistula. Her hospitalization was lengthy, and she required several operations. Over several months her condition worsened, and her parents were prepared for the fact that she would eventually die. Finally, the physician told the parents that no further heroic measures would be carried out to prolong their baby's life. During their subsequent visits the parents vacillated between the attitude that they hoped for her death to come soon and questioning why the staff was not doing more for her to prolong her life.

These feelings are natural for parents who feel guilty over the decision to discontinue heroic measures. For this reason, parents should never be forced to make the decision about discontinuing heroic measures.

Kennell and co-workers[7] pose the question of whether the mother should be allowed to handle her newborn if there is a chance he will die. This study concluded that regardless of whether a mother had physical contact with her infant, she would still exhibit mourning responses at his death. There was perhaps a higher degree of mourning in mothers who had touched their infants before death because these mothers had a higher degree of affectional bonding with their infants. (According to Lindemann, a high degree of mourning is preferred to an underreaction, since with underreaction the griever may just postpone his grieving and mourning and do himself harm in this manner.)

Kennell's study gives several practical suggestions for staff who are involved with parents of dying infants or infants who have already expired. These suggestions are based on information gained during the study of twenty mothers whose infants had died.

1. Mothers whose babies have died should be moved from the obstetrical unit away from mothers of healthy infants.

2. There should be good communication between the staff in the nursery and the staff on the postpartum floor, so that all are informed when an infant dies.

3. At the time of an infant's death the nursery team should discuss with the parents the usual reactions related to the death of a child and the approximate length of most mourning responses.

4. Both parents need to discuss their feelings openly with one another; fathers especially may need to be encouraged to express their feelings of grief.

5. Approximately four months after the infant's death the parents should be interviewed again to find out how they are working through their grief, to discuss autopsy findings, and to answer any further questions.

Dealing with parents whose infant has just died is perhaps the most difficult area in which nurses must be involved. The nurse has feelings about death and may be emotionally involved with the infant who has expired and with his parents, which makes it extremely difficult. It is not easy to be objective in this emotionally charged patient situation, yet this is what is expected of personnel who work in many NICUs.

ETHICAL-LEGAL PROBLEMS

Anyone who is involved with the care of any critically ill patient is aware of the ethical-legal problems that arise. Which treatments can be described as heroic measures and which are used to keep the patient alive are difficult questions to answer. Following are some of the questions that arise: When should a respirator be discontinued? Should a patient be given the intravenous therapy known as total parenteral alimentation if he will eventually die when it is discontinued? Should surgery be performed to relieve the bowel obstruction of a neonate with Down's syndrome? What types of experimental drugs should be used? When should the decision be made to not utilize resuscitative measures and why? The final decisions in all these problems rests with the physician in charge of the case, but before making a decision, he would be wise to gather information from the rest of the staff who care for the infant. Group meetings, discussed later in this chapter, can be worthwhile in helping to make these types of decisions.

Difficult situations inevitably arise for nurses who care for critically ill infants. Based on their own personalities and on information about the ethical-legal ramifications of certain methods of treatment, nurses must determine their own philosophy of care. One means of accomplishing the second objective is to have a panel, which includes a physician, a social worker, a lawyer, and a clergyman, discuss the ethical-legal issues involved in caring for critically ill infants. After each member of the panel presents his information, a discussion period should follow in which the staff of the NICU can ask questions about specific cases or situations. In addition to this formal panel discussion, the sessions described on p. 101 may be used to discuss ethical-legal problems as they occur.

EMOTIONAL STRESSES
ON THE STAFF

The staff involved in the care of high-risk infants is continually placed in emotionally stressful situations such as the death of an infant or the despair caused by the knowledge that an infant who received optimal care is nonetheless brain damaged. The "Mother Surrogate Syndrome,"[6] in which young nurses become emotionally attached to the neonates in their care to the point of having difficulty relinquishing them when the time comes for their discharge, is also a form of stress. The stress produced by parents who are belligerent or grieving over their newborn who has died is bound to have an effect on the nurses who were involved in the infant's care.

The emotional energy required for all these problems, coupled with the demanding physical work load of most NICUs, can produce a volatile situation. One way to cope with these circumstances is to have group sessions with a psychiatrist or social worker or both in which personnel are encouraged to speak openly about their feelings. Hostility and anger are expressed in some sessions, whereas at others frustration and despair may be the primary emotions displayed. At the conclusion of the session the psychiatrist or group leader should summarize what has been said and try to propose possible solutions to the problems discussed.

Every effort should be made to form a cohesive staff that involves all the nurses and physicians in the unit. Intershift rivalries should be discouraged, since they frequently have a demoralizing effect on the nursing staff. Frequent staff meetings among the nurses to pass on information

and to discuss "pet peeves" should be held to keep an open, sharing atmosphere within the NICU. In most nurseries, due to the physical layout, the nurses are in close proximity at all times, thus conflicts can occur easily. The suggestions just given are offered as partial solutions to the stressful situations that confront the personnel who work in a neonatal intensive care unit.

SUMMARY

This chapter has dealt with some of the specific social problems inherent in the care of the high-risk newborn. Some of the problems are directly related to the infant and his parents, but many involve the staff who care for the infants. The solutions that have been suggested are a combination of those which have proved beneficial in my experience and those which come from clinical studies by investigators in other centers. These suggestions are offered as "food for thought" to all nurses involved in NICUs. An awareness of all the problems that surround the high-risk newborn is necessary for nurses who work in an NICU, perceive the high-risk infant as an individual patient, and attempt to give family-centered care.

References

1. Babson, S. G., and Benson, R. C.: Management of high-risk pregnancy and intensive care of the neonate, ed. 2, St. Louis, 1971, The C. V. Mosby Co.
2. Barnett, C., Leiderman, P. H., Grobstein, R., and Klaus, M. H.: Neonatal separation: the maternal side of interactional deprivation, Pediatrics 45:197, 1970.
3. Bowlby, J.: Child care and the growth of love, Harmondsworth, England, 1961, Penguin Books, Ltd.
4. Engel, G. L.: Psychological development in health and disease, Philadelphia, 1962, W. B. Saunders Co.
5. Faranoff, A. A., Kennell, J. H., and Klaus, M. H.: Follow-up of low birth weight infants —the predictive value of maternal visiting patterns, Pediatrics 49:287, 1972.
6. Harris, C. H.: Nursing care of high-risk infants. In Duffey, M., Anderson, E. H., Bergersen, B. S., Lohr, M., and Rose, M. H., editors: Current concepts in clinical nursing, St. Louis, 1971, The C. V. Mosby Co., pp. 71-85.
7. Kennell, J. H., Slyter, H., and Klaus, M. H.: The mourning response of parents to the death of a newborn infant, N. Engl. J. Med. 283:344, 1970.

8. Lindemann, E.: Symptomatology and management of acute grief, Am. J. Psychiatry **101:**141, 1944.

9. Redmann, R. E.: Black child—white nurse: a nursing challenge and privilege. In Duffey, M., Anderson, E. H., Bergersen, B. S., Lohr, M., and Rose, M. H., editors: Current concepts in clinical nursing, St. Louis, 1971, The C. V. Mosby Co., pp. 106-114.

10. Rheingold, H. L.: The effect of environmental stimulation upon social and exploratory behaviour in the human infant, Determinants of Infant Behaviour **1:**143, 1961.

11. Rhymes, J. P.: Working with mothers and babies who fail to thrive, Am. J. Nurs. **66:**1972, 1966.

12. Robson, K. S.: The role of eye-to-eye contact in maternal-infant attachment, J. Child Psychol. Psychiatry **8:**13, 1967.

13. Sagar, M.: A mother's ability to love her child. In Duffey, M., Anderson, E. H., Bergersen, B. S., Lohr, M., and Rose, M. H., editors: Current concepts in clinical nursing, St. Louis, 1971, The C. V. Mosby Co., pp. 141-148.

13

A study of a parent care and instructional unit

Beverly Shea

Over the past several years pediatric units in which parents "room-in" with their hospitalized children and assume responsibility for the semiprofessional tasks of caring for them have developed. The results generally are a better satisfied child, a better informed and less anxious parent, and a smoother transition home after discharge. Usually in these instances such a unit is minimally staffed with ancillary nursing personnel but has professional nursing service available, should the need arise. Commonly located in a geographical area apart from the pediatric acute care section and its associated facilities, the cost of overhead is less. The combination of (1) decreased and lesser-paid staff and (2) decreased cost of unit maintenance enables many hospitals to pass on to the patient substantial savings in the room rate.

Children's Medical Center in Dallas, Texas, has recently completed a nursing study of a similar type of unit. However, the emphasis there was on both intensive parental instruction and administration of care under nursing supervision until the parent learned to perform the procedure well and was comfortable in doing so alone and unassisted. Not only technical procedures but also the basics about the nature of the child's illness were taught. Knowing the "whys" for treatments and medications gave impetus to parental follow-through, both during and after hospitalization.

To accomplish these goals, a full-time professional nurse was with patient and parents from 8 A.M. until 4:30 P.M. Working with her were two experienced nursing assistants, one working from 6:30 A.M. until 3 P.M. and the other, from 2:30 until 11 P.M.

During the night no Parent Care Unit staff was present for three reasons: (1) not being acutely ill, the patients slept most of the night and did not require much care; (2) being alone with the child helped the parent gain self-confidence, and, if assistance was needed, the mother had only to notify the nurses' desk by intercom; and (3) discouraging the admission of children who were too ill for this type of service was emphasized.

A second difference in this unit, as compared to many others, was its setting. Located on an acute pediatric floor, the Parent Care Unit rooms were not only intermingled on a given corridor but also were used interchangeably, which at times created confusion between the two staffs on that corridor.

Each Parent Care Unit patient was assigned a private room containing a television set, telephone, desk, bulletin board, and adjoining bathroom. A Barker lounge could be made into a comfortable bed for the parent at night. Other facilities, such as the playroom, treatment room, and utility rooms, were shared with the patients on the traditional unit. Meals for parents were provided at a cost of $1.50 a meal.

Prior to the opening of this unit, an effort was made to determine the needs of our patients. Questionnaires (pp. 111 and 112) were mailed to 129 attending physicians and to 100 parents. A stratified random sample was taken from parents whose children had been hospitalized at Children's Medical Center during the year 1970. The questionnaires were used to decide on criteria for selection of patients and of staff who could meet their needs. It was assumed from the outset that assessing teaching needs, providing emotional support, and utilizing professional judgment would be basic requirements for the staff. However, more specific information was sought from the questionnaire.

Admission criteria established from collected data were (1) availability of a suitable and willing parent, (2) simple nursing care requirements, (3) preferably at least a two-day period of hospitalization, and (4) an illness of such a nature that the patient would benefit from having his parents familiar with his care.

Admissions to the Parent Care and Instructional Unit were made directly or by transfer from an acute-care unit. Transfers were fluid both into and out of the Parent Care Unit. Should a child's condition deteriorate or his parents become unable to stay with him, he would be transferred to general floor care.

The objectives of our Parent Care Unit were several. First, by enabling a parent to take over the care himself, the hospital staff might be able to shorten the patient's stay. Furthermore, not only was there greater security for the child in having his parent caring for him, but also the parent was provided with a constructive outlet for his energy. A "family-centered" environment was created in which the parent was included as an important member of the health team. Finally, by familiarizing the parent with the child's care, the staff probably would make his transition home easier.

QUESTIONNAIRE FOR PHYSICIANS

Please check the appropriate answers in the spaces provided. If you have comments, please state them. Should you need additional space, you may use the back of this page.

1. In circumstances whenever it is necessary for you to hospitalize a child, would you prefer that the parent remain with the patient?

   Yes____No____Undecided____
   Comments:

2. Do you feel that the presence of a parent generally makes hospitalization less difficult for the child?

   Yes____No____Undecided____

   For the mother?

   Yes____No____Undecided____

   Does the age of the child enter into this question?

   Yes____No____Undecided____

   If so, at what age?

   _____

   Comments:

3. Would you be interested in having the mothers of your patients be taught to give care to their children under nursing supervision?

   Yes____No____Undecided____
   Comments:

4. Do you feel that teaching parents to care for their hospitalized child will result in better care at home following discharge?

   Yes____No____Undecided____
   Comments:

5. If a Child Parent-Care Unit were available, would you be interested in utilizing it for some of your patients?

   Yes____No____Undecided____

   Specifically which type of patient?

   _____

   Comments:

QUESTIONNAIRE FOR PARENTS

Please check the appropriate answers in the spaces provided. If you have comments, please state them. Should you need additional space, you may use the back of this page.

1. If your child had to go to the hospital, would you choose to "room in" with him?

    Yes____No____Undecided____
    Comments:

2. Do you feel that your being with your child during his hospitalization would make him happier? (List the age(s) of your child or children in the squares provided and indicate for each whether or not you feel your presence would make him happier.)

    ☐ Yes____No____Undecided____
    ☐ Yes____No____Undecided____
    ☐ Yes____No____Undecided____
    ☐ Yes____No____Undecided____

   Would your remaining with your child while he is in the hospital make you happier?

    Yes____No____Undecided____
    Comments:

3. While your child is in the hospital, would you be interested in learning about health care?

    Yes____No____Undecided____
    Comments:

4. Do you think that by learning to care for your sick child in the hospital, you would be better able to care for him at home after discharge?

    Yes____No____Undecided____
    Comments:

5. If your child were hospitalized, would you be interested in his being on a unit where you could actively participate in caring for him?

    Yes____No____Undecided____
    Comments:

In the study answers were sought to the following questions:

1. Will a Parent Care Unit meet the needs of those patients and parents who utilize Children's Medical Center?

2. If so, in what activities will nursing personnel need to be involved?

3. What can these parents be taught to do in the area of nursing care?

4. What quality of care does the patient receive from the parents?

5. What are the best criteria for selecting candidates for this unit?

Sixty-three patients participated in the study. Although there were a variety of diagnoses, cystic fibrosis and eye conditions were the most common, followed closely by convulsive disorders. Both medical and surgical problems were included, with the former holding a slight majority. Patients ranged in age from 3 days to 17½ years.

After being given adequate instruction and emotional support by the staff, the mothers themselves were able to perform a wide variety of necessary nursing procedures for their children. Although the activities shared by staff and parents de-

pended on the complexity of care, it was both surprising and rewarding to learn what parents were capable of doing. Most of the mothers gained skill and confidence quickly.

Once every twenty-four hours a mother was given a daily work sheet on which were recorded medications and anticipated activities for that day, such as laboratory work and the making of tests and roentgenograms (p. 113). Each test was explained to her. She also recorded the medications (oral unless there was a vital need to learn to give injections) that she gave her child at designated times. Before the administration of a drug, its action, use, side effects, and dosage were carefully explained to the mother. After giving the drug under supervision, the parent administered it by herself. If assistance was needed, professional help was always available. The daily record also provided space for the parent to record any observations that she thought were pertinent—how well the diet was taken, vital signs, and stools and voiding. If a mother did not know how to take a temperature, she was taught to do so. Mon-

---

CHILDREN'S MEDICAL CENTER
Parent care unit daily record

Date _____   Room _____

Name _____

Breakfast _____

Lunch _____

Dinner _____

Liquids _____

Urine _____

B.M. _____

Temp. 8:00 _____   Appointments: _____

       12:00 _____   _____

        4:00 _____   _____

        8:00 _____   _____

Treatments: _____

_____

_____

Medicine _____   Time _____

_____   _____

_____   _____

_____   _____

Observations:

---

itoring of pulse and respiration was also taught to reliable parents whose children's conditions necessitated these procedures.

PATIENTS' REACTIONS

Children generally appeared to make better progress with their parents administering to them because they were less frightened. Good rapport was readily established with the Parent Care Unit staff because the children did not experience frequent traumatic encounters with them. Care given by parents, although not always liked, was accepted, since care by the mother had been the child's experience from birth. If the child was old enough and the situation appropriate, he was taught and encouraged to participate in his own care. An example of this was the diabetic child's administering his own insulin and checking his urine.

The mean age for the patient on this unit was 6.9 years. However, it must be noted that this figure was skewed because of one 17½-year-old patient and the fact that this statistical computation was based on months of age. Only twenty-one members of the study population were over 2 years old.

PARENTS' REACTIONS

With the exception of one father all parents participating were mothers. However, the fathers visited regularly and frequently "relieved" on weekends. They, too, were taught to care for the children. Whenever treatment had to be continued at home (e.g., in the case of cystic fibrosis), the effort was made to involve both parents. It was not unusual to have grandmothers and even baby-sitters come to the hospital for training sessions.

Parents readily admitted to feeling "scared" and "awkward" at first. However, after performing a procedure a few times they quickly gained confidence and skill. They were noted to exercise extreme care in the accuracy of a given activity. None of the sixty-three participants could be classified as "incompetent" or "unreliable" in the care of his child.

Evaluations of the Parent Care Unit were elicited from the parents at the time of their children's discharge. In an effort not to bias the responses in a positive direction, the parents were asked to give suggestions that would assist the Parent Care Unit in meeting the needs of its patients. The parents' comments were highly favorable and included such items as the following:

1. They liked being involved in their children's care and "knowing what's going on."

2. They believed that their children were better satisfied.

3. They liked the special interest and attention shown by the Parent Care Unit staff.

4. They preferred being busy as opposed to "just sitting."

5. They felt more secure and after discharge knew what to look for and what to do.

The few complaints were about the parents' getting tired and bored, especially after three days. Several suggested group sessions, but lack of space and the physical layout prevented implementation of this idea. However, several informal sessions were held in the hall.

It was evident from their comments that parents strongly preferred this system to the traditional one. Several patients in the study were readmitted to the hospital while the study was still in progress, and in all but two instances the parents requested to have their children reassigned to the Parent Care Unit. Of the two instances cited, one child was placed in the intensive care unit, and the other, a teenager, preferred assignment to a floor for older children, so as not to be annoyed by the sound of crying infants. After the study was concluded, two other previous Parent Care Unit patients were readmitted to the hospital, and in both cases the mothers expressed disappointment that they were unable to participate in the nursing care as before.

Follow-up interviews revealed that the transition home had proceeded smoothly, and much of this seemed to be attributed to the security the parents had felt. One mother wrote six weeks after discharge of her child that, had it not been for the Parent Care Unit, she did not believe that she would ever have been able to take home her infant son, who required demanding and complex care. Two other parents wrote as follows:

I enjoyed being in the Parent Care Unit. If I had my choice, I wouldn't stay anywhere else . . . This prepares me; I know what to do when I go home and I have confidence in myself that I'm doing everything right. If I'm ever to be back at Children's, I will request to be back on the Parent Care Unit.

I feel the Parent Care Unit is most beneficial. Though my son is now well and no further treatment is required, I found it quite satisfying to be able to do something for him while he was ill no matter how small. I think the worst part of his illness is the absolute feeling of helplessness a parent has. Any involvement in his care is a step in the proper direction of alleviating to some degree this feeling. It brings the mother closer to the situation and not totally in the dark.

PHYSICIANS' REACTIONS

When questionnaires (p. 111) were sent out to 120 staff physicians during the planning phase of the Parent Care Unit, eighty-seven, or 72.5%, responded. Of this number, seventy-nine indicated that they would be interested in utilizing the unit for some of their patients. During the period the unit was in operation, however, only twenty-eight physicians (three of whom were house officers) assigned patients to the unit. Furthermore, thirty-one of the sixty-three patients comprising the research population (49.2%) were admitted to Parent Care Unit by only three physicians—a pediatrician, a surgeon, and an ophthalmologist.

After completion of the active parent-participation phase of the study, questionnaires (p. 116) were sent to those physicians who had had patients on the study unit. Their opinions and suggestions concerning this unit were considered important. Seventeen, or 60.7%, returned the questionnaires; however, two failed to respond, being unaware of the function of the Parent Care Unit.

Ten physicians rated the care given by parents as "excellent" and five as "good" on a Likert-type scale. No responses were made to the choices of "average" and "poor."

Care given by parents at home after discharge was considered by ten of the physicians to be "better" than that usually given by parents whose children were on the traditional unit, "about the same" by four, and "not as good" by one.

Seven physicians were of the opinion that they received fewer telephone calls after discharge from parents who had participated in the study; five saw no difference; none said that there were more; and three had drawn no conclusions at that time.

Eleven considered that parents understood follow-up care "very well," and "fairly well" was the judgment of four physicians. The choices on either end of the continuum, "very little" and "thoroughly," were not selected by any of the respondents.

Understanding by parents of the nature of their child's illness was viewed as "adequate" by twelve physicians and as "thorough" by three. The choices "limited" and "none at all" were not selected.

Physicians cited a number of what they considered to be advantages of the Parent

Care Unit. In summary, the following comments were included:

1. Families received more time and attention.
2. Better communication resulted, and the parents were more informed.
3. Parents developed a better knowledge and understanding of their child's illness, which assisted in the management of his problem.
4. Physicians liked having the families involved and were of the opinion that it smoothed the transition from hospital to home.
5. Parents whose children were having diagnostic work-ups were involved.
6. Both mother and child were believed by these physicians to be more comfortable.
7. The unit, as a "limited-care facility," was a step in the right direction, and the respondents would like to see it continued.

Note that twenty of the twenty-eight participating physicians had had only one patient in the study group. Furthermore, the small number of patients on the Parent Care Unit during any given period provided ample time to work in depth with them and their parents. However, even at a point when the census rose to nine, the Parent Care Unit staff appeared to be able to provide their usual high-quality performance. Furthermore, the staff expressed a strong preference for having a larger number of patients.

Each of the fifteen physicians respondents indicated that, should a Parent Care Unit be established on a permanent basis, they would continue to utilize it for their patients. Some cited specific types of patients as being suitable; others thought that all types could benefit, but generally those children with chronic diseases, e.g., with colostomies were listed more frequently as the best candidates.

Many physicians did not recall any specific comments made by parents pertaining to hospitalization, but those who did (approximately one half) replied that responses were favorable.

STAFF NURSES' REACTIONS

At best communication with the regular hospital nursing staff was less than desirable. The unit to which these nurses and the Parent Care patients were assigned was

PARENT CARE UNIT

QUESTIONNAIRE FOR PHYSICIANS

1. What quality of care do you feel the child received on the Parent Care Unit? Please check the appropriate choice.

    ____Poor   ____Average   ____Good   ____Excellent

2. Generally, do you feel that the quality of care the Parent Care Unit child received at home after discharge was better or worse than that afforded the child discharged from the traditional unit?

    ____Not as good   ____About the same   ____Better

3. Was there a difference in the number of phone calls you received from Parent Care Unit parents after their child's discharge as compared to those received from parents whose child had been on the traditional hospital unit?

    ____More   ____About the same   ____Fewer   ____No conclusion

4. In your opinion, how thoroughly did the parents understand their child's follow-up care?

    ____Very little   ____Fairly well   ____Very well   ____Thoroughly

5. Do you feel that generally the parents participating in this project developed an understanding of the nature of their child's illness?

    ____Not at all   ____Very limited   ____Adequate understanding

    ____Thorough understanding

6. What do you feel were the advantages of the Parent Care Unit, if any?

7. What type of comments have you heard from parents (and/or patients) pertaining to this unit, if any?

8. If a Parent Care Unit were established on a permanent basis, would you continue to utilize it for your patients?

    ____No   ____Yes

    Only for specific types of patients. If so, please specify general type.

9. Please state any additional comments you would care to make pertaining to the Parent Care Unit.

geared to crisis care, although these patients were not acutely ill. Therefore the Parent Care nursing staff was operating from a nursing station with different responsibilities and emphases. The parent-care and the nurse-care systems were operating concurrently. Because each group was absorbed in its own activities, little time or incentive was available for adequate communication. When one group made efforts to initiate a dialogue, the time that they suggested for it was often not convenient for the other staff. In my opinion the function of the Parent Care Unit was never fully understood by the total nursing staff, despite group and individual explanations by the Parent Care Unit staff and the nursing administration.

After five weeks of operation the unit moved to a different floor. Three reasons were cited for this decision:

1. An increase in the rate of admissions to the original floor at the close of the school year made getting rooms for possible Parent Care Unit patients difficult. On one occasion the unit, occupying only two rooms, had three patients waiting who were never admitted because of lack of available rooms.

2. It was deemed advisable from a research point of view to explore the effects, if any, of a different ward environment on the Parent Care Unit.

3. The majority of patients admitted to the Parent Care Unit were under 2 years of age (a ratio of 30:17) and would ordinarily have been assigned to the second floor utilized in this study.

One nursing assistant resigned from the Parent Care Unit staff because working relief made it too difficult for her to fulfill her family responsibilities. Because of this decrease in staff and the low occupancy on weekends, it was deemed necessary and feasible to operate the unit Mondays through Fridays. Whenever weekend coverage was indicated, a part-time professional nurse and I provided service. At times well-instructed parents were able to care for their children under the guidance of the floor personnel.

Since many staff nurses were involved with patients on the Parent Care Unit, questionnaires (p. 118) were given to twenty-four nurses who had worked at Children's Medical Center while the experimental unit was in operation on the floor where they worked. These questionnaires were handed directly to those nurses who were working on a day chosen at random, and care was taken to ensure that each was given the same orientation. It was requested that the questionnaires be completed at the respondents' convenience and, since they were supposed to remain anonymous, be put in an inconspicuously located box.

Of the twenty-four questionnaires distributed, thirteen were returned. Eight of these respondents worked on the second floor used in the study and five on the first. Responses are grouped by floors because activity on the original floor was confined to the first five weeks of operation and on the one in later use, from the sixth week until termination of the program.

Length of employment among the nurse respondents ranged from seven months to twenty years, and all indicated that they had had contact with Parent Care Unit patients. The vast majority had made this contact on the day shift. Only four individuals reported contact with Parent Care Unit patients on the evening and night shifts, and these were divided equally between the floors 1 and 2. In relation to the number of patients with whom this contact was made, the approximate number ranged from three to sixty-three.

Regarding the quality of care given by parents, four nurses on floor 1 saw "no difference" as opposed to seven on floor 2: four of them rated the care as "good," one as "excellent," and one as "average." One respondent on floor 1, viewing the care given by parents as different, rated their care as "good." No question was asked to determine how the nurses would rate the quality of care that they themselves gave. (It is interesting to note that the nurse respondent who had seen all sixty-three patients was the only one who rated care by parents as "excellent.")

Seven nurse respondents on floor 2 indicated that the child benefited "very favorably" psychologically by having his parents care for him, whereas one selected the "somewhat" response. Four respondents

QUESTIONNAIRE FOR NURSES

1. Approximately how long have you been employed at Children's Medical Center as a professional nurse?

2. Have you had contact with any of the patients while they were assigned to the Parent Care Unit?

   ____Yes   ____No

   If so, which shift(s) primarily?

   ____6:30 to 3:00   ____2:30 to 11:00   ____10:30 to 7:00

   Approximately how many patients have been involved?

3. Generally, did you notice any difference in the care the patients received?

   ____Yes   ____No

4. If your answer to the question above was yes, then how do you view the care given by parents?

   ____Excellent   ____Good   ____Average   ____Poor

   ____Inadequate

5. From your observations of specific patients, do you feel that the child generally benefited psychologically by having his parents care for him?

   ____Very favorably   ____Somewhat   ____None

6. Check those adjectives that you feel may be generally descriptive of those parents participating in the Parent Care Unit study.

____Capable	____Confident	____Conscientious
____Incapable	____Dependent	____Careless
____Dependable	____Emotional	____Enthusiastic
____Irresponsible	____Stable	____Bored
____Excitable	____Fearful	____Impulsive
____Calm	____Self-confident	____Cautious

from floor 1 chose the response indicating that the child benefited "somewhat" psychologically by having his parents care for him, and one stated "no difference."

Adjectives checked by nurse respondents as being generally descriptive of parents were favorable for the most part. Except for the "self-confident" category (3), a majority of nurses who checked the list of adjectives saw the parents as capable (9), dependable (11), calm (6), confident (6), stable (7), conscientious (10), enthusiastic (9), and cautious (9). In seven of the nine categories both the favorable and less favorable adjectives were checked, thus neutralizing the response. These were therefore not included in the numbers previously tabulated. Furthermore, two respondents did not check the list of adjectives.

It is of interest to note that six nurse respondents viewed the parents as being fearful. I believe that much of this anxiety was alleviated through practice while the child was hospitalized. This opinion is based on comments made by parents both at the time of and after discharge. This was the only category in which the less-desirable adjective was checked a substantial number of times. Others included incapable (0), irresponsible (0), excitable (2), dependent (2), emotional (2), careless (0),

bored (1), and impulsive (1). (See responses on this page.)

Six nurse respondents reported that their nursing responsibilities were not affected by the Parent Care Unit. Five others replied that their activity was affected to a "minimal degree" and two to a "large degree." Ways in which nursing activity was affected were listed as "creating confusion in giving medications" and "not being sure of their role" in relation to patients on the Parent Care Unit. Others responded that the Parent Care Unit lessened their responsibility, giving them more time for their own patients; made them more aware of the necessity of instruction for all patients before discharge; and decreased the amount of time that they spent in teaching if they knew a patient was being transferred to the Parent Care Unit. One questionnaire contained no reply to this question.

Nine nurses indicated that they had made referrals to the Parent Care Unit, and four stated that they had not. Reasons cited for making referrals included recognition of a need for intensive teaching; a belief that such a unit would be beneficial to parent and child; a lack of need for intensive nursing care; a recognition of the need for guidance, instruction, confidence,

---

RESPONSES BY STAFF NURSES CONCERNING GENERAL DESCRIPTION OF STUDY PARENTS
N = 11

9 Capable	6 Confident	10 Conscientious
0 Incapable	2 Dependent	0 Careless
2 Both checked	2 Both checked	1 Both checked
0 No answer	1 No answer	0 No answer
11 Dependable	2 Emotional	9 Enthusiastic
0 Irresponsible	7 Stable	1 Bored
0 Both checked	2 Both checked	0 Both checked
0 No answer	0 No answer	1 No answer
2 Excitable	6 Fearful	1 Impulsive
6 Calm	3 Self-confident	9 Cautious
2 Both checked	1 Both checked	1 Both checked
1 No answer	1 No answer	0 No answer

and intervention; and a desire to help the Parent Care Unit get started. Two respondents gave no reasons.

To the question, "If given the opportunity, would you work on a unit of this type?" six nurses responded "yes" and seven "no."

The respondents evidenced by their written comments a strong opinion that the Parent Care Unit should have its own separate location, staff, and policies. Generally they thought that such a service was a good idea, and they indicated that they would like to see such a facility continued. Benefits for both parent and child derived through the Parent Care Unit were cited, and one respondent stated that she missed the unit after the program was terminated. After caring for a previous Parent Care Unit patient and seeing what the mother was capable and willing to do, this nurse stated that she became aware of other families who could have benefited from such a service. Previously mentioned problems that related to the two systems' functioning within the same locational confines were frequently cited.

Nurses, both on the questionnaire and in informal conversations throughout the study, expressed the opinion that room rates should be reduced. This group, at least in terms of expressing their feelings, stressed this point far more often than did either physicians or parents.

PARENT CARE UNIT STAFF'S REACTIONS

The staff on the Parent Care Unit (whose composition has already been described) faced a difficult and at times frustrating task. Challenged with keeping abreast of the pathology, treatment techniques, laboratory tests, medications, diagnostic tests, and x-ray films of any patient admitted to the Parent Care Unit, in addition the nurse had to be well enough informed to give parents accurate information and answers to their questions. Also, to work at maximum effectiveness required close communication and interaction with the physicians. Such close communication was difficult if not impossible in most instances. Despite letters explaining the Parent Care Unit to attending physicians and a detailed Parent Care presentation given at a medical staff meeting, the majority of physicians seemed to lack interest or not to understand the functions of this unit. Furthermore, many physicians possibly were not comfortable in a situation in which the parents were well informed and dealt with as health team members. In contrast, however, a few physicians participated fully.

Unfortunately, the house staff apparently was not officially informed of the existence of the Parent Care Unit. The nursing administration and I unsuccessfully requested time, on several occasions, to explain the function of the Parent Care Unit to the residents. However, many of the house staff became acquainted with the unit through working with Parent Care patients to whom they had been assigned. Several house physicians even transferred some of their parents to the Parent Care Unit. Generally speaking, however, the house staff did not appear to be so receptive to the new unit as did the attending staff.

Probably the greatest frustration of the Parent Care Unit staff resulted from the difficulty in getting patients. Although the unit was initially set up to contain twelve beds, nine was the maximum number that was ever accommodated, and for only one day out of the five-month period. The end result was a mean occupancy of 2.19 patients per hospital day. Patients remained an average of 4.3 days on the Parent Care Unit. This apparent discrepancy in figures was a result of those times when no patients were assigned to the unit and of the frequently low weekend occupancy. Parent Care Unit staff reached a point at which recruiting patients became a struggle. Staffing was a problem, since the number of patients served did not warrant the hiring of additional staff. It became necessary to give days off on weekends because the unit was less likely to have patients at this time. Whenever weekend coverage was needed for patients whose parents were well instructed, these patients were placed on floor care with the understanding that their parents could continue to care for them. When it was believed that parents were not adequately instructed, the Parent Care Unit professional nurses provided weekend coverage on the day shift. Patients were placed on floor care during the evenings in these instances. When the 2:30 to 11:00 shift nursing assistant was ill during the week, no relief was available for her, and again patients on this unit were placed on floor care. No doubt this was confusing for patients, parents, floor personnel, and the Parent Care Unit staff. This was probably one of the major reasons that the Parent Care Unit never gained autonomy but remained dependent on the traditional unit. I believe this dependency created varying degrees of alienation between members of both staffs.

Because the Parent Care Unit had "no place of its own and was housed within the quarters of others," flexibility and creativity were thwarted. Developing policies of its own while functioning within the rigid structure of a crisis-oriented unit was both limited and difficult. At times various members of the Parent Care Unit expressed the feeling of being "in the way."

On the more positive side, working on such a unit afforded one the opportunity to perform "total nursing." Relationships between families and staff were unusually good, and each patient and his parents became "special." Former patients frequently returned to visit after discharge, and some called the staff to ask questions.

Activities of the Parent Care Unit staff included orienting the parent to the ward; presenting the basic facts about the child's illness to the parent; instructing parents on the "hows" and "whys" of treatments and the action, dosage, administration, and side effects of medications; and explaining any test pending. Anxiety appeared to diminish markedly, and this fact was so remarked on a number of occasions. The mother and the nurse together prepared a nursing care plan, which was altered when indicated by a change in the child's condition.

In cases in which the child was old enough, he was taught and encouraged to participate in his own care. For example, two diabetic patients, 8 and 9½ years of age, were taught the basic facts about their illness, insulin administration, and testing of their urine for sugar and acetone.

The Parent Care Unit staff also worked closely and coordinated efforts with the inhalation therapy, dietary, social service, and home care coordinators when patient need was indicated. Through these collaborative efforts, total patient care was accomplished.

From the parents' point of view, attempts to meet the emotional needs of patients through counseling and exhibiting sincere interest contributed greatly to the success of the unit. In my opinion this aspect proved to be the major source of job satisfaction for the staff. Until trust and a good rapport with families were established, the ability to fulfill other functions was limited.

SUMMARY AND CONCLUSIONS

On January 11, 1971, I arrived at Children's Medical Center and began preliminary work on a nursing study of a Parent Care Unit. A survey of the literature and a visit to the University of Kentucky Medical Center where a Care by Parent Unit is in operation were made in an attempt to learn what was being done in this area of patient care. Questionnaires were then designed and administered to Dallas area physicians and parents for the purpose of obtaining some guidelines to use in meeting the needs of our patients and their families. On April 12, 1971, the first patient was admitted to the Parent Care and Instructional Unit. The actual "care by parent" phase of the nursing study was concluded August 27, 1971. From that date until October 15, 1971, the evaluative phase of the study was in progress.

Sixty-three patients, a mean of 2.19 patients per hospital day, were admitted to this unit during its operation. Failure to achieve the desired progress in terms of the number of patients admitted, a lack of economic feasibility, and evidence that such a unit could not develop fully within the rigid structure of a crisis-oriented hospital brought about termination of the Parent Care Unit, as such.

Difficulty in obtaining patients was viewed as a major detriment and was largely considered to be the result of a lack of general medical support. Some physicians participated wholeheartedly, but it must be noted that, from 120 staff physicians, only twenty-eight (some of whom were house officers) had patients assigned to this unit. One might conclude that at the time of the study the vast majority of physicians at Children's Medical Center were not ready to take this approach to pediatric patient care.

Another obstacle to such a unit was the high cost of rooms. Professional nurses and house physicians voiced their objections to this most frequently, seeing failure to reduce room rates as a deterrent. Comments by some of these individuals indicated that they interpreted the assigning of a patient to the Parent Care Unit as a disservice, in that they saw the parent doing all the work, being left alone at night, and paying the highest room rates on the floor. No doubt, for some, what they thought could be gained did not seem to be worth the cost.

The Parent Care Unit operated on both of the existing medical-surgical floors at Children's Medical Center. No significant difference was noted in the effect that either environment exerted on the Parent Care Unit; rather the implications on both of utilizing a crisis-oriented hospital had to be considered. The general opinion was that more interest was demonstrated by nursing personnel on floor 2 than on floor 1; this was substantiated in the number of referrals made by each (a ratio of 3:12).

It was both pleasing and rewarding to Parent Care Unit staff to learn how much parents were able and willing to do for their children. The parents were highly motivated, and with practice they performed treatments correctly and smoothly, administered medications accurately and on time, and made pertinent and consistent observations of their children. Both parents and children appeared more comfortable than those in the customary situation.

The parents who participated made highly favorable comments about the study. In general, their written statements indicated that they preferred this system to the traditional one, that they liked being involved in their children's care, and that they felt better prepared and more secure in caring for the children at home at the time of discharge. A follow-up interview was attempted on every patient, and I was successful in reaching all but six. Comments during the interview further substantiated the original statements. The parents indicated that they would like to see the program continued. The children responded more favorably when their care was given by their mothers.

The reactions of physicians whose patients had participated in the study were favorable, as evidenced by questionnaire and verbal expression. All who responded indicated that they would continue to use such a facility if it were continued on a permanent basis. One physician commented that he was "sick because the Parent Care Unit was being discontinued."

The conclusion, based on comments made by parents and observations by Parent Care Unit staff, was that the psychological aspects were particularly important. For example, how can the parent of a child with cystic fibrosis effectively deal with treatment procedures, medications, and diet if he is not ready emotionally and intellectually to accept the fact that his child has a fatal disease? Counseling by Parent Care Unit staff proved helpful in these instances; to counsel effectively, a good rapport with the parent was necessary. To gain the trust of the parent was a major ingredient in gaining the trust of the child.

RECOMMENDATIONS

To have a successful, operational Parent Care and Instructional Unit, one of my recommendations, based on comments made by nursing personnel and Parent Care Unit staff, is that a unit located apart from any acute-care facility be designated for this purpose. Such a unit should contain some convenience facilities for the parents remaining with the child, such as a lounge for sitting and talking, a kitchenette, and laundry facilities. Ideally, the kitchen could be so equipped that demonstrations of food or formula preparation would be possible and snacks could be prepared. Meals for participating parents should be served with the child's and the cost absorbed in the daily room rate. One might question the advisability of placing television sets in every room; however, during the process of this study we observed that television did not appear to interfere with parent-child interaction to any appreciable degree.

Room rates for those children assigned to the Parent Care and Instructional Unit should also be proportionately decreased. The study demonstrated that a good quality of patient care can be administered by parents with sufficient instruction and supervision; thus the number of nursing staff can probably be decreased. On the day shift a professional nurse and a well-qualified nursing assistant would probably be sufficient. One professional nurse would be needed for the evening shift. The staff for such a unit should be carefully selected. The nurses' questionnaires indicated that about half of them would not like this type of nursing and might not be well suited for it. No staff would need to be assigned to this unit during the night, although professional help should be readily available if the need arises. The staff already mentioned—two professional nurses and one nursing assistant—might be adequate to accommodate twelve patients over a twenty-four–hour period. Weekend occupancy patterns would need further study; however, one additional professional nurse working relief would possibly prove adequate.

Furthermore, opening of a Parent Care and Instructional Unit should be a joint undertaking of medicine and nursing. An interested and involved physician should serve as its medical director and work closely with the two professional nurses assigned to this unit. Together this group and interested other professionals could develop policies necessary for the effective functioning of the unit. Both medical and nursing students could utilize such a unit as a valuable learning experience.

The fact that parents get bored was evident. Some accommodations to alleviate boredom would be helpful. Having available sewing machines, puzzles, magazines, and other supplies for diversion is suggested. Furthermore, parental discussion groups with the professional nurse as leader would prove emotionally and intellectually beneficial and would tend to create interaction among parents at other

times during the day. A larger and better equipped playroom should be provided.

At the present time, Children's Medical Center does not have the space to accommodate a Parent Care and Instructional Unit; therefore the following recommendations, based on what was learned from the study, are being made. Some of them are being implemented at this time by the Department of Nursing.

1. A clinical nurse specialist could be employed to work with those families who are in need of her assistance. To meet the needs of patients, this nurse should have a rich pediatric background. Additional experience in public health would also prove beneficial. Nursing leaders reserve the title of *nurse specialist* to those professional nurses who have a master's degree in their nursing specialty.

2. This nurse should be a free-floating agent who can arrange her time to meet the needs of her patients.

3. Her responsibilities at this time would consist of instructing parents and children in the technical and theoretical aspects of the patient's illness, including such things as treatment procedures and medications. She would also assist in making referrals when indicated for such services as dietary, home care follow-up, and social service. Since establishing rapport with the patient and parents and assisting them in emotional acceptance of difficult situations is an integral part of the job, skill in counseling is important. Preparation for discharge should begin at the time of admission.

4. Furthermore, this nurse must work closely with each patient's physician. A coordinated team approach by parent, nurse, and physician would appear to work well.

5. The mechanics of coordinating floor care and parent care need to be designed carefully to prevent duplication of services or failure to give medications, treatments, and other aspects of care.

• • •

Even though the project at the Children's Medical Center in Dallas did not continue in its original form, the idea of the project is being continued by a pediatric nurse who is employed full time as a parent teacher and counselor. She is a free-wheeling agent serving any family whose child is hospitalized at Children's Medical Center. Her patient load is increasing rapidly, and both medical and nursing staff are requesting her services. The original project as described in this chapter was financed by private donors, and at present the parent teacher and counselor is also paid by private funds. However, it seems likely that the position will be supported by the hospital once the grant funds have been exhausted.*

---

*Editor's note: Personal communication from Trude R. Aufhauser, R.N., Director of Nursing, Children's Medical Center of Dallas, and Professor of Nursing, Texas Woman's University College of Nursing.

14

Pica practice in childhood

Paulette Robischon

The magpie (genus *Pica*) is a bird whose omnivorous habits include stealing and swallowing objects that cannot be considered food. Thus derives use of the term *pica* to denote the practice in man of repeatedly ingesting substances that are considered nonedible.

Adults as well as children practice pica. Nurses are most likely to be familiar with the practice when it appears in some of their pregnant patients or when they encounter children hospitalized for poisoning due to the ingestion of a noxious substance. My interest in pica practice in children stemmed from an interest in childhood accidental poisoning. Pica is the usual forerunner of lead poisoning, which occurs when lead-containing paint that has flaked or chipped off the walls, ceilings, windowsills, and other woodwork of old buildings is eaten by children, usually preschoolers.

Pica is more prevalent than is generally known and has potential for grave effects on well being and future health. In some children it may be an innocuous practice that is outgrown before it brings them harm. Although pica may receive attention from health workers when it is the forerunner of lead poisoning, it often otherwise goes unnoticed. Yet many children who ingest toxic substances other than those containing lead also practice pica. The probability of serious permanent sequelae after poisoning is great. Children who practice pica are also prone to ingest nontoxic substances that may adversely affect their health. Furthermore, childhood pica may be carried over into adulthood and in that case, if practiced in pregnancy, may have direct implications for the health of the mother and infant.

What is this condition called *pica* (pronounced pee-ka by some, pie-ka by others—I prefer the former)? Why is so little known about it? Why does it often come to light only when a health worker, often a nurse, questions parents about their children's hand-mouth behavior or when accidental poisoning occurs because of its practice? This chapter will deal with these questions as it explores pica terminology, history, incidence, divergent views of its etiology, pica studies and findings, and implications for nursing.

TERMINOLOGY

There is general agreement as to the definition of pica insofar as it is considered a "perversion" of the appetite manifesting itself in the ingestion of substances usually considered nonedible. Beyond this general agreement are found differences in terminology and definition as to types of substances ingested, age at which the ingestion is considered abnormal behavior, severity of the condition, and other criteria, some of which deal with the etiological basis of the behavior.

Pica, which derives from Latin, has also been called *kitta,* the Greek word for the magpie or jay. Other terms under which pica has been known in various parts of the world include *allotriophagy, malacia, mal d'estomac, erdessen, geophagy,* and *cachexia.* Some of the terms have meant and are still used today to mean a specific type of pica, for example, geophagy means the eating of dirt or clay. Cachexia, also referred to as malignant cachexia and cachetic pica, is found in association with extremely inadequate diets; its victims often die of malnutrition. Writers of the early 1900's differentiated among pica, an appetite for substances that are not foods such as chalk, clay, and earth; malacia, a craving for highly spiced foods, found mainly in chlorosis and pregnancy; and allotriophagy, a desire for decomposed substances such as urine and feces. Although most contemporary writers use the term *pica* in a broad sense to include all abnormal ingestion, some differentiate among pica, coprophagy, and geophagy, with pica denoting the practice of habitually eating nonfood substances, coprophagy the rare inclusion of feces in the pica habit of the seriously retarded or psychotic, and geophagy the clay-eating custom found in various cultures.

Geophagy and trichophagy, the eating of hair, are sometimes dealt with as entities distinct from pica or as unique practices under the general topic of pica. Dirt eating has been known in many cultures and is believed to be endemic in many parts of the world. Dirt has been used in the diet for various reasons: in times of famine to allay the pangs of hunger, as a condiment or relish with food, mixed with acrid foods to improve their taste, as a delicacy for its own sake, as a medicine, and as part of religious rites. A deficiency of mineral substances is not always implicated, contrary to popular belief, since the clays consumed often contain negligible amounts of salts.[13] However, in one investigator's view geophagy in regions where iron-deficiency anemia is prevalent represents a state of specific hunger, since clays eaten in Brazil contain for the most part high proportions of iron salts.[2] Others also note the high yield of minerals in the ashes used as food condiments by salt-deficient tribes of Central Africa.[31] One wonders, however, why geophagy occurs when seemingly adequate quantities of food are available.

From the United States have come reports of the eating of clay and laundry starch. These were recently summarized in the nursing literature.[6] This is an especially prevalent practice among children whose mothers ingest these substances and whose mothers have come from communities where the practice is part of the cultural pattern.[14]

Trichobezoars, or hair masses of the stomach, are the result of the habitual ingestion of hair. Reports of trichophagy occasionally appear in the pediatric and psychiatric literature. Most standard texts include hair eating in discussing pica, whereas others include hair and textile fibers in the list of substances eaten in pica but treat trichobezoar as a separate topic, mainly because of the unique and dramatic problem of surgical intervention often necessary in its treatment.

A recent paper that defined pica as the "habit of chewing non-edible materials with or without ingestion" resulted in a flurry of letters to the editor.[25] In this instance the author had not distinguished between chewing on hard materials (e.g., a wooden chewing stick used in some African cultures) and the habitual *ingestion* of nonedible materials. It seems likely that differences in definition and terminology have tended to confound the picture of pica practice and have rendered difficult the search for etiological factors.

HISTORY

Discussions of pica practice are found in the literature of ancient and medieval authors, explorers, anthropologists, and colonial physicians and in the literature of the late nineteenth and twentieth century in Europe and America.[5,12] My review of the nineteenth and early twentieth century literature on pica revealed mainly single case reports. An exception to this was a pioneering study in Scotland in 1896 of eleven children with pica who were described from a physical, emotional, and environmental standpoint in which the investigator ruled out physiological causes and concluded that pica was a type of mild psychosis.[30]

Beginning in the 1920's references to pica in the United States literature are found in occasional reports concerning incidents of lead poisoning. As early as 1924 pica was found to be one of the most important etiological factors in lead poisoning in children.[28] In the 1950's and 1960's a spurt of interest in and publicity about lead poisoning appeared, accompanying its recognition as a preventable disease properly belonging in the domain of public health. The occurrence of lead poisoning appeared to parallel interest in and publicity about the disease. The federal government disseminated publications on lead poisoning in children aimed at parents and health workers. At the same time reports began emanating from hospitals and health departments of major cities. Concomitant with this interest in lead poisoning was an expected increase in references to pica practice.

Over a period of years it was found that pica persisting for several months was the usual forerunner of lead encephalopathy, screening for pica practice proved an effective casefinding method for lead poisoning, and a history of pica gave a higher correlation with abnormal blood lead levels than any other test or symptom. Thus the repetitive ingestion of leaded paint was found to be the common denominator in lead poisoning.[4,16]

In the 1970's reports continue to corroborate the fact that the known incidence of lead poisoning parallels the alertness of health personnel to the problem and thus the reporting of cases. In 1971 Public Law 91-695, the Lead-based Paint Poisoning Prevention Act, was enacted,[15] the United States Public Health Service issued a policy statement relative to childhood lead poisoning,[21] and crash programs were instituted to find the estimated 225,000 children in the United States who have lead poisoning.[19] Pica continues to come to light as poisoning cases are investigated carefully. Yet little study has been undertaken to discover the underlying cause of pica itself.

INCIDENCE

The relatively scanty reports of pica in the literature do not reflect its incidence. Mothers generally do not complain spontaneously of pica in their children; it may be considered insignificant by the child's parents, or they may be reluctant to volunteer information about what others may believe are their children's bizarre appetites. Therefore nurses, medical practitioners, and other health workers may be largely unaware of its existence. Yet incidence rates are reported as high as 50% in certain groups of children. A study of 635 children in a low-income area showed pica present in 51% of the children 1 to 2 years of age. The presence of pica decreased stepwise with advancing age, but a history of eating nonfood items other than paint was obtained in approximately one third of the children 1 to 5 years of age. This study population was 92% to 96% black.[7] In another study of children 1 to 6 years old the incidence of pica ranged from a high of 56.5% in the 1- to 2-year age group to 17% in the 5- to 6-year age group in the black children and from 28.3% in the 1- to 2-year age group down to 2.2% in the 5- to 6-year-olds in the white "private patient" group.[22]

In a study of children 1 to 6 years old randomly selected from birth records, the overall pica prevalence rate was found to be 18.5% in white and black children studied by parental interview and 32.1% in white children studied by mailed parental questionnaire. There was a slight preponderance of blacks with pica as compared with whites, but the difference was not statistically significant.[1] In a longitudinal study of premature infants from the lowest socioeconomic class in New York City, mostly black but some white and Puerto Rican, fifty-nine of 272 children (21.7%) had pica when examined between 30 and 33 months of age. The incidence was slightly higher in the black group as compared to the white and least prevalent in the Puerto Rican.[32] In my study of 130 low-income black children between 19 and 24 months of age there was a pica incidence of 37%.[26]

DIVERGENT VIEWS OF ETIOLOGY

In most old reports anemia, malnutrition, and parasitic infestation were consistently incriminated in pica causation. Treatment consisted of iron preparations, a plentiful and varied diet, and healthy living conditions. In contemporary reports some of these etiological factors and modes of therapy still appear as of primary importance in pica. In current pediatric texts anemia, malnutrition, behavior disorders, alimentary disorders, neuroses, compulsive eating, and inadequate adult supervision are variously incriminated in pica causation. The wide disparity of viewpoints ranges from the opinion that ingestion of foreign material in childhood is a normal practice and to call it pica implies that it is an abnormal manifestation to the other extreme, which holds that severe psychopathological factors are operative in pica cases.

Despite differing points of view concerning etiology, there is general agreement on the following:

1. It is normal behavior for a child to mouth and sometimes to swallow nonedible substances in the first year and part of the second year of life, whereas habitual ingestion of nonedible material after this age is considered the practice of pica.

2. Although pica is found in mentally defective children, it is also found in the mentally normal.

3. Pica tends to be a self-limiting condition in many instances; in these cases it disappears at the end of the preschool period, except in the mentally defective or psychotic child.

4. Pica is commonly of a general nature, with numerous types of substances ingested.

5. Pica appears to be equally distributed between the sexes.

PICA STUDIES

Pica studies have yielded inconclusive data. Several studies reported findings suggesting emotional elements in pica—excessive desire for attention, lack of a stimulating environment, feelings of aggression, disturbed mother-child relationship, and an "oral fixation."[3,11,17,23,24] A survey of environmental factors in pica showed no significant correlations between a history of pica and the child's sex, type of dwelling, number of siblings, size of apartment, and person responsible for the child's daytime care.[7] In a lead poisoning study investigators reported that pica was not a racial characteristic but rather that the high rate of lead poisoning found in black and Puerto Rican families was due to the fact that they lived in substandard housing and the health districts in which the greatest interest was shown were predominantly populated by these two groups.[10] In another study statistically significant correlations were found between pica and frequency of physical defects and illness and between pica and the occurrence of feeding problems.[5]

Several nutritional studies revealed conflicting data; two of them concluded that iron deficiency causes a physiologic urge initiating pica and that iron therapy is curative.[12,20] Two double-blind, controlled experiments showed that iron, vitamins, and minerals were no more effective than placebos in curing or improving pica practice.[8,9] In a randomly selected population of children from 1 to 6 years of age there was no common factor in the variety of substances ingested, but it was found that selectivity increases with age. It was concluded that increasing discrimination was more consistent with the developmental process than with an attempt to offset a dietary deficiency by self-selection.[1] A survey of accidentally poisoned children found correlated behavior in the area of hyperactivity, negativism, limited parent-child relations, and a tense and distant family atmosphere. It was also found that poisoning repeaters ate far less bizarre but more toxic items than did children with pica.[18,29] The longitudinal study of prematurely born children suggested the existence of developmental discrepancies prior to, as well as after, pica practice began.[32] There is no convergence of viewpoints toward either a psychosocial or biophysical theory of pica. Elements of physiological causation still persist, and the psychological dimension is only beginning to be explored experimentally. It seems likely that a combination of factors is operative in pica, that multiple variables are interacting to affect the child's behavior, as is the case in many deviations in health.

DEVELOPMENTAL STUDY

Since pica is commonly of a general nature with a variety of substances ingested and since many children practice pica when adequate food is available, it does not seem likely that it is a craving caused by a nutritional deficiency. The fact that pica practice tends to decrease with age as does other hand-mouth behavior lends credence to the idea that pica may be evidence of a developmental lag. It may be the prolongation of an infantile behavior pattern, a pattern that has not yet been relinquished and replaced with behavior more appropriate to the child's age. It is in this context that I carried out a pica study.

It was hypothesized that children who practice pica and those who have other persistent hand-mouth behavior have a lower developmental level than those children who do not exhibit these behaviors. The study sample consisted of three groups (pica, hand-mouth, and control) of thirty children each who were between 19 and 24 months of age. Their parents were United States' mainland-born blacks of the lower socioeconomic class. These were well children who had no history of twin birth, low birth weight, birth injury, congenital anomaly, psychosis, lead poisoning, or other major deviations in health, since these conditions may be associated with deviations in development. Also excluded from the study were children who were known to ingest or to have ingested in the past substances such as paint, plaster, or putty because their blood lead levels may have reached a point of toxicity such that development was affected although poisoning was not diagnosed.

In a large city child health station I interviewed parents to select children for the study groups. Each group was matched for age. Two testers who had no knowledge of the children's group assignment performed a developmental test that assessed four areas of behavior: gross motor, fine motor–adaptive, language, and personal-social.

Developmental findings

The gross motor data yielded significant differences among the three study groups. Differences among the groups in the fine motor–adaptive, language, and personal-social areas were not significant. Further analysis revealed that children practicing pica and children in the hand-mouth group both had significantly lower gross motor scores than did children in the control group, although there was no significant difference in the scores of the pica and hand-mouth groups. Details of the study methodology and findings have been published elsewhere.[27]

It has been speculated that the child with pica may be one who is restricted in activity by being denied normal play opportunities and who therefore practices pica as an outlet. It may be that the control children in my study, busier because of higher motor activity, were too occupied to practice pica or other persistent hand-mouth behavior. In all gross motor items the control children passed items ahead of age more frequently than the pica and hand-mouth children. They balanced on one foot, jumped in place, and were able to do the broad jump more frequently than the other children. They also passed fine motor–adaptive items more frequently than the other two study groups. The children in the control group were generally more skilled than the pica and hand-mouth children in the area of personal-social behavior as well, which means that they were kept busier with self-help activities.

A view of pica and other persistent hand-mouth activity as a lag in the normal progression of development of hand-mouth behavior tends to be supported by findings of this study, particularly in the gross motor area. The child with persistent hand-mouth activity may not yet have experienced increased response to auditory and visual stimuli, his manipulation of objects is still limited, he still participates little in imitative play, and his motor abilities do not yet permit him to widely explore his environment. No study children were found to have obvious motor disabilities. The items failed in the motor area were probable evidence of motor retardation, which implied a performance normal in quality and abnormal only as to age. The items passed ahead of age were probable evidence of developmental acceleration, a quickened tempo as measured by the standardized test age norms.

It was not surprising to find a lag in only one developmental area in the pica and hand-mouth groups. These children, as well as the children in the control group, were considered intellectually normal and had been under rather close health supervision since birth. Had gross deviations been present, these would have been observed previously and would have rendered the children ineligible for inclusion in the study. An unevenness in one aspect of the child's total development may be due to maturational and environmental factors interacting in complex ways. The persistence of this behavior is gradually overcome by the operation of normal maturational processes and behavior patterns more appropriate to the child's age that replace the hand-mouth behavior.

Sex difference

In the literature there is no report of marked difference in sex distribution among pica practitioners. Yet in this study there was an unexpected and unexplained finding. Although there was an almost equal sex distribution in the total sample—forty-three boys and forty-seven girls—there was a statistically significant higher incidence of pica in girls than in boys. Sex differences in the hand-mouth and control groups were statistically nonsignificant. Does the sex difference indicate that hand-mouth behavior is perceived and therefore handled differently by parents in girls than in boys? Might this behavior be condoned by parents in their daughters and not in their sons? Might some of these study mothers be encouraging or at least condoning pica practice in their daughters on a cultural basis? This sex difference finding requires further study.

Pica group

The pica practitioners ate a great variety of nonedible substances. Among common items eaten were paper, matches, ashtray contents, baby powder, string, thread, pencil erasers, and crayons. A few children were selective, preferring certain substances to others, for example, a child who was observed to eat huge quantities of toilet tissue and a child who had a preference for brown paper. Only a few habitually ate only one nonedible substance. The finding that pica was of a general nature in the great majority of children corroborates other reports. This nonselectivity lends credence to the theory that pica in this age group is not a craving but rather a persistent hand-mouth activity. The children seemed to consume whatever was accessible; often the substances consumed were items they could pick at or pluck and easily reach and handle.

Persistence of a cultural practice was seen in the instances of consumption of laundry starch, in which mothers volunteered information that their grandmothers, mothers, sisters, themselves, and now their children consumed this substance. One child who ate laundry starch exclusively as a pica item and was fed this by his mother was eliminated from the study, since he was

not considered to have pica as defined in the study.

Trichophagy was seen in three children who also consumed other nonedible items. One child had been in danger of developing a trichobezoar. Her mother had removed a large hair mass from the child's rectum the week before. Only five children practiced geophagy; all five ate the dirt from flowerpots. Few families had house plants, thus soil was not easily accessible in this manner to the study children. The investigation was carried out in late winter and early spring; therefore the children were not playing outdoors where earth may have been within reach. Furthermore, even in a warmer season earth would not have been readily accessible, since the children lived in a congested urban area, few had yards, and there were few unpaved park areas. Factors like these must account for the more frequent reports of geophagy emanating from rural as compared with urban areas. Two mothers, recently returned from vacations spent in rural areas in a warmer climate, said that their children had eaten earth while there. It is likely that the dirt eaters in this investigation ate dirt because it was accessible as a nonfood substance they could pick at and bring to their mouth, rather than to meet a physiological need.

Of the thirty children practicing pica, mothers found the pica substance in the stool in 63% of the children. The substances found in the stool were paper, thread and string, hair, leaves, tobacco, ashes, crayons, powder puffs, and rubber balloons.

Almost three fourths of the children practicing pica also displayed persistent hand-mouth behavior other than pica. This finding is in keeping with that of some other studies, in that children with pica had a high degree of other oral activity as well. The children in this investigation often sucked and mouthed pacifiers, their fingers, clothing, empty nursing bottles, and their toys, among other items.

Most mothers showed an attitude of resignation toward their children's pica practice; only a few showed exasperation. Those who tolerated it indicated that there was not much that could be done about it, that the child would cease the activity eventually. This is the attitude found among mothers in several other studies as well.

Hand-mouth group

The incidence of persistent hand-mouth behavior, excluding children with pica who also had a high degree of other hand-mouth behavior, was 32% in the 130 children considered for this study. To be assigned to the hand-mouth group meant that a child mouthed and sucked objects daily on different occasions. The mother's report of this behavior was corroborated in all instances by investigator observation or evidence of the behavior. Of the children in this group, almost one half also occasionally ingested nonfood items but were not considered to have habitual pica. The objects mouthed by the children in the hand-mouth group were much the same as those mouthed by the children with pica who had a high hand-mouth rating. The objects were all easily accessible to the children. Most common were toys, empty nursing bottles, fingers, pacifiers, paper, and clothes.

Generally, mothers seemed more concerned and showed more annoyance and embarrassment about thumbsucking, fingersucking, and use of pacifiers than they did about pica practice. This may be because mothers view pica as a passing phase, whereas they perceive mouthing and sucking as a habit that will persist into later life. It is also possible that sucking and mouthing have sexual connotations that may be absent in pica practice. Furthermore, mothers may recall their own childhood, in which they were reprimanded for sucking activities but perhaps not for the ingestion of nonedible substances that they may have eaten secretively or with adults in the case of clay or laundry starch.

The children's diets

This study did not focus on the children's diets, but the nutritional area was explored with the mother as a preface to the questions about nonnutritional hand-mouth behavior. The nutritional findings tend to substantiate what is well known about the low-income diet and its deficiencies. Many of the children consumed excessive quantities of milk—as much as two and one-half quarts daily. Often the nursing bottle containing milk was used as a pacifier. As would be expected, the children who practiced pica and those who had other persistent hand-mouth behavior had not relinquished use of the nursing bottle as readily as the control children. Excessive milk consumption due to clinging to the nursing bottle may explain the link between pica and anemia that some investigators have found. It may also suggest why efforts to cure pica with iron are often unsuccessful. The children in the control group manifested excessive milk consumption to the least degree. Other dietary patterns were similar among the three study groups.

Familial pica and lead poisoning

Mothers were not questioned as to the presence of pica or lead poisoning in siblings or other relatives of the study children, but several volunteered this type of information. Among the study children, two mothers reported that siblings had been deleaded, one at 1½ and the other at 3 years of age. Another mother reported that a study child's cousin had died of lead poisoning at 3½ years of age and a cousin in another family was presently being treated for it. Still another mother reported that three years previously two of the study child's siblings had had lead poisoning; the 2 year old had died, the 3 year old had recovered. Another mother reported that a sibling, then 5 years old had had lead poisoning at 2 and again at 4½ years of age with residual disability. There undoubtedly were other incidents of sibling or relative pica and poisoning not reported by mothers and not included in the health records.

Of the 130 children who were subjects of the interview, 37% had pica, and of these children, 25% consumed substances containing lead. Naturally, this figure was determined by the accessibility of lead-containing substances because the children's environment varied from housing with old crumbling interior walls with leaded paint to public housing in which lead-free paint was used. The fifteen children known to consume lead were eliminated from the study and referred to the child health station personnel for follow-up care. Four were found to be free of poisoning, although of these, three had borderline blood lead levels nearing toxicity, in six the level of toxicity was as yet undetermined when the study ended, and five were found to have lead poisoning. Add to this last figure the probability of siblings and other relatives with borderline or toxic blood lead levels, and it becomes obvious that lead poisoning is indeed a "silent epidemic."

IMPLICATIONS FOR NURSING

Nurses can engage in further study of pica practitioners. The sex difference needs to be substantiated or refuted. Serial studies could determine whether pica and other persistent hand-mouth activity decrease in relation to increased motor activity. Longitudinal studies could determine whether abnormal hand-mouth behavior is an antecedent of delayed motor development, whether the reverse is true, or whether they tend to occur simultaneously. Further exploration of delayed development in all types of persistent hand-mouth behavior is needed, since the children in the hand-mouth group (nonpica) in my study fared even worse in the developmental test than did the children who practiced pica.

If further research were to substantiate that development and pica were indeed related, the nurse might help to develop children's motor skills as a primary preventive measure. With children in whom pica practice or other persistent hand-mouth behaviors already exist, the nurse might help to develop the child's motor skills as a replacement for these behaviors.

Based on what is already known about pica, there are steps that nurses can take now. Since children with pica are not as easily identified as those with other persistent hand-mouth behavior and since mothers generally do not share information spontaneously about their child's pica, improved interviewing techniques have to be developed. The nurse, as the health worker most involved with parents and their infants and preschool children, is in a highly favorable position to detect pica through interviews with parents or other caretakers. Nurses must develop alertness to the possibility of pica and develop ob-

servational skills to identify the child who practices it. This would include observation of parental behavior, for example, how the mother deals with the child's oral behavior, as well as observation of the child's behavior, the degree of the child's hand-mouth activity. Many opportunities exist for nursing observation of children's behavior in both formal and informal ways, in all types of settings. Nurses can institute effective follow-up of children lagging in motor development and those displaying an excessive amount of hand-mouth activity because these behaviors may be clues to deviations in health or to the child's vulnerability to environmental hazards. Nurses can improve methods of parental education concerning the development of hand-mouth behavior and pica in particular, since present modes of dissemination of information about the hazards of pica are not sufficiently effective. Last, nurses can increase their knowledge about pica and the development of hand-mouth behavior and share this knowledge with other personnel with whom they work on behalf of child health.

References

1. Barltrop, D.: The prevalence of pica, Am. J. Dis. Child. 112:116, Aug., 1966.
2. Castro, J.: The geography of hunger, Boston, 1952, Little, Brown & Co.
3. Chisolm, J. J., Jr., and Harrison, H. E.: Exposure of children to lead, Pediatrics 18:943, 1956.
4. Chisolm, J. J., Jr., and Kaplan, E.: Lead poisoning in childhood: comprehensive management and prevention, J. Pediatr. 73:942, 1968.
5. Cooper, M.: Pica, Springfield, Ill., 1957, Charles C Thomas, Publisher.
6. Dunston, B. N.: Pica during pregnancy. In Bergersen, B. S., Anderson, E. H., Duffey, M., Lohr, M., and Rose, M. H., editors: Current concepts in clinical nursing, vol. 2, St. Louis, 1969, The C. V. Mosby Co., pp. 268-279.
7. Griggs, R. C., Sunshine, I., Newill, V. A., Newton, B. W., Buchanan, S., and Rasch, C. A.: Environmental factors in childhood lead poisoning, J. A. M. A. 187:703, 1964.
8. Gutelius, M. F., Millican, F. K., Layman, E. M., Cohen, G. J., and Dublin, C. C.: Nutritional studies of children with pica. I. Controlled study evaluating nutritional status. II. Treatment of pica with iron given intramuscularly, Pediatrics 29:1012, 1962.
9. Gutelius, M. F., Millican, F. K., Layman, E. M., Cohen, G. J., and Dublin, C. C.: Treatment of pica with a vitamin and mineral supplement, Am. J. Clin. Nutr. 12:388, 1963.

10. Jacobziner, H., and Raybin, H. W.: The epidemiology of lead poisoning in children, Arch. Pediatr. **79:**72, Feb., 1962.

11. Jenkins, C. D., and Mellins, R. B.: Lead poisoning in children, Arch. Neurol. Psychiatry **77:**70, Jan., 1957.

12. Lanzkowsky, P.: Investigation into the aetiology and treatment of pica, Arch. Dis. Child. **34:**140, April, 1959.

13. Laufer, B.: Geophagy, Chicago, Field Museum of Natural History, Anthropological Series, Publication No. 280, **18** (2), 1930.

14. Layman, E. M., Millican, F. K., Lourie, R. S., and Takahashi, L. V.: Cultural influences and symptom choice—clay eating customs in relation to the etiology of pica, Psychol. Record **13:**249, July, 1963.

15. Lead peril solution: A beginning, The Nation's Health, Nov., 1971.

16. Lin-Fu, J. S.: Childhood lead poisoning: An eradicable disease, Children **17:**2, Jan.-Feb., 1970.

17. Lourie, R. S., Layman, E. M., and Millican, F. K.: Why children eat things that are not food, Children **10:**143, July-Aug., 1963.

18. Margolis, J. A.: Psychosocial study of childhood poisoning: A 5-year follow-up, Pediatrics **47:**439, 1971.

19. Mass lead testing, The Nation's Health, Feb., 1971.

20. McDonald, R., and Marshall, S. R.: The value of iron therapy in pica, Pediatrics **34:**558, 1964.

21. Medical aspects of childhood lead poisoning (policy statement), HSMHA Health Reports **86:**140, Feb., 1971.

22. Millican, F. K., Layman, E. M., Lourie, R. S., Takahashi, L. Y., and Dublin, C. C.: The prevalence of ingestion and mouthing of nonedible substances by children, Clin. Proc. Child. Hosp. D. C. **18:**207, Aug., 1962.

23. Millican, F. K., Layman, E. M., Lourie, R. S., and Takahashi, L. V.: Study of an oral fixation: pica, J. Am. Acad. Child Psychiatry **7:**79, Jan., 1968.

24. Millican, F. K., Lourie, R. S., and Layman, E. M.: Emotional factors in the etiology and treatment of lead poisoning, Am. J. Dis. Child. **91:**144, Feb., 1956.

25. Neumann, H. H.: Pica—symptom or vestigial instinct? Pediatrics **46:**441, 1970.

26. Robischon, P.: A study of the relationship between children's developmental level, pica practice, and other hand-mouth behavior, doctoral dissertation, School of Education, New York University, 1970.

27. Robischon, P.: Pica practice and other hand-mouth behavior and children's developmental level, Nurs. Res. **20:**4, Jan.-Feb., 1971.

28. Ruddock, J. C.: Lead poisoning in children with special reference to pica, J.A.M.A. **82:**1682, 1924.

29. Sobel, R., and Margolis, J. A.: Repetitive poisoning in children: A psychological study, Pediatrics **35:**641, 1965.

30. Thompson, J.: On pica, or dirt eating, in children, Arch. Pediatr. **13:**154, Feb., 1896.

31. Trowell, H. C., and Jelliffe, D. B.: Diseases of children in the subtropics and tropics, London, 1958, Edward Arnold, Ltd.

32. Wortis, H., Rue, R., Heimer, C., Braine, M., Redlo, M., and Freedman, A. M.: Children who eat noxious substances, J. Am. Acad. Child Psychiatry **1:**536, 1962.

15

A 5-year-old child controls his aggressive response to body intrusion

Eileen Gallagher Nahigian

Freddie was a white boy with flirting brown eyes, wind-tossed brown hair, a conspicuous soft rubber tracheostomy tube, and a voice quality that varied from muffled to whispering to squawking. He was the third son in a family of four children, whose ages ranged from 9 to 4 years. His only sister was the youngest sibling. He celebrated his sixth birthday anniversary two months after our initial contact.

It was during his thirty-second and thirty-third hospitalizations for removal of respiratory papillomas that I cared for Freddie. He had a history of juvenile papillomatosis of the larynx. This diagnosis, established at the age of 18 months, followed repeated respiratory infections throughout infancy. Surgical removal of the papillomas was initiated at the time of diagnosis; tracheostomy was necessary at the age of 25 months, in addition to repeated excision of the polyps. Thereafter, tracheostomy continued to constitute a threat to Freddie's life.

The disease and the tracheostomy provided real danger of asphyxiation. In fact, despite frequent tracheal aspirations, his mother (Mrs. F) was forced on several occasions to remove and replace the tracheostomy tube because of mucous obstructions in its lumen. Furthermore, a consistently patent airway could be assured only by surgical intervention every two to five weeks. Additionally, severe respiratory infections required interim hospitalizations elsewhere. The severity of these infections was illustrated during one conversation with Mrs. F when she related that Freddie had been so near death that his nurses had been praying for his recovery.

Mrs. F focused most of her attention on Freddie; she restricted her son's activity and seldom allowed him out of her sight. One year prior to the events recorded in this chapter, Mrs. F's doting care was violently interrupted for several months. Since the cause of this separation figures significantly in Freddie's interpretation of his life, it is shared here for further reference. One afternoon Mrs. F discovered the children outside playing with paint. Angrily she threw their clothes into the bathtub with gasoline. The bathtub was near the kitchen; the gas stove pilot light ignited the fumes, setting off an explosive fire that destroyed the F family's house. In the fire Mrs. F sustained extensive burns necessitating lengthy hospitalization and separation from Freddie.

Freddie's father maintained two full-time jobs as a semiskilled worker, and even when he was not working he spent little time at home. When at home, he often expressed disgust at Freddie's coughing, and he openly refused to eat at the same table with his son. He had promised Freddie that when he became 6 years old he could accompany his father on occasional hunting and fishing trips. However, this promise was never realized, since the parents separated within days of Freddie's sixth birthday.

Hospital personnel considered Freddie hyperactive; some were also repelled by his behavior, which was further complicated by the "disgusting cough" described by his father. This situation became clear to me as I began to work with Freddie and tried to understand him. The observations excited me perhaps because this preschool child unwittingly illustrated what required me to do almost endless library research to grasp—the significant interrelationship of his behavior, medical and family history, and developmental milestones. Freddie prompted me to far-reaching study on a variety of topics, including development, body image and associated concepts, ambivalence, aggression, ego defenses, fantasy, reaction to intrusive procedures, and the effect of body defects on behavior.

THE CHILD'S CONTROLLED AGGRESSION

As participant-observer in his care, I collected a quantity of data from encounters with Freddie and his parents. Subsequent analysis of the data revealed patterns by which he controlled and defended himself against aggression, which might have been precipitated by his composite life circumstances. An appreciation of Freddie's controlled aggression and defenses can be achieved only after one understands the need for aggression and its control.

What necessitated aggression in this child's behavior?

First, remember that Freddie was still within the limits of the preschool years, also known as the Oedipal phase of psychosexual development. Intrusive behavior, evidenced by generally irruptive activity as well as by physical attack against a person or thing, is characteristic of the preschool-aged child.[5]

Second, an individual exposed repeatedly to enforced passivity, loss of autonomy, or danger of attack may either succumb to it or struggle against it. Fear of attack is not an uncommon component of the Oedipal phase of development. Josselyn[10] describes how a boy's unconsciously romantic feelings toward his mother and rivalry toward his father result in heightened castration fears. The castration fear has been expanded by Schilder[15] to include a generalized fear of being either attacked or dismembered. Anna Freud[28] further notes the easy displacement of castration fears to other body parts under appropriate circumstances such as surgery.

Third, weak body boundaries create the sensation of vulnerability to external danger.[6] "Body boundary" means the psychic boundary that separates the self from the object world. Persons who sustain disturbances of the body's interior

are especially likely to experience weak and easily penetrable boundaries.[6,26] This concept has direct relevance for Freddie, since he was regularly attacked by surgery, tracheostomy aspirations, and administration of medicines, all of which intrude and therefore threaten the body's boundary. Erickson[25] reports that hospitalized preschool children consider most treatments as hostile invasions. Furthermore, Sylvester[23] states that ill and hospitalized children respond negatively when subjected to clinical equipment because these experiences interfere with differentiation of self from others. With the distortion of ego structures and body image, the consequent sensation of vulnerability must be met either by withdrawal or active resistance.

Aggression may also be precipitated in response to uncertainty. Uncertainty may occur, along with lowered self-esteem and a feeling of being neglected, from the psychic reflection of organ inferiority.[1] Undoubtedly the most menacing aspect of Freddie's constitution was his respiratory inferiority.

A child's aggression might also be aroused by threats to self-preservation,[21,27,35] or by an adult's initial aggression toward him.[19] Surely the constant specter of asphyxiation was foreboding, as were the required therapeutic intrusions.

Aggression, although often considered an undesirable behavior, has many positive and constructive uses. Following are some of the positive outcomes of aggression:

1. It allows for catharsis, or dissipation of affect such as resentment.[4,13]

2. It provides a degree of socialization via the ability to reach and grasp the object world.[7]

3. It expresses the child's efforts to achieve ego consciousness.[1]

4. It contributes significantly to the individual's differentiation of self from environment.[30]

Freddie's need to be aggressive might have been a reaction to repeated intrusions, to rejection by his father, to his own role as the object of repeated assaults, or to self-blame for his imperfections and for the instability of his parents' marriage. Even a superficial look at Freddie's life situation renders the need for aggressiveness in this child's behavior blatantly obvious.

Why did this child maintain control on his expression of aggression?

How an individual discharges aggression is essentially determined by his appraisal of the threat presented.[11] Direct attack may be displaced because of situational constraints, which may be experienced by the young child by means of rather subtle lessons designed to check aggression in accord with society's inhibitions.[4,15] Control by defensive behavior may serve the individual's simultaneous needs to restrict internal drives while allowing adaptation to the external environment.[7] Control may also originate in the normal ambivalence derived from early life experiences. This ambivalence is apparent in day-to-day interrelationships in which hostile feelings are tempered with affection.[33] As with anyone, then, much of Freddie's control occurred without conscious effort or design.

What distinguishes controlled aggression?

Fundamental to answering this question is a definition of the term *aggression* itself. A review of the literature on the topic reveals no single or precise definition, but rather a series of connotations. For one author, aggression indicates only the directing of an action toward an object. For some, the emphasis is positive; for others, the act is negative, or undesirable. Bender,[3] for example, states that destruction is exhibited only secondarily, and even this may vary in degree from pushing or throwing objects to inflicting pain. One study specifies purposeful intent between the aggressive act and the resultant injury, destruction, or depreciation.[37]

In this chapter, *aggression* denotes any behavior in which an attack is either threatened or performed against another in such a way as to provoke retaliation. In contrast, *controlled aggression* is any behavior that threatens, performs, or suggests aggression while limiting the probability of direct physical retaliation. It is this *controlled aggression* that constitutes a significant force in Freddie's life.

Defense measures may exert restraint over expressions of aggression. Such defenses include fantasy, which has been described as one component in a hierarchical sequence of aggressive activities[37] and may be exhibited through the media of doll play,[18,31,36,39] games, toys, cars, or artistic creations.[2,16] Ambivalence,[9] as well as inhibition, restitution, projection, denial, undoing, and use of body functions,[17,35] has been implicated as a defense against aggression. All these function rather like a lid on a boiling pot; the differentiation between controlled aggression and aggression occurs at the point when the water boils over despite the lid.

How did the child control his aggression?

The answer to the question "How did Freddie control his aggression?" rendered his behavior understandable. Since he was permitted behavioral expression without recrimination, nursing care took on meaning by facilitating his ability to cope with cumulative stresses.

Freddie's controlled aggression was exercised through a variety of channels. He effectively employed motor behavior, physical contact, orality, verbalizations, fantasy, and artistic creativity toward a common end.

He was fortunate to have been in a clinical setting that provided space for *gross motor behavior*. Accordingly, he was able to vent his internal struggle as he exploited large toys, such as a tricycle and a tractor. Characteristically he first maneuvered these vehicles slowly and then accelerated to a peak of activity. He also feigned a vehicular crash and then promoted an actual collision between the tractor and tricycle. Similar behavior appeared in ball play; he began quietly and easily, perhaps rolling or tossing the ball before rapidly progressing to bouncing or kicking the ball or both. At such times he played with so much intensity that his presence could not be ignored.

Pearson[35] relates that since the motor system provides a vehicle for aggressiveness, motor activity may be an indication of the amount of the child's aggressiveness. Another author has specifically described *epinemesis,*[17] in which play spreads outward from a circumscribed area as it becomes more aggressive, a description of activity similar to Freddie's. Fortunately Freddie was able to maintain ego control within this pattern, thus obviating the need of external controls for protection from the id. His independent control afforded support coincident with the passivity enforced by the intimidation of the adult world.

During periods of *less active play*, Freddie further capitalized on the opportunity for aggressiveness. During these play periods he accentuated the vigor of the play in a table hockey game by pounding his fist hard and loud on the tabletop, by allowing as well as causing a crash of two toy jets, and by handling most toys roughly. More directly, he smashed, flattened, and threw his Play-Doh against the play surface, and he pinched his balloon repeatedly until it burst.

Freddie participated in several play interviews[24] that allowed him to express his feelings with impunity in my presence through nondirective play. During the first two interviews over a period of less than two hours, fifty-five instances of physical attack were recorded. The "victims" of these attacks were all the dolls in the toy kit, cotton balls, pillow, car, pillbox, pills, and miniature house furniture. Freddie was similarly resourceful in his selection of methods of attack: injecting, cutting, tearing, pushing, slamming the toy refrigerator into the doctor doll's face, and restraining, anesthetizing, and flushing the boy doll down the toilet.

Twice he attempted to choke me. The first time, as he sat on my lap, he grabbed and quickly pressed his fingers into my neck with force sufficient to hurt; the second attempt was less direct. A still more subtle attack occurred in *fantasy*, when he identified his truck as a fire engine and then announced that I was sitting on the fire and would have to save myself without his assistance.

What do all these behavioral expressions mean? The literature reflects a meaning far beyond playfulness. Fantasy attacks against nonthreatening or nonretaliating objects constitute indirect expressions of aggression, restricted because of fear of retaliation.[15] Within fantasy the level of safety appears proportionate to the absence of

symbolic relevance to the actual feared person or event. According to this idea, the least threatening object would be the least symbolic one. This being true, Freddie could employ an array of safe objects, such as the Play-Doh, ball, or games, without fear.

Furthermore, fantasy allows a degree of aggression against symbolic representatives of real people in an atmosphere of greater permissiveness than is possible in an anxiety-laden real situation. That Freddie's intrusive injections of the dolls and other objects were indeed aggressive seems to be supported by the findings that children have equated hypodermic syringes with guns, daggers, and bombs.[24]

The instances of controlled aggression toward the nurse—classified as such because they were neither obvious retaliations against the person, nor provocations to retaliation—present an interesting phenomenon in Freddie's coping behavior. Perhaps he was responding in part with "revenge fantasies,"[34,38] which represent not only anger at those who are directly responsible or blamed for the defect but also the wish similarly to stigmatize them. Freddie's apparent choking of the nurse seemed to express a desire to inflict a wound comparable to his own tracheostomy. Perhaps having others look like himself might contribute to his feelings of security.[29] One might also conjecture that this child approached persons as he approached objects, meaning that he would have exploited both animate and inanimate objects in a more or less mechanized type of relationship. This idea, suggested by Sylvester,[23] would imply that Freddie was unaware of any associated aggressiveness.

Displaced aggression was further expressed in Freddie's oral sadistic ingestion of food. Such *oral sadism* was evidenced by his manner of devouring solid and liquid foods. He consistently gobbled his food and drink. A few times he allowed his spoon to dangle from his clenched teeth; once he was observed to gulp his soup directly from the bowl. This orality may have been useful in assuring him of his masculinity, or it may have been in accord with Keiser's[32] concept of body orifices as being basic to the creation of body boundaries. In other words, Freddie was repeatedly reminded of the penetrability of his body; confronted with this dilemma, he reinforced himself by active oral assertiveness.

Freddie also proved to be *verbally aggressive* in both reality and fantasy. His verbalizations evidenced an attempt to master and a concentration on attack, as well as destructive, critical, or injurious thoughts about himself or others. Verbal anger in real situations was communicated by demands on the nurse, by scolding the nurse who infringed on his private game rules, and by name-calling, such as "lazybones" (muttered about his mother when she failed to answer his repeated phone calls). He also complained about the nurse's repeated tracheal aspirations, crying, "Ow! You hurt me!" and "You're a brat! I don't like you!" Ability to attack the nurse verbally in a way that approached direct aggression and yet to maintain the relationship demonstrated a certain strength in Freddie's personality.

In fantasy he revealed anger at what he may have believed were arbitrary verbal and physical attacks by others. In the second play interview (p. 139) he fiercely rammed the father doll's abdomen with a needle and added, "It's gonna stay there forever and ever. Now we can see if he cries every day!" There were other examples of displaced, and possibly distorted, verbal aggression in fantasy; one such instance was Freddie's administration of medicine to the sink with the explanation that medicine "kills" either germs or bad breath. Correspondingly, it has been recorded that children interpret administration of both oral and parenteral medication as aggressive attacks.[28]

That Freddie had dammed up and refused direct release of his aggressive feelings was suggested by repeated mention of bombs and fires, which are destructive if unleashed. He built a castle and then destroyed it with a "bomb." He fantasied a fire in the sink's overflow drain, caused by "gasoline and paint and bombs." This last fantasy holds special interest in view of his history.

In a play sequence with two toy jets, he crashed the jets, killing all the German passengers but not the American pilot. To his tale about the "crash" he added incidentally that Indians kill people with their tomahawks. Interestingly, Schilder[14] found that children who have been forced to suppress aggression express violent tendencies toward groups such as Germans or Indians. Also in play, a truck carrying soldiers was headed toward Freddie's hometown to attack everyone and everything there because ". . .I don't like them."

Bender[2] relates that when a child uses *creative media* he draws what he sees and knows about the object and that in clay modeling he finds a means to solve some of his problems. Application of this concept to Freddie is intriguing. His chalk drawings were of a "monster," a "ghost monster," and a "200-legger," which he later dubbed a "five-legged octopus." Initially, the only crayon drawing he could produce was a red "ghost town with a ghost in it." When given Play-Doh at another time he modeled a "monster" and a "snake hole."

A child's conflicts may be discovered by an interpretation of his art, but a valid explanation requires that his entire life situation be considered along with the art. A monster, for instance, might be more readily identified with aggression than might a ghost; however, in view of Freddie's total situation both productions betray controlled aggression. His creatures were ugly and fear inspiring. He not only less than adequately endowed his Play-Doh monster, but he also dismembered it: "The monster got no eyes, and got no mouth, and got no peek! I'm gonna take his heart out!" Perhaps this expression revealed Freddie's self-concept or his desire to attack the "monsters" who continually assaulted him! His red ghost and ghost town conjured up the picture of an angry, insubstantial, penetrable, and therefore vulnerable being. The common connotation of a ghost might also suggest that Freddie's drawing and his aggressiveness were also an attempt to prevail over an underlying fear of death.

What defenses did the child employ against the expression of aggression?

As already indicated, most of Freddie's aggression was controlled and indirect.

EXCERPTS FROM SECOND PLAY INTERVIEW

He took the baby doll and laid it flat in the tub saying, "Baby in tub! Now baby's gonna get shot right in the mouth!" He poked the needle firmly into the doll's eye. "I mean right in the eye! You're gonna get a whole bunch of shots!" He poked the chest. "Right in the heart! Yegh!" He tried to open the diaper pin, could not, and asked for assistance. The nurse opened the pin and removed it but did not remove the diaper.

As Freddie removed the diaper, he made an expression of disgust and remarked, "He didn't wipe his (pointing to his own bottom) heinie . . . . That's why he's gettin' a shot! Right through him!" As he said this, the needle pierced the doll's buttocks and exited through the penis.

Next the baby's abdomen was injected. He removed the needle and then thrust it into the abdomen again as if it were a dagger; then he hammered at the syringe. "Somebody put in a bow and arrow! I think I will." He started to put the needle into the doll's abdomen but then pushed it into the doll's face instead. He suspended the doll by the syringe and said, "See where it is?" Then he thrust the needle into the doll's forehead so that it exited through the back of the head.

With the needle still in place he flung the baby into the tub, and as he pulled the needle out he said, "I gotta go to hospital."

"Now the brother!" He changed needles and, without bothering the brother, paused to ask what noise he had heard.

He had placed the boy doll on a counter, which he said was the doctor's place. He took the alcohol wipe and rubbed the doll's foot with it. He said, "You gonna get shot right in your foot!" He injected the foot. He started to cough nonproductively and turned away; he returned to the desk.

"I feel like goin' back to my room." He started to push the toys into the kit. He found the Band-Aid. He held it up. "A Band-Aid?" The nurse nodded. He took it to the "doctor's place," opened it very deliberately, and applied it over the doll's arm so that it restrained the arm to the countertop. He returned to the table in search of another Band-Aid. The nurse explained that she had brought no more.

He brought the mask to the doctor's place. He said, "Gonna make him go to sleep." He put the mask over the doll's face and instructed, "Count to three in there!" (He spoke this instruction directly through the mask.) He removed it, said, "He's asleep!" and put the mask on the table. He returned to the doll, pounded on its head and neck, and said, "Shot, shot, shot, shot, shot!" He picked up the doll and said, "Ow!"

Once more he said that he wanted to return to his own room.

Nevertheless, further control was exerted by eight patterns of defensive behavior. These were comparable to those identified by Albino[17] and Pearson[35] as behaviors used by children to prevent aggression or to terminate play.

Id impulses do not achieve gratification unless the ego assents. If the ego instead applies controls, the id impulses must conform to reality, to ethical and moral standards enforced by the superego. To this end, the ego employs defensive measures that secure its boundaries.[8] Such was the case with Freddie as he effected an orches-tration of defenses that precluded pathological reliance on a single mechanism, as well as a pathological, id-governed state.

An examination of this child's defenses readily illustrates that he utilized all his energy and every moment of his waking life to exclude direct aggression from his behavioral repertoire. Further examination reveals a feature common to most of the following defenses—ambivalence:

1. Freddie's *body and bodily functions* defended him, as when he stiffened and extended his arms in an apparent effort to resist striking the nurse during tracheal as-

pirations. He also cleverly utilized coughing as a defense. Although he frequently required encouragement to cough productively to clear his airway, at other times he interrupted mounting aggressive activity to initiate an apparently unnecessary and nonproductive cough. On other occasions he was observed to escape similar involvement by excusing himself to go to the bathroom, thereby removing himself from the threatening situation.

2. As if prevention of intrusion might diminish the need for retaliation, he *resisted intrusion* several times by verbal and physical refusal to allow aspiration of secretions from his tracheostomy. He was resourceful in resisting. At least four separate attempts were observed: he placed his finger over the tracheal orifice; he rested his chin over the orifice; he lay on his abdomen as the nurse approached; and he delayed the nurse by complaining that her technique varied in minor detail from his mother's technique.

3. *Undoing* was also much in evidence. He apologized before or after an act; for example, he clung to and hugged me after his feigned choking effort, he patted the cotton ball tenderly after having injected it, and he announced to the boy doll, "Sorry, fella, but you gotta get a shot in the arm." This same defense was demonstrated in his need to alternate the pretty with the ugly or the good with the bad; for example, he wanted to make a lamb after having made a monster, and he drew a rainbow after having drawn a ghost town. On another occasion he frantically sought an eraser and removed his chalk drawing of a monster.

4. He *inhibited play* as still another protection against even fantasy aggression. This termination was achieved by at least three maneuvers: pausing temporarily within a game, replacing one game with another, and stating an absolute preference to discontinue the game.

5. Another common defense was *retreat*, escape, or withdrawal from threatening aggression. This, too, he managed in several ways, as became increasingly obvious during successive observations. Several times he expressed a desire to leave the scene of activity, for example, having repeatedly

injected the dolls, he said, "I wanna go back to my room." . . . "I feel like goin' back to my room." At other times he moved the aggression-generating toys either by setting them away from himself or by moving them and himself to a new location. A third mode of retreat was actually to walk away from the area of activity or to leave the room entirely.

6. Freddie's genius was still more evident in his successful *enlistment of external aid* during his aggressive play. As in other defenses, several variations of this theme were apparent. Among these variations were the use of one implement to push another, the solicitation of the nurse's approval or assistance, and the assumption of the doctor's identity during a fantasy of administering an anesthetic and performing surgery on a doll.

7. During the recorded encounters, Freddie also exhibited several instances of endeavoring to understand his aggression. This attempted *cognitive mastery* over aggressiveness was exemplified by the following verbalizations: (1) Freddie was cautioned not to throw dishes because they would break. He replied, "Dishes break. Do all dishes break?" (2) He injected the mother doll's and the boy doll's legs and fantasied: "Oh, oh, some blood come out. Some blood always come out of legs?" (3) When the father doll could not be stabilized in an upright position, Freddie queried, "Guess I gave him too much shots?"

8. Another defense, *reparation-restitution,* implied a turning of aggression against himself. He directed the affront "Cheat!" toward himself at the end of a ringtoss game; he disrupted his play with a question suggesting self-retaliation: "If the hospital was on fire, would all the kids get died?" More directly, he interrupted his oxygen supply by blocking his tracheostomy against his pillow and by depriving himself of the prescribed oxygen-mist collar.

SUMMARY AND CONCLUSIONS

The cumulative effect of ill-timed events in the physical and psychic development of one child has been described in this chapter. The child, Freddie, was almost 6 years old at the time of data collection for this study. He was at that time experiencing his thirty-second and thirty-third hospitalizations for removal of respiratory papillomas, which had plagued him since the age of 18 months. At the age of 25 months a tracheostomy was done, and since then he had required frequent tracheostomy aspirations for maintenance of a patent airway. Because Freddie exhibited a continually active level of behavior, an attempt was made to elucidate his activity as it related to his life situation.

The literature supports the idea that children view surgical intervention and intrusive procedures as hostile invasions, the possible responses to which might be either flight or fight. A review of Freddie's home life suggested cause for a similar response.

It became obvious that Freddie did, in fact, experience many events in his life as a threatening assault. His response to these circumstances, however, could hardly have been termed purely flight or fight; it was instead a unique combination of attempts to fight and to withdraw. The aggressive component of his behavior was largely evidenced by irruptive activity in excess of that which characterized his preschool-aged peers. This aggression was primarily of a controlled nature, but, nevertheless, it intimidated him so that he exerted a series of defenses against its expression. In addition, a theme of ambivalence was repeated sufficiently to warrant investigation.

The interrelationship of ambivalence and aggression was discovered to be especially influential in shaping this child's development. Because of his age at the time of diagnosis and institution of treatment and the body penetration achieved by each surgical procedure and tracheostomy aspiration, ambivalence actually became an integral part of Freddie's personality. The significance of this interrelationship is explained by Brody[22] and Mahler.[12] Brody states that ambivalence originates developmentally when the infant begins to replace passive with active libidinal attitudes. This is a salient concept because at just this crucial time, between the ages of 18 and 25 months, Freddie's developmental progress was interrupted by a subjection to enforced passivity and intrusive assault. These attacks were further perpetuated throughout a period when the toddler's delusional

magical powers and self-esteem ordinarily are vulnerable to exposure, a period in which physical contact is usually replaced by word and gesture in the toddler's rapprochement with his mother.[12]

This study was undertaken in an attempt to understand Freddie's behavior. This understanding provided several implications for nursing care. At least three implications can be recognized and are suggested here for implementation: (1) that the nurse should acknowledge the existence of forces operating within the patient, even though unable to identify each force precisely; (2) that the nurse should deliberately attempt to understand the forces governing the patient's behavior; and (3) that the nurse ought to allow the patient to exhibit his coping behavior, assisting and supporting him in this when indicated.

References
Books

1. Adler, A. E.: The neurotic constitution, translated by Glueck, B., and Lind, J. E., New York, 1930, Dodd, Mead, & Co.
2. Bender, L.: Child psychiatric techniques, Springfield, Ill., 1952, Charles C Thomas, Publisher.
3. Bender, L.: Aggression, hostility, and anxiety in children, Springfield, Ill., 1953, Charles C Thomas, Publisher.
4. Buss, A. H.: The psychology of aggression, New York, 1961, John Wiley & Sons, Inc.
5. Erikson, E. H.: Childhood and society, ed. 2, New York, 1964, W. W. Norton & Co., Inc., Publishers.
6. Fisher, S., and Cleveland, S. E.: Body image and personality, Toronto, 1958, D. Van Nostrand Co., Ltd.
7. Freud, A.: Normality and pathology in childhood, New York, 1965, International Universities Press, Inc.
8. Freud, A.: The writings of Anna Freud; the ego and the mechanisms of defense, rev. ed., based on translation by Baines, C., vol. II, New York, 1966, International Universities Press, Inc.
9. Freud, S.: A general introduction of psychoanalysis, translated by J. Rivere, New York, 1949, Garden City Publishing Co., Inc.
10. Josselyn, I.: Psychosocial development of children, New York, 1948, Family Service Association of America.
11. Lazarus, R. S.: Psychological stress and the coping process, New York, 1966, McGraw-Hill Book Co., Inc.
12. Mahler, M. S., and Furer, M.: On human symbiosis and the vicissitudes of individuation. Vol. I. Infantile psychosis, New York, 1968, International Universities Press, Inc.

13. Murphy, L. B.: The widening world of childhood, New York, 1962, Basic Books, Inc., Publishers.

14. Schilder, P.: Psychoanalysis, man and society, New York, 1951, W. W. Norton & Co., Inc., Publishers.

15. Schilder, P.: Contributions to developmental neuropsychiatry, New York, 1965, International Universities Press, Inc.

Periodicals

16. Aarons, Z. A.: Effects of the birth of a sister on a boy in his fourth year, Psychoanal. Q. **22:**372, 1953.

17. Albino, R. C.: Defences against aggression in the play of young children, Br. J. Med. Psychol. **27** (parts 1 and 2):61, 1954.

18. Baruch, D. W.: Aggression during doll play in a preschool, Am. J. Orthopsychiatry **11:**252, 1941.

19. Bender, L.: Aggression in children, Am. J. Orthopsychiatry **13:**392, 1943.

20. Bender, L., Keiser, S., and Schilder, P.: Studies in aggressiveness, Genet. Psychol. Monogr. **18** (5,6):357, 1936.

21. Bonaparte, M.: Some palaeobiological and biopsychical reflections, Int. J. Psychoanal. **19:**214, 1938.

22. Brody, M. W.: Clinical manifestations of ambivalence, Psychoanal. Q. **25:**505, 1956.

23. Calef, V.: Psychological consequences of physical illness in childhood, J. Am. Psychoanal. Assoc. **7:**155, 1959.

24. Erickson, F. H.: Play interviews for four-year-old hospitalized children, Monogr. Soc. Res. Child Dev., Inc. **23** (3), 1958.

25. Erickson, F. H.: Reactions of children to hospital experience, Nurs. Outlook **6:**501, 1958.

26. Fisher, S., and Cleveland, S. E.: Body image boundaries and style of life, J. Abnorm. Soc. Psychol. **102:**373, 1956.

27. Fodor, N.: Varieties of castration, Am. Imago **4:**32, Aug., 1946-Dec., 1947.

28. Freud, A.: The role of bodily illness in the mental life of children, Psychoanal. Study Child **7:**69, 1952.

29. Greenacre, P.: Early physical determinants in the development of the sense of identity, J. Am. Psychoanal. Assoc. **7:**612, 1958.

30. Hartmann, H., Kris, E., Loewenstein, R. M.: Notes on the theory of aggression, Psychoanal. Study Child. **3/4:**9, 1949.

31. Hollensberg, E., and Sperry, M.: Some antecedents of aggression and effects of frustration in doll play, Personality **1:**32, Jan., 1951.

32. Keiser, S.: Body ego during orgasm, Psychoanal. Q. **21:**152, 1952.

33. Loewald, H. W.: Internalization, separation, mourning, and the superego, Psychoanal. Q. **31:**483, 1962.

34. Neiderland, W.: Narcissistic ego impairment in patients with early physical malformations, Psychoanal. Study Child **20:**518, 1965.

35. Pearson, G. H. J.: The chronically aggressive child, Psychoanal. Rev. **26:**485, 1939.

36. Sears, R. R.: Effects of frustration and anxiety on fantasy aggression, Am. J. Orthopsychiatry **21:**498, 1951.

37. Sears, R. R., Pintler, M. H., Sears, P. S.: Effects of father separation on preschool children's doll play aggression, Child Dev. **17:**219, Dec., 1946.

38. Watson, E. J., and Johnson, A.: The emotional significance of acquired physical disfigurement in children, Am. J. Orthopsychiatry **28:**85, Jan., 1958.

39. Wurtz, K. R.: Some theory and data concerning the attenuation of aggression, J. Abnorm. Soc. Psychol. **60:**134, Jan., 1960.

16

Anne copes with open heart surgery

Marion H. Rose

Children's reactions to hospitalization have been the subject of many articles and books; however, there are few published descriptions of the behavior of children actually undergoing the experience of hospitalization. One notable exception is the classic study by Blake.[1]

In this chapter I will present excerpts from observations made on a child who had open heart surgery. These observations were made as part of a study of fourteen children who were hospitalized for surgery in a university teaching hospital in a large midwestern city. The propositions underlying the study were that most children have the capacity to cope with hospitalization and that changes seen in behavior during hospitalization would be temporary. The purpose of the study was to investigate how children cope with the experience of hospitalization.

In the study, data were collected on the fourteen children by naturalistic observations at home and in the hospital. Two prehospital and two posthospital observations were made on each child. The prehospital observations were made one to three weeks before the child was hospitalized, depending on how long before hospitalization the admission was scheduled. The posthospital observations were made during the second and fourth weeks after each child's discharge from the hospital. Each home observation was one-half hour in length. During hospitalization, two fifteen-minute observations were made each day; one in the morning and one in the afternoon. The observations, both at home and in the hospital, were made in five-minute segments interspersed by five minutes when the child's behavior was not recorded. Thus the half-hour home observations extended over an hour and the hospital observations over a half-hour period. Additional information about each child was obtained by interviewing the parents before and after hospitalization.

The study, which has been reported in detail elsewhere,[3,4] demonstrated that children, although different from each other, showed similar changes in behavior in the hospital, even though the magnitude of change was different from child to child. After hospitalization they reverted back to their prehospital patterns of behavior.

In most of the previous studies, hospitalization has been looked on as a total experience that was considered to be stressful. However, hospitalization is made up of a variety of experiences, some of which can be considered highly stressful and others much less stressful or even enjoyable. A number of factors contribute to the amount of stress children encounter. Some experiences are probably inherently stressful, such as those which produce a great deal of physical discomfort; however, the child's perception of the situation, his previous experiences, and the amount of support available to him also contribute to the amount of stress he actually experiences and to the behaviors he selects to deal with it.

The descriptions in this chapter illustrate how one child, Anne, coped with a very stressful hospitalization and how the behavior of others both supported and undermined these coping efforts. They also illustrate consistency in Anne's behavior under stress, both at home and in the hospital.

Anne, 4 years and 4 months of age, was a thin, pale, shy little girl. She lived with her parents and her two older brothers in a quiet middle-class neighborhood. Her maternal grandparents lived nearby. During the prehospital interview her mother said that Anne's usual reaction to strangers was as follows: "Very shy. Even if she meets them the second time, she will be shy. She has to know someone well to talk to them. If a person talks to her, she will hang onto my skirt and hide behind me."

With persons she knew well she was friendly and happy, and with her brothers she could be aggressive. She had very little appetite and still drank her milk from a bottle. Occasionally she used the bottle as a source of comfort, but usually she drank milk as she rested on the couch after physical activity.

Brief conversations from prehospital and posthospital observations will be quoted to illustrate Anne's behavior in her familiar home environment. The excerpts of hospital observations have been selected to show how Anne reacted during the periods of stress before and immediately after surgery, usually by retreating behind a wall of silence while still being aware of the world around her. However, the observations also show that as she physically recovered and was subjected to fewer procedures, she became increasingly more independent and animated, although she was quick to retreat to silence when she perceived someone or something in the environment to be threatening.

The following excerpt is from the first prehospital observation and demonstrates her silent but alert initial assessment of me.

> The observation begins in Anne's bedroom. She is sitting at a small table and has a headband from a nurse's kit in her hand. She looks at it and twists it around in her hand. Anne looks at the observer briefly, then back at the band.
>
> She leans her head on her arm and then sits up and puts the nurse's band across her eyes. She looks briefly at the observer over the top of the band. She holds the band to her eyes as if she is trying to see through it. She glances at the observer over the top of the band.
>
> This behavior continued throughout the first five minutes of observation.

Anne usually was an undemanding child. At times she disobeyed, but without making an issue of it. Following is an incident from prehospital observation 1. Other examples of this same type of behavior recur throughout hospitalization and during the posthospital period.

> Anne and her mother are in the kitchen. Mother is cleaning the refrigerator, and the door is standing open. Anne is playing with the light switch.

> Mother in a matter-of-fact way: "Don't do that, Anne."
>
> Anne stands and looks calmly in the refrigerator and then looks at her mother.
>
> Mother: "Leave the light alone—you'll get shocked."
>
> Anne turns and presses the switch and watches with interest as the light goes off and on.
>
> Mother calmly: "I know what you can do, you can put some things away."
>
> Anne stands and stares, then plays with the light switch again.
>
> Mother matter-of-factly: "Do you like to play with the light?"
>
> Anne: "Yes," and continues to play with it. Then she puts her foot into the refrigerator.
>
> Mother: "Don't put your foot there."
>
> Anne smiles at her mother and says in a teasing way: "I did already."

An excerpt from prehospital observation 2 illustrates Anne's behavior with her friend Vicky (about the same age) and her older brother Bert.

> Anne and Vicky are in the backyard playing. They climb up on a picnic table and stomp around and grin at each other.
>
> Vicky: "I'm on the yellow." (The bench is painted yellow.) Anne puts a foot on the other bench and says, "I'm on the yellow." They both seem to be enjoying this play.
>
> Vicky jumps down; Anne says, "I can do that," and climbs down from the table, but slowly and with some caution. Vicky jumps up and down but Anne just sort of wanders around.
>
> Anne: "Can you do this?" and climbs into the swing. Vicky is not paying any attention to her. Then Vicky goes over and begins to swing her. (It is a two-seater garden swing.)
>
> Bert walks over and begins to swing Anne vigorously. At first Anne seems to enjoy this, then she says emphatically, "Stop it." Bert stops, then pushes Vicky. Anne screams vigorously and angrily, "Stop it." Bert gives Vicky another shove, then goes back to pushing the swing. Vicky also comes and pushes, and Anne giggles happily.

Anne was hospitalized twice during the study. She was hospitalized for three days for a cardiac catheterization, which confirmed the diagnosis of atrial septal defect. After the cardiac catheterization Anne went home for the weekend and then was readmitted for open heart surgery. This second hospitalization lasted for twelve days.

Anne had little preparation for hospitalization. Before she was admitted for the cardiac catheterization, her mother told her that she had to go to the hospital to have a test before she could go to school. Prior to being readmitted for surgery, Anne's mother told her that she had to go back to the hospital to "have her heart fixed." Some preparation for surgery was done by the nurses and the inhalation therapist. This consisted primarily of explaining various procedures that she would be subjected to after surgery. She also had the opportunity to practice using the various pieces of inhalation equipment that she would need after surgery.

The hospital observations are in sequence over the period of the two hospitalizations and show how the pressures of hospitalization build up. What was tolerated the first time was anticipated and dreaded the next time. The difference in Anne's reactions to the initial finger stick for a blood count and her reaction to the same procedure at the beginning of the second hospitalization illustrates this point. But pleasant things also happened and could be anticipated and savored. Anne's pleasure with the doll she received from her father illustrates this point. The examples here show that Anne was both helped and hindered in her coping efforts.

The following two observations illustrate the difference between Anne's reaction to having her finger stuck at the beginning of the first hospitalization and at the beginning of the second hospitalization.

From hospital observation 1, first hospitalization:
Anne is in the laboratory, and her mother is in the adjacent waiting room.

Anne sits quietly, watching curiously as the technician gets the equipment ready.

The technician says gently, "I'm going to give you a little stick in your finger, O.K.?"

Anne shakes her head yes but without enthusiasm.

Technician says, "You remember that from before, don't you?"

Anne again shakes her head yes.

The technician wipes off Anne's finger, and Anne watches somewhat apprehensively. She looks up at the technician very briefly.

The technician says, "Say ouch," and sticks Anne's finger.

Anne sits tensely but does not say ouch.

The technician draws the blood up in the tubes, and Anne watches her intently, a slight frown on her face. She holds her hand out rigidly.

Throughout the remainder of the procedure, Anne sat quietly but very stiffly.

From hospital observation 1, second hospitalization:
Anne is in the laboratory waiting room with her mother. She is about to have her finger stuck for a blood count.

The technician calls for Anne to come into the laboratory. Anne backs away and cries. Her mother picks her up and carries her into the laboratory. Mother sits in the chair with Anne in her lap. Anne looks at the technician and cries, then leans back against her mother and whines quietly.

Anne sits up, and her mother says gently, "It'll be all right." Anne shakes her head no and whines.

The technician walks past her, and Anne looks at her apprehensively, then leans against her mother and whines quietly. Anne watches the technician get the equipment ready and cries.

The technician reaches for Anne's finger, and Anne pulls away. The technician takes Anne's hand and begins to wipe her finger. Anne cries loudly.

Mother puts her hand gently on Anne's forehead.

The technician sticks Anne's finger, and Anne cries loudly and jerks away.

The technician draws some blood into the tube. Anne watches her with a fearful expression and continues to cry. She snuggles against her mother, but she seems very tense.

Anne continued to cry throughout the remainder of the procedure.

The following excerpts are from observation 3 of the second hospitalization. During her first hospitalization Anne's father had brought her a doll, and Anne expresses her pleasure in her doll. This observation also demonstrates Anne's change in behavior when approached by potentially threatening persons.

Anne is lying in bed turned to one side. She is cuddling her baby doll and smiles affectionately. She looks at the observer and says, "My daddy bought the doll for me," and smiles proudly.

Observer smiles and says, "Didn't he buy it the last day you were here before?"

Anne shakes her head yes, looks pleased, and repeats, "My daddy bought it for me." She pulls the cord to make the doll talk, cuddles it, puts it at her side, and looks at it fondly. . . .

Later in the observation the nurse is in the room making Anne's bed. They have been discussing Anne's dog.

Nurse: "Is he bigger than you?" Anne replies proudly, "Yes. He's my dog."

Nurse: "Does he bite." Anne says hesitantly, "Yes, sometimes."

Anne smiles and looks around thoughtfully as the nurse makes the bed. Some doctors come in, and Anne looks at them curiously. . . .

A doctor says, "Can you smile?" Anne scoots back in the chair, looks slightly apprehensive, and looks down. Then she scoots around in her chair and looks at the doctors with a wide-eyed expression as they talk to each other.

One doctor leans over and feels her neck. Anne sits very quietly and tensely.

The doctor says, "Can you open your mouth?" Anne opens her mouth but sits quietly and stiffly.

The doctors say goodbye and leave. Anne sits quietly and watches them.

The nurse says in a gentle tone, "That's quite a few people." Anne smiles slightly and looks out the door.

Nurse says gently, "Wasn't there?" Anne smiles slightly and scratches her head.

All of hospital observation 4 is quoted, since it demonstrates how Anne became more and more distraught as the unsuccessful blood drawing continued and more and more demands were placed on her. It shows too that although not very happy about it, she could cooperate and even respond a little to the dentist who demanded little of her and did not hurt her. This observation takes place on the morning of the day before Anne is to have heart surgery.

> Anne is sitting in a wheelchair at the nurse's station. A doctor walks up to her and says, "Anne, there's something I've got to do. Let's take you down there [to Anne's room]."
>
> Anne gets out of the wheelchair and looks at the observer with a worried expression.
>
> The doctor says, "Why don't you go down to your room, and I'll be right down."
>
> Anne walks to her room and sits in the chair. She picks up a bracelet and looks at it.
>
> The doctor comes in, tells Anne he is going to draw some blood, and says gently. "It doesn't hurt too much." Anne looks like she is going to cry.
>
> The nurse comes in and says, "O.K., Anne, c'mon honey, just going to hurt for a little bit."

Anne begins to cry, and the nurse picks her up and puts her in bed, where Anne sits rigidly.

Doctor says kindly, "You're going to be a big girl." Anne continues to cry.

The nurse says something about Anne's bracelet, then "Here, do you want to wear it?" Anne continues to cry and look frightened.

The nurse says "Lay down," and gently pushes Anne to get her to lie down. Anne resists momentarily, then lies down and curls up as if to protect herself. She cries loudly.

The doctor says gently, "Hey," but Anne continues to scream loudly. She seems very frightened.

The doctor and nurse hold her and straighten her arm. The doctor says loudly, "Be real still." Anne cries loudly and looks at the observer, then at the nurse with a frightened expression.

The doctor feels her arm, and Anne watches him apprehensively. She is still crying.

The doctor says, "If you hold real still, it will be over faster." Anne screams louder and looks at her arm with a panicky expression, then looks toward the observer briefly.

The doctor says kindly, "Why don't you close your eyes?" Anne nods her head but continues to look and scream.

The doctor says, "Close your eyes." Anne watches with a panicked expression and screams as he pushes the needle in. He probes for the vein, and she watches him and continues to cry, but more quietly.

Anne looks at the doctor briefly, then at the observer, then back at the doctor. She cries loudly and seems very frightened.

The doctor gets the needle in the vein and says, "There we go." Anne looks at the doctor and continues to cry, but it is quieter and more mournful than before. She looks at the observer with a sad expression and sobs.

The nurse says in a soothing tone, "O.K., honey, that's the worst part." Anne continues to cry sadly, looking at the doctor, then the observer.

The nurse says, "Where did you get the pretty earrings?" Anne doesn't answer. She continues to sob.

The doctor and nurse change blood tubes. Anne cries louder, then looks around her with a sober expression.

The doctor takes the tourniquet off and says, "O.K., honey, I'm sorry." (He has not gotten enough blood and will have to stick her again.)

The nurse says gently, "One more time." Anne has stopped crying but looks soberly at the nurse and nods her head.

The nurse says, "Where did you go in the

wheelchair?" Anne stares at her sadly but does not say anything. She looks briefly at the observer.

Nurse repeats, "Where did you go?" Anne just looks at her soberly and cries quietly. She looks at her arm with a sad expression. She looks at the observer and cries sadly.

The nurse says gently, "C'mon, you want to sit up for a little while?" and picks her up and cuddles her. Anne sits quietly, then glances toward the observer. Someone walks past the room, and Anne glances out the door.

The nurse says in a concerned tone, "Are you still bleeding?" Anne does not answer, but she has almost stopped crying. The nurse gently rubs Anne's forehead as Anne sits quietly, looking very sad.

This ends the first five minutes of observation.

At the beginning of the second five minutes of observation the doctor and nurse are holding Anne as she lies in bed. The doctor is again trying to draw some blood.

The doctor inserts the needle, and Anne cries loudly and looks at the observer with a very sad expression on her face.

The doctor says, "O.K. now, we're in there. You hold still, and it'll be over in a minute." Anne looks at him briefly, then at the nurse. She cries loudly and seems sad and hurt.

The doctor repeats, "You hold real still now." Anne looks at him, then at her arm, then at the nurse. She continues to cry sadly. She glances briefly at the observer, then out into the hall, then back at the doctor. She cries sadly.

Anne continues to look around, into the hall, at the observer, at her arm, and at the nurse. She sobs sadly, then begins to cry loudly.

The doctor has not been able to get the blood; he takes the tourniquet off and says, "No."

Another nurse walks into the room, and Anne looks at her with a sober expression, then at the doctor, then back at the nurse. The nurse says, "O.K." in a gentle tone. Anne wiggles around and looks at the doctor with an apprehensive expression.

The doctor says, "I'll have to do it again." Anne cries loudly. The nurse says, "Now?" The doctor says apologetically, "I'm sorry, Anne," and prepares to stick her again. Anne cries loudly, looks briefly at the nurse, the observer, and out into the hall. She stares at the doctor with an apprehensive look.

The messenger comes to take Anne for another test, but the doctor tells him to come back later. Another nurse comes into the room. Anne looks apprehensively at the doctor and then the nurse.

The doctor says, "Let me try the other side." Anne cries. The nurse says in a teasing way, "Anne doesn't want to give us any blood." Anne does not answer and looks at the second nurse with a sad expression.

Anne watches the doctor as he gets a syringe. She looks frightened. Anne looks at the nurse with a sad expression. The nurse bends down and says something to her in a quiet tone. The two nurses talk, and Anne stares at the doctor with a wide-eyed expression as he walks around the bed.

The doctor says, "I just want to look at this other one again. I'll tell you before I stick you." Anne sits up in bed and cries loudly. The nurse sits beside her on the bed and lays her down. Anne lets her do this.

The nurse asks when surgery is going to be done. The doctor says, "Tomorrow, so we have no choice but to get the blood."

Anne looks first at the nurse and then at the doctor and cries. Doctor says gently, "I'm sorry." Anne cries.

The doctor feels for a vein, and Anne cries. She looks scared.

The doctor says, "I'll tell you if I'm going to do anything. Just going to look here." Anne continues to cry and looks toward the ceiling.

This ends the second five minutes of observation.

At the beginning of the third five minutes of observation the doctor is still trying to draw some blood from Anne. Anne is lying on the bed. The nurse is leaning across Anne to keep her from kicking, and she is holding Anne's hand.

Anne screams loudly and frantically and is lying stiffly.

The doctor says, "We're almost through." Anne looks at him and continues to cry.

The doctor takes off the tourniquet and says to the nurse, "I'll get someone else to try." Anne stops crying and stares at the nurse with an apprehensive expression.

The doctor says, "Sorry, Anne." Anne looks at him apprehensively and wiggles one foot up and down.

The nurse says, "Are you finished with Anne?" Doctor replies, "I'll send someone else in."

A nurse walks into the room; Anne looks at her with a frightened look and then looks at the observer briefly.

The nurse says, "I'll see if I can send her to pulmonary function studies." Anne sobs.

The nurse says in a gentle tone, "Here, let me go get a Band-Aid. Can you hold it [a piece of cotton on her arm]?" Anne holds the cotton on her arm. The doctor gives the nurse a Band-Aid, and she puts it on Anne's arm.

Two men walk in, and one says, "Hi there, big girl." Anne looks at him with an apprehensive expression and sits up.

The man says, "Have you been a big girl?" Anne stares at him with a sober expression.

He says with a smile, "I'm Dr. ————, the dentist. I want to count your teeth to see how many are there." Anne looks at him very soberly. He says gently. "I'm just going to look in your mouth. You don't have to worry." Anne looks at him with a wary expression.

The dentist says, "Is that a new bracelet?" Anne shakes her head yes and looks sober. He says, "Is it yours?" Anne shakes her head and says, "Yes." He says encouragingly, "Put it on for me so I can see how you wear it." Anne just looks at him with a sad expression.

The dentist says, "You don't want to, O.K." He touches her very gently as he says, "Don't you worry, we just want to look at your teeth, and we'll be all done. O.K.?" Anne just looks at him with a sad expression. The dentist pats her gently.

The nurse comes to the door and says to Anne, "The next time you need to go potty you come tell us first, O.K.?" Anne shakes her head yes.

The dentist says, "You want to lie down. It won't take very long," and reaches over and lays her down. She lets him do this, and he says gently, "That's a big girl."

The dentist looks in her mouth and says, "Some silver teeth. Where did you get those? They are nice." Anne looks at him soberly.

The dentist says, "Will you open wide?" and extends the tongue blade. Anne opens her mouth, and he looks in her mouth. He says in a gentle tone, "You've got 20 teeth. Did you know that?" She shakes her head yes. Smiling he says, "One for every finger and every toe." Anne nods her head. She looks very sad.

The dentist says, "Open wide again." She opens her mouth wide. He pushes at her front teeth and says, "Does that hurt?" Anne shakes her head no. Dentist, "Do any of your teeth ever hurt?" Anne shakes her head no.

The dentist tells her that he wants her to come to the clinic sometime, "O.K.?" Anne looks at him with a sad expression.

The dentist says gently, "You've been a big girl. Bye Bye, I'll see you later." Anne looks at him solemnly. He gives her a tongue blade on which he has drawn a face. Anne takes it and watches him with a solemn expression.

The afternoon of the day before surgery, the doctor accompanied by a laboratory technician returned to obtain the blood that he had been unable to get in the morning. Although Anne could not prevent them from drawing blood, she effectively delayed the procedure for several minutes. Following is the last five minutes of observation 5.

A laboratory technician and the doctor who had tried to draw blood in the morning come into Anne's room. Anne is sitting on her bed.

The doctor says matter-of-factly, "Why don't you lie down." Anne begins to cry, and the doctor lays Anne down in bed. Anne continues to cry, and she looks scared.

The technician says, "Would you like to have a lollipop?" Anne cries sadly.

The technician and doctor talk about how to draw the blood. Anne stares at them apprehensively and whimpers. Anne glances at the observer.

Technician says, "Did it hurt to put the holes in your ears?" (Anne has pierced ears.) Anne shakes her head "no." She is very tense. Technician says, "You probably don't remember when the holes were put in your ears." Anne looks at her sadly as if she is going to cry.

The technician says in a calm voice, "Make a fist." Anne makes a fist as she looks apprehensively at the technician who is feeling her arm. . . . The technician says, "I have to feel around down here." "Make a fist. Make it real tight." Anne makes a fist and continues to stare apprehensively at the technician.

The technician says calmly, "I have to give you a little prick, O.K.?" Anne shakes her head "yes," but looks sad. Technician says, "Then I'll get you a lollipop." Anne tries to smile but begins to cry slightly. She sits up.

Anne looks toward the end of the bed and then at her coloring book. She looks as if she is trying to keep from crying.

The doctor says, "How are you feeling this afternoon. Are you still coughing?" Anne shakes her head "no." The doctor says, "How's your nose. A little better?"

Anne suddenly gets out of bed and goes toward the bathroom. The doctor says, surprised, "Where are you going, Anne?" Anne says matter-of-factly, "To the toilet."

Anne stayed in the toilet for four minutes. The observation continues when she comes out.

Anne is lying down in bed. The doctor and the technician sit on the bed in preparation for drawing blood. Anne sits up and cries. She seems frightened.

The technician says, "You want a lollipop?" Anne does not answer. The doctor tries to lay her down, and Anne struggles and cries fearfully and loudly. The technician puts her down, and Anne screams loudly and seems very frightened. The doctor holds her so that she can't move her arm. The technician wipes Anne's arm, and Anne screams loudly and moves around in bed. She is obviously very upset.

The technician prepares to stick Anne with the needle. Anne looks very frightened and screams loudly and thrashes around. The doctor leans across her to keep her from moving and holds her arm firmly. The technician sticks Anne's arm with the needle, and Anne screams loudly. The technician begins to draw the blood into the syringe. Anne cries sadly but not so loudly as before; the tears roll down her face. She lies quietly but is very tense.

For the first few days after surgery, Anne was almost completely nonverbal. She was usually cooperative, although she resisted some treatments such as suctioning and the positive-pressure breathing machine. Following is an excerpt from hospital observation 8 when Anne was still in the pediatric intensive care unit; it is typical of her behavior throughout her stay in intensive care. She was in an oxygen tent, had intravenous fluids running, and was attached to a cardiac monitor. She had a stuffed cat in bed with her.

The nurse walks around the bed, and Anne watches her with a sober expression. A doctor walks into the room, and Anne looks at him soberly.

The nurse says cheerfully, "How are you, Anne?" Anne looks at her with a sober expression. The nurse asks Anne to cough. Anne looks at her with a sad expression.

The nurse rearranges the pillow and says gently, "Let's try that. Were you sleeping?" Anne does not answer. She sits quietly, then looks into the hall.

The nurse says in a cheerful tone, "Who gave you the cat?" Anne looks sober and does not answer.

The nurse rearranges the pillow and asks Anne to cough. Anne sits quietly with her eyes downcast toward the bed.

The following excerpt from hospital observation 10 demonstrates that Anne continued to use quiet persistent behavior that was very similar to her behavior during the prehospital observations.

Anne had heart surgery a couple of days ago and is still in an oxygen tent. Her father is visiting with her but has stepped out into the hall for a few minutes.

Anne is sitting in bed, leaning toward the door, apparently looking for her father. She is very solemn. Little by little she inches her way out of the oxygen tent.

The nurse comes over and puts Anne back in the tent, telling her gently that she has to stay in the tent.

Anne moans and frowns but allows herself to be put back in the tent. She sits very still, looking resigned and very unhappy about the whole matter. She gazes at nothing in particular and fingers her blanket. This behavior continues for a couple of minutes.

Anne looks around the room with a solemn expression, then she lifts up the edge of the oxygen tent.

She glances at the observer with a "wonder if you will let me do it" expression on her face. The observer does not respond.

Anne crawls out of the tent and to the front of the bed where she can have a better view.

Two days later Anne was out of the intensive care unit, but she was still in an oxygen tent and attached to the cardiac monitor. She remained wary of doctors, but when left to her own devices was beginning to recover her sense of humor and interest in her surroundings.

A group of doctors walk into the room. One of them smiles and says, "How are you doing?" Anne looks at him, a little glum and wide-eyed, and doesn't answer.

The doctor gently takes Anne's gown off. Anne lies very still, wide-eyed, watching him.

The doctor gently takes the bandage off her incision. . . .

Anne looks at her incision. She seems concerned but interested. Anne looks at the doctor and frowns. The doctor fixes an electrode on her chest, which is connected to the monitor. Anne looks at him and frowns. She glances at the group of doctors. She is frowning and looks very glum. . . .

The doctor puts her gown back on and asks her gently, "What's your name?" Anne does not answer and looks away from him.

The following episode took place ten minutes after the doctors left.

Anne is sitting up in bed, dangling her legs. A toddler is standing by the door.

Anne looks at the toddler and smiles widely. She glances at the observer and smiles widely. Observer smiles at Anne.

Anne looks at the toddler with a big smile. The toddler stands at the door watching Anne.

Anne glances at the T.V. For the first time since surgery she looks relaxed and happy.

The toddler walks in the room a few steps. Anne looks over at the toddler with a happy, wondering look.

The toddler scurries out of the room very fast (probably in awe of all the machinery).

Anne looks at the observer and grins. The observer smiles at Anne.

Later that day when her parents were there, Anne was animated and happy. However, when they left, life became difficult again, even with support from the observer and a nurse.

Anne's father tells her very gently that he and her mother have to leave. Anne immediately begins to cry and look sad. Her parents talk to her softly, trying to reassure her that they will return. Anne continues to cry softly.

Her parents leave, and Anne struggles to get out of bed. She is crying very hard and seems to be afraid. Since she is still attached to the cardiac monitor, the observer sits beside Anne and holds her hand. Anne continues to cry very hard, but remains in bed.

After a couple of minutes a nurse walks into the room, sits beside Anne on the bed, and talks to her in a soothing tone, "I know how you feel; when parents leave, all little girls cry."

Anne continues to cry, then she begins to whimper softly. The nurse takes her hand and holds it. Anne lies quietly but continues to whimper.

The next afternoon when her mother and grandmother came, Anne was again animated, talkative, and involved in play activities, but when they got ready to leave, Anne again became very sad. However, this day she was able to accept her mother's suggestions and take refuge in other activities.

Mother tells Anne that they are leaving. Anne begins to cry quietly. Mother says, "You're not to cry," and talks to her in a comforting tone. Then she says, "Papa will be here in an hour or two, O.K.? The boys will be home soon." Anne looks at her mother with a sad expression.

Grandmother kisses Anne. Mother pats Anne gently and kisses her. Anne sits quietly.

Mother says, "Miss Rose will play with you a little." Observer says she will when she finishes the observation.

Grandmother kisses Anne again and says, "Uncle Fred will come later." Anne looks around with a sober expression. . . .

Mother and grandmother say, "Bye," and leave. Anne says, "Bye," quietly but doesn't look at them.

Anne begins to paint and looks at the paint book with interest. Someone walks down the hall, and Anne looks up quickly. She screws her face up, as if disappointed that it is not her mother.

Anne stares at the book then begins to paint. She looks at the observer several times but continues to paint. Finally she says to the observer, "Later you can go around with me." Observer says, "I will."

Anne repeats, "Later you can go around with me." (She apparently wants to go for a walk.) Observer says, "O.K."

When the observation period was over, Anne remarked to the observer in a happy voice, "Almost don't see me in the hospital any more." The observer laughed and said, "That's right." Anne smiled and said, "Not going to be here long."

Two days later Anne was up and about most of the day; she was cheerful and appeared to be happy most of the time. However, she was still wary of unfamiliar people.

Anne has been walking around the halls, just looking and exploring the various rooms and equipment. She looks at a chair in the hall, smiles, and says something to herself about it. She looks into a room and says, "They're painting." She continues on down the hall looking around her curiously as she walks.

There is a boy sitting in a wheelchair, crying. Anne looks at him and puts her hand to her face as if she is distressed.

Anne walks down the hall, stops, and peers into a laundry hamper. She looks back at the boy in the wheelchair as if concerned, then wanders down the hall.

There is a boy, about 9 years old, in a wheelchair. Anne looks at him with a guarded expression. The boy says, "Hi," in a cheerful tone. Anne looks away and smiles at the observer uncertainly.

Anne looks coyly at the boy and then looks back at the observer. She backs around the chair away from the boy—still looking uncertain.

The boy says, "You want to play ball?" Anne looks down at the barrette in her hand. He says again pleasantly, "You want to play ball?" Anne smiles briefly at him and then turns away.

The boy picks up a ball and says again, "Want to play ball?" Anne looks at him shyly, twisting the edge of her gown. He says again, "You want to play ball?" Anne looks at him coyly and then looks at the observer uncertainly and twists her gown.

He says, "Come on." He seems to be puzzled by her lack of response. Anne looks at him with a shy smile, then looks down again. She moves cautiously away from him and walks down the hall.

Anne looks back at the boy, then wanders down the hall looking around her curiously. Anne walks to the nursery and stands on her tiptoes to try to see the babies. She wanders down the hall, peers into a laundry hamper. She looks at the observer and grins.

Later on the same day Anne again was happy and excited when her mother was there. Although still sad to see her mother leave, she accepted reassurances and looked forward to going to the playroom. She also seemed eager to show the observer her toys as her mother had suggested.

Mother and grandmother are getting ready to leave. Anne looks at her mother with a sad expression, as if she might cry.

Mother says, "You can go to the playroom. Miss Rose is with you". . . . Anne looks at her mother sadly.

Mother kisses Anne and says, "After supper your Daddy comes." Anne replies, "Are you coming again?" Mother says, "I come tomorrow." Mother pinches her affectionately on the cheek and leaves.

Anne yells, "Bye," then gets out of bed and runs out into the hall. Her mother is talking to the nurse, and Anne stands and watches her mother. Then she walks over to her mother and hangs on to her sweater. Mother reaches down and pats Anne's head as she continues to talk to the nurse. Anne leans against her mother, and mother strokes Anne's head.

Anne and her mother walk to the elevator. Mother says to grandmother, "Anne's going to push the button for us," and picks her up. Anne says, "Let me do it," and pushes the button.

Mother puts her down, kisses her, and says, "Now you show Miss Rose your toys." Anne smiles and says, "O.K." Mother smiles and says, "Papa will come in a few hours."

Mother says, "Bye," and she and grandmother get on the elevator. Anne waves and smiles. She walks back to her room and says to the observer, "I'm going to show you all my toys."

By the next day Anne had found a friend, a boy her own age named Lon. The following brief excerpt is from an observation made in the playroom.

Anne runs over to the slide and climbs on the barrellike top. Then she gets down and says, "I can't climb the horse." Anne says to Lon, "Move down, and then I can get on." Lon calmly moves down.

Anne tries to get on the barrel but does not make it and says matter-of-factly, "I didn't make it." Anne climbs up again and sits on the barrel sideways. She seems to be content. . . . Anne says, "Like the ladies." (She may be referring to ladies riding horses sidesaddle.)

Anne straddles the barrel and acts like she is riding a horse; she says happily, "I'm riding a horse," and smiles broadly. Anne says to Lon (sitting in front of her on the barrel), "C'mon, ride the horse," and touches him. Lon says, "O.K. Don't push me off." Anne bounces up and down and says, "Hey, this is fun, ain't it?" and laughs. Lon and Anne continue to ride the "horse," both laughing happily.

Even though the last few days of hospitalization were fairly pleasant, going home was eagerly anticipated. Throughout the last hospital observation Anne ran up and down the halls chatting happily with people and pursuing one of her favorite hospital activities, looking at and peering into things. When a mother of another child asked her "What are you going to have at home?" Anne smiled and said in a proud voice, "I'm going to see my big dog." Another mother said, "She is going to have a ball when she gets home." Anne replied, "I sure will and my cat, too."

Anne was more active and had a better appetite after than before hospitalization, both probably due to improved heart functioning. The following excerpt from the first posthospital observation demonstrates that Anne continued to act as if she were going to comply with directions but in fact frequently did as she wished.

Mother has been trying to get Anne and her brother to clean up the toys and papers they left lying around the living room.

Mother to Anne in a firm tone, "You clean up your mess too. Did you make your bed?"

Anne: "Yes." (It is not made.)

Mother says, "Go on, fix it up."

Anne says something about her brother cleaning up the living room.

Mother: "You clean it up. You made the mess."

Anne runs to the living room and watches her brother for a while; she then goes to her bedroom and begins to play.

Anne's mother reported that Anne was still concerned about the incision and insisted that it be covered by a bandage, even though medically there was no need for this. However, the following excerpt from the second posthospital observation shows a predominantly happy child.

> Anne and her friend Vicky are in the backyard on the swing. It is a very hot day, and the sprinkler is on underneath the swing, soaking both children.
>
> Anne cries out, "Let me down, let me down." (She is obviously uncomfortable because of the sprinkler.) Vicky does not stop the swing. Anne stands up and tries to stop the swing by dragging her foot in the mud. She cries out, "Let me down," and takes a towel from Vicky. The swing stops, and Anne gets off.
>
> Anne runs and hides behind a door, and both she and Vicky laugh. Anne runs to the basement, climbs on a tricycle, and rides around. She cries out in great glee, "It's slippery, it's slippery." She almost collides with her brother and screams, but it seems to be a put-on scream.
>
> Anne rides around the basement, a look of delight on her face. She turns to see if Vicky is still there. She continues riding; she seems to be enjoying this.
>
> She looks at her brother's bicycle and says to Vicky, "For sure you can't ride that one, it's Ron's." Vicky looks suitably impressed but does not answer.
>
> Anne continues riding, screeching with pleasure as she rides. She rides fast and says, "Whee-ee-ee!" She continues riding around very fast. She looks a little tired, but she is singing happily.
>
> Anne says to Vicky, "Follow me." Vicky follows her. Anne says, "I can do it [ride] better than you," and continues to ride around singing, "Speedy, speedy."

• • •

The preceding observations illustrate how one child coped with the experience of hospitalization and surgery. Casual observation of Anne might lead one to think that Anne would be completely devastated by this experience. However, consistent, long-term observations show that Anne had the persistence and resilience to effectively cope with hospitalization.

It is interesting to note the consistency with which Anne retreated to silent but alert behavior when faced with unfamiliar and threatening situations. Murphy[2] notes that children "stow away observations" to be used when circumstances are favorable

for an active response. Anne spent a large amount of time in the hospital looking, as if trying to get her bearings and to identify sources of threat. However, she also looked and then investigated because there were new and different things to see and feel, such as trash cans with swinging lids, wheelchairs, and babies in the nursery.

There were times though when Anne was not allowed to look and then to enter into activities as she desired. Observation 4 is an excellent example of how procedures took precedence over the desires and feelings of the child. Anne was obviously distraught, yet within a period of one-half hour she was stuck with a needle several times, told she would have another test as soon as the blood was drawn, asked to tell the nurse when she needed to go to the bathroom, and visited by the dentist. However, observation 5 demonstrates that even in a very stressful situation Anne tried to exert some control—in this case by disappearing into the bathroom. Since the physicians did not leave, Anne eventually had to submit to being stuck again; however, the important point is that Anne made some attempt to control what was being done to her.

Murphy[2] emphasized the importance of gratification as a means of tiding oneself over periods of threat or loss. Even though Anne was often alone, sources of gratification and support were available to her. Anne's parents and grandparents visited her daily, and when they were not there, she was able to find gratification in other activities such as playing with toys brought to her by her parents. Hospital personnel were another, although somewhat inconsistent, source of support. Anne particularly enjoyed her trips to the large, well-equipped, and well-staffed playroom. But most important of all was Anne's own ability to enjoy the world around her. Her frequent exploratory walks around the ward provided Anne with a constant source of stimulation and pleasure.

This chapter has presented descriptive data to illustrate how one child coped with a hospital experience. The other thirteen children in the study also coped with hospitalization in their own unique ways. It is apparent that the findings of this study based on fourteen children in one hospital cannot offset the findings of many studies that adverse psychological changes in children result from hospitalization. Nevertheless, the consistency with which the children in this study showed changes during hospitalization but reverted toward their prehospital pattern of behavior after hospitalization indicates that children do have the capacity to cope with stressful situations provided that they have some help and support.

References

1. Blake, F. G.: Open heart surgery in children, Washington, D. C., 1964, Children's Bureau, Department of Health, Education, and Welfare.
2. Murphy, L. B.: The widening world of childhood, New York, 1962, Basic Books, Inc.
3. Rose, M. H.: The effects of hospitalization on the coping behaviors of children, unpublished doctoral dissertation, University of Chicago, 1972.
4. Rose, M. H.: The effects of hospitalization on the coping behaviors of children. In Batey, M., editor: Communicating nursing research: The many sources of nursing knowledge, Boulder, Colo., 1972, Western Interstate Commission for Higher Education.

17

The prehospitalization visit to help a child cope with stress

Julina P. Rhymes

As a pediatric nurse, I have been repeatedly dismayed by the severe and unnecessary psychological stresses thrust on children in the hospital and by the seeming insensitivity of the staff in not providing protection. Sometimes health professionals seem to be habituated to children's distress and to the erroneous assumption that hospitalization must be traumatic. This chapter will address itself to one way of reducing some of these stresses for both the child and the parent.

Stressful experiences are difficult and potentially dangerous for everyone, but exposure to extreme or prolonged stress imposes a double hazard for a child. Unlike the adult, who has reached some physical, mental, and emotional maturity, the child is in danger of having his continuing development blocked or distorted by disintegrative reactions to stress. Physical illness or stressful experiences that make demands on a child that are greater than he can handle with his usual resources can interfere with the process of growth itself.[13] Moreover, unsolved childhood problems and unsuccessful attempts to cope with stress can cripple a child in his ability to handle future stress.[2]

All children experience stressful situations, even crises, while growing up. Even if protection from stress were possible, it would not be desirable. Growing up includes developing the capactiy to cope with stress and crisis. One's success in developing this capacity during childhood largely determines one's later ability to withstand life's inevitable problems. Successful coping not only permits continued growth but also helps the child to develop increasing capacity for struggle, triumph, and mastery.[13]

Many childhood stresses are part of normal growth and development—the usual difficulties of growing up. Experiences such as weaning, separation from home and mother to move into the larger world of neighborhood and school, and learning to tolerate disappointments are examples of these normal stresses. Others are out of the ordinary and carry a greater threat. Some are so great that a child exposed to them is in jeopardy. Hospitalization is one of the extraordinary stresses.

Whether a stress such as hospitalization becomes traumatic for a child will depend on his ability to cope with it. His coping ability in turn will depend on many factors: the nature and severity of the stress; his age and stage of development; his past experiences with stress and the degree of success of his past coping efforts; his understanding of the situation, as well as his interpretation of it; his ability to communicate his feelings about it; his ability to protest or turn away from danger; his overall vulnerability, resilience, and coping resources, including the use of defense mechanisms; and last, but not least, the effectiveness of human support available to him.[13]

Since hospitalization carries with it a potential for grave psychological trauma, those who are responsible for a child's care in the hospital have a twofold task: first, to reduce the destructive impact of the hospital as much as possible, and second, to help the child strengthen his resources for coping with stress. Ideally one should seek to make hospitalization beneficial rather than traumatic—a growth-promoting, integrative experience, rather than a disintegrative one. The idea of the possibility of hospitalization's being a helpful experience for a child is foreign to many people; nevertheless, handled creatively, hospitalization in some instances can be beneficial.[22]

The dual goals of reducing the danger of hospitalization and helping children to strengthen their resources for coping with it can be approached in two ways: (1) by manipulating, or changing, the hospital environment to make it as supportive and nonthreatening as possible and (2) by working with, or changing, the child in ways that will get him involved in his own behalf. For example, if a child is anesthetized in his room before being taken to surgery, the stress of the trip to the operating room is removed by a change in the environment. If, on the other hand, a child is prepared for the trip and supported along the way, change is being effected in him by the encouragement of his coping resources.

Admittedly a child and his environment cannot be separated, but an artificial distinction will be made here for the purpose of organizing the discussion.

CHANGING THE ENVIRONMENT

Gradually over the past twenty years, the hospital environment has been widely improved, especially with regard to liberalizing visiting hours, allowing mothers to room in, instituting play and educational programs, and, in an increasing number of hospitals, enlarging the staffs to include Child Life Workers.[8] However, only the beginning of an effort has been made to focus on ways to help the child utilize his own resources. Play programs, for example, whose goal used to be primarily to provide entertainment, are now becoming therapeutically oriented and are being used as part of the child's treatment.

INVOLVING THE CHILD

In working with the child, the nurse wants to encourage and to enable him to become an active participant in his treatment, rather than a passive, helpless victim of it. Using play to help a child express his feelings is one way to get him actively involved. Play is especially useful after a child has suffered a painful treatment or procedure. Another way to involve him

actively is to permit him some control over what happens to him, even if only by giving him a choice of which finger is to be stuck by a needle or letting him help to put a Band-Aid on it. Still another way is to help him mobilize his inner resources by giving him appropriate information before a stressful experience to prepare him psychologically.

RATIONALE FOR PSYCHOLOGICAL PREPARATION

Most authors who have written about or done research in the area of the psychological aspects of pediatric care agree that the child who is about to be hospitalized or undergo some upsetting medical procedure should be told what will happen, why it will happen, and what he will probably feel and that this should be done in a simple, honest, reassuring way in language that he can understand. The rationale for advance preparation is that unexpected stress is more upsetting than expected stress for which the child has had an opportunity to mobilize inner defenses. Misinformation or vague, undefined threats that are likely to stimulate frightening fantasies are more upsetting than threats that are understood.[23] Fear of the unknown is often terrifying. A hospitalized child may think that he has been abandoned or is being punished for some misdeed or that his body is being mutilated. Petrillo and Sanger[15] give an example of a 7-year-old boy, hospitalized for diagnostic tests, who believed that his eyes were going to be removed.

Even though children are, of course, made anxious by being informed of impending stressful experiences, the anxiety is based on awareness. Appropriate information diminishes the diffuse, bewildering quality of anxiety, making it more explicit. Being forewarned permits a child to look at his anxiety, acknowledge it, and thus make use of it. Although too much anxiety can overwhelm a child and be disintegrative, children, too, have defenses that can be mobilized to keep anxiety within bounds. One of our tasks is to help them use their defenses.

The manner in which coping is carried out varies with age and the individual. A child, in a healthy effort to master fears and other stresses, may use a variety of methods. He may make overt, direct attempts to escape or turn away from danger or he may seek help or support from others. He may cope intellectually, if he is old enough, by using acquired information to gain understanding of what is going on around him or use defense mechanisms such as denial, regression, or projection, or he might escape into fantasy. According to Hartmann,[9] one way of defining fantasy is as "a detour to the mastery of reality," and it is a useful one. These various methods of coping may be used singly or in combination to help a child maintain his integrity.[14]

In the hospital a child's attempts to cope with danger by actively turning away from it or fending it off are almost always thwarted in a crushing, destructive way, when he is forced by others bigger and stronger to submit to terrifying, often demoralizing manipulations. By offering the right kind of preparation and support, it is often possible, even with very young children, to enlist their active cooperation in treatment, thus eliminating the need to forcibly restrain and victimize them. Unfortunately, the majority of people who care for children in hospitals do not use preventive techniques. One wonders why, with our present knowledge of the emotional needs and responses of children, these practices are permitted to continue. Care of the whole child has always lagged behind advances in physical care and treatment, but some heartening changes are beginning to appear and are being made available as models.

Clearly, a new trend in pediatric care is emerging in which some of this knowledge is being applied. The child's intellect and emotions are being taken into account. The concept is not new, but the practice is. Imaginative play techniques using dolls and real and miniature replicas of hospital equipment, creative encouragement of self-expression in children, and enlightened techniques of supportive care are being used in a few hospitals.

Cited here are, in my opinion, some of the most valuable currently available statements regarding improvement of patient care. They are the result of pioneering work done by a few persons. Notable among these is the work of Petrillo and Sanger,[15] a nurse-psychiatrist team at New York Hospital. Working together, they have designed and implemented a therapeutic environment for hospitalized children. The account of their experience has recently been published. This is one of the few sources giving specific details about how to prepare and support children psychologically. The book is valuable not only for its clarity in spelling out the nature of hospitalized children's needs and describing specific techniques for care, but also for the authors' tactful, forthright account of their difficulties in overcoming staff resistance to innovation and change.

Another excellent guide to child care is the information contained in Plank's[16,17] recently revised book. Still another valuable document that describes ways a nurse can support and encourage active coping in a child is Blake's[1] beautifully written account of her nursing care of a child after open heart surgery. An additional source of information is the relatively new and rapidly growing national organization that addresses itself to improvement of the hospital care of children. It is open to all professionals working with children in medical settings. The organization, The Association of Child Care in Hospitals,* has annual meetings and publishes a newsletter in which members share new information and ideas.

PERSONALIZED PREPARATION FOR PARENTS AND CHILDREN

Another venture in the improvement of pediatric care, is that of providing personalized preparation for hospitalization. Giving a child information about the hospital before he is admitted is not a new practice, but the use of personalized visits of parents and children to the pediatric ward to which the child will be assigned is new. Following is a discussion of the experience of a group in which I was involved during 1966 through 1967. We brought 105 children and their parents to the hospital for highly specific, individualized preparation.

*Formerly The American Association of Child Care in Hospitals.

The program was instituted by a nurse, in collaboration with an interdisciplinary group attempting to improve pediatric care. Our aim was improved patient care and not research. However, to determine whether visits were beneficial, some information about the children was collected from observations, conversations with parents and staff, and questionnaires sent to parents after the visits.

From a review of the available literature and on visits to a score of pediatric hospitals on the Eastern Seaboard, I* found that prehospitalization preparation, when it was done at all, was most often done by parents and the admitting physician. In preparation they used books, brochures from the hospital, pictures, and verbal explanation. Not all physicians were adept at or interested in this type of preparation, and information given by parents is frequently inadequate or misleading. Moreover, the parents' anxiety may color the presentation of the facts, so that the child's apprehension is heightened rather than diminished.

Some hospitals take groups of school children who are not expecting to be hospitalized on educational tours similar to those of other community enterprises or service institutions. Other hospitals sponsor periodic tours for groups of children who are scheduled for admission. Some of these programs include puppet shows or other formalized presentations to familiarize the children with the hospital. Many programs are conducted by volunteers. Although these group visits are undoubtedly useful, they neither permit direct verbal exchange, nor take into account each child's unique needs and concerns. Because of the wide variation in children's adaptive abilities and life situations, even among those of the same age who are scheduled to undergo the same kinds of surgery, we must tailor our intervention to fit each family. We reasoned that individualized preparation is therefore preferable to group orientation and planned our program on this basis.

For personalized preparation to be effective the individual doing the conditioning needs to have a certain amount of knowledge, skill, sensitivity, and basic understanding of children. One needs knowledge of child development to know what a child of a given age is likely to be able to comprehend and to tolerate. Being able to "read" children is necessary to be aware of what a child is feeling and to learn enough about him in a short time to specialize the preparation for him. A certain quality of understanding—perhaps the ability to "feel with" the child—is needed for the skillful and supportive transmission of this kind of information.

In our program we brought each of 105 children who were scheduled for elective admission to visit the hospital ward to which they would subsequently be admitted. We excluded children who were scheduled for complex, intensive procedures such as cardiac surgery because these procedures require a different kind of processing. We were aware that the pediatric ward is a feared and, in reality, fearful place to visit. There were some very sick children and some frightening sights in this pediatric division. The child's eye would see other children hooked up to tubes and bottles, children with their hair shaved off, children with casted legs tied to overhanging frames, and children with holes in their windpipes who were fastened to machines. Although we fully expected these visits to be beneficial, we were not sure what the actual impact would be. At that time we knew of no one else who had used this method of preparation. Long before the 105 visits had been completed, we were satisfied that a trip to the ward prior to admission could be a positive, rather than a negative experience for children and their families.

A first consideration in planning a program of preadmission visits was to decide which children should be included and how long before admittance to schedule the trips. We arbitrarily limited our age group to children between 3 and 13 years old, not because younger children and adolescents would not benefit, but only to make our task manageable.

Timing also depends on the child's age. The younger the child, the shorter the time span required between the visit and his admission. Regarding this, Anna Freud[7]

---

*As the nurse member of the group, I conducted the visits.

makes the point that two factors need to be considered in deciding on the length of time between preparation and operation. If the preparatory period is too long, there is too much room for spreading out of id fantasies. However, if the time between preparation and surgery is short, the ego does not have sufficient time for preparing its defenses. After trying different time intervals, we concluded that, on the whole, children over 5 years old benefited most by coming in no earlier than two days before. The younger children were often brought in to visit the day before entering the hospital with good results.

Children were invited to come in by letters sent to their parents explaining the purpose of the visit and inviting them to telephone for an appointment. At the appointed time, they were met in the lobby of the hospital by the nurse who conducted the tours. Individualization began at the front door. We found that meeting the child in the lobby before he had a chance to see any other part of the hospital seemed to dilute the threat and in some way to make the visit safer. It also seemed to help the child to establish trust in the guide.

Since the tour was essentially for the child, remarks were directed to him. His mother was included in the discussion whenever it was appropriate, instead of the usual other way around. After the initial exchange of pleasantries, each child was asked when he would be admitted to the hospital and why. This was done early in the visit, not only because information of this kind is useful to the person doing the preparation, but also because it is a way of taking the child seriously, thus helping to establish trust.

From the lobby the child was escorted to the ward along the same route that he would follow on the day of admission. One of the chief benefits of this procedure is the confidence that the child gains when his admission proceeds exactly the way that it has been rehearsed.

Initially, we omitted the trip to the laboratory where capillary blood drawing is a routine part of admission. We were operating on the premise that the time to tell a child about a painful procedure is shortly before it occurs, not several days in advance. We subsequently learned that it is less upsetting to a child to be told that he will have his finger pricked than to omit a step in the admission procedure. This is exemplified by the following comments from returned questionnaires:

I should have liked to be warned about the blood count before admission to the ward. Having explained carefully to Peter the full admittance procedure, we were both thrown by this unexpected journey to the third floor and the wait outside a room in which another child suddenly screamed out in protest (as his finger was pricked). However, after that was over, everything went well.

He was not told about the blood test and felt that he should have been warned.

I'm sure I too would have overlooked the blood count as it was done on our visit; however, it turned out to be upsetting to Stacey.

Along the way to the pediatric ward, various items of interest were brought to the child's attention: the coffee shop where his parents would eat, a stretcher or wheelchair, staff members in various uniforms. It is helpful and less confusing to a child if he can identify workers by the color of their clothing—if he knows that the woman who serves the food wears yellow; housekeeping people, blue; and doctors and nurses, white.

On arrival at the ward, the child and his mother were introduced to the persons who were to have principal responsibility for his care. From there, starting where the child would start on his admission day, he was shown around the ward. While he was being shown the scale, thermometer, and blood pressure equipment, the procedure that goes with each was briefly explained. If temperatures are to be taken rectally, it should be explained at this time. This is important because, if he is unfamiliar with rectal temperatures, he can view this as an assault on his body.

He was then taken to a room similar to the one he was to occupy. If it was a four-bed unit, he was introduced to the other children, to whom the reason for his being there was explained. Children often remembered each other. Some initial contacts carried over after admission. Younger children whose mothers planned to stay with them were shown a room with a cot near the bed, and it was explained to the child that his mother would sleep near him while he stayed in the hospital.

Children were encouraged to examine and manipulate as much of the equipment as they wanted to. They enjoyed rolling the bed up and down, pushing the call light, talking over the intercom, and examining the standard contents of a bedside stand. These explorations, in addition to providing valuable information, contribute to a positive acceptance of the hospital. Most of the children who visited looked forward, perhaps with a mixture of apprehensiveness and anticipation of the now-known environment, to being admitted. After admission, they expressed enjoyment of many aspects of the hospital. A mother wrote the following in a letter:

Of course Gary [8 years old] did not care for the shots and the postoperative vomiting that he was subject to and would prefer not to have another operation, but the experience on the whole was good. On his first day, while being wheeled down the fascinating corridors to have an x-ray, he remarked to me, "I knew hospital would be fun, but I didn't know it would be this fun."

In 8-year-old Gary's statement is conveyed the feeling of being able to cope with what was happening to him, even though he knew it would not all be pleasant. For him, it was an eminently successful experience.

When visiting the playroom, schoolroom, and craft room, relevant equipment seen along the way was casually introduced. A trip to the ward kitchen to look at the food cart and trays is helpful. If the child will be eating in bed, it is important for him to know how this will be accomplished.

The bathroom is an especially significant room to hospitalized children. It is important to show them how to identify and differentiate it from other rooms (the door with the light over it or the second door from the end). A look inside the bathroom is useful too, especially if it has cubicles, which may be new and strange to a child.

It is important to show a child any toileting equipment that will be used in bed: bedpan, urinal, toilet paper, basin, soap, comb, toothbrush. He should also know how to close the curtain for privacy. Children are often fearful of using a bedpan, lest they wet or soil the bed. They need a simple, reassuring explanation of the way toileting in bed is handled.

The adult does not always realize that what he considers to be commonplace, inconsequential details of his surroundings are of great consequence to children. Knowledge about mundane items is essential if children are to feel able to manage themselves, and feeling able to manage is one of the basic elements of coping. There is a sizable discrepancy between what hospital staff considers important and what children consider important. The child worries little or not at all about whether the infusion has the right ingredients and a great deal about how to get to the bathroom, about wetting himself, or about how he will get help if he needs it. We need to pay much more attention to the things children worry about.

While the tour was in progress, the nurse was observing the verbal and nonverbal reactions of the child as he explored the area and equipment. She used these observations as a guide in talking to him later. The visit to the ward was treated more or less as a sight-seeing event, during which information was gathered and given, but not discussed. Clarification of what he had seen and a discussion of the events that would actually occur on the day of admission took place after the tour in a small private office. At that time, the child was invited to comment or ask questions. If he chose not to respond, as was often the case, an offer was made to tell him a little about what it would be like when he came to the hospital. At that point, children often changed the subject or in other ways signified that they did not want to hear it. The conversation, when that happened, was shifted to his mother or to nonthreatening, reassuring subjects, such as his right to bring his own pajamas and slippers or something of his own to play with—books, a radio, a favorite toy, or anything not too big to fit on his bedside stand. Many children wanted to talk about what they would bring from home. The information given the child from that point depended on his age, personality, reason for hospitalization, and his behavioral cues at that time. No two children were given the same information. In most instances, however, it was again made clear, even though the child had been told before, that his stay in the hospital would be temporary, that his mother would visit him or stay with him if that was the plan, and that the people in the hospital were there to help him.

In general, during this conference, the child was told, step-by-step, in a brief, nonthreatening, matter-of-fact way what would happen on admission to the ward, beginning with the initial screening by a nurse who would weigh him and take his temperature and blood pressure. From there, he was told, he would go to his room and get into his pajamas, not because it would be bedtime, but because the physician would come to examine him. It is good to let him know that he does not have to get into bed and that he can go to the playroom. A child needs a brief explanation of what the physician will do, and, if several other persons are expected to examine him, he should know that also. It is helpful to have a stethoscope, blood pressure cuff, and other equipment available in the conference room for him to examine. During the conference, all the routine activities and events that he was expected to encounter after admission were covered briefly, one step at a time: the examination in his room followed by activity in the playroom; a visit from the anesthesiologist; supper and bedtime, with juice before bed; his early rising and morning fast; his preoperative medication to make him sleepy; and a ride on the stretcher to the operating room.

If the operating room is not included in the tour, it should be described. Some of the books written to prepare children to enter the hospital are useful for this purpose.[3-5,12,18-20,24] Books of this kind should be carefully selected and are most effective when used in combination with direct discussion.

Children need to be acquainted with the clothing worn by operating room personnel. We gave our visiting children disposable masks to make the masks familiar and therefore less awesome and threatening. Anesthesia must be explained as simply and reassuringly as possible. One approach is to tell the child that he will breathe a strong-smelling gas that has an odor like that of airplane glue, through an apparatus that resembles a space mask and that the physician will ask him to count. He can be told that most children only count up to three or four before they go to sleep. It is important to reassure a child that he will remain asleep throughout the operation and that he will wake up afterward. He also needs to be reassured that no other part of his body will be operated on. A child who is scheduled for intensive complex surgery requiring that he wake up in an intensive care unit needs special preparation that must be done in stages, over a period of days.[19,22] This fact influenced us to exclude from this pilot program children who were to undergo cardiac surgery and other very complicated procedures.

None of our children was scheduled to wake up in the intensive care unit, but, if a child was to awaken in the recovery room, he was prepared by being told that he would wake up in a room different from his hospital room, that he would stay there only for a little while, and that then he would be brought back to his own room, where his mother would be waiting. He was told that he would probably be very sleepy for the rest of the day. Children who underwent surgery were informed about postoperative pain and told that the nurse would give them something that would make them feel better. We have found in preparing children for tonsillectomy that it is helpful for a child to be told that his throat will hurt so much that he will not want to drink but that, if he tries hard to drink little sips one at a time even if it hurts, his throat will improve faster. In our experience, most children who are prepared in this way become much involved by making a valiant effort and do have less trouble drinking after tonsillectomy than children who are told that they will have "sore throats" and be given ice cream. A positive note can be introduced by telling the child that he can have a choice of liquids, enumerating the possible choices. Allowing a child to make a choice is a way of encouraging active participation and lessening the victimizing aspect of hospitalization.

The specific way that each child is prepared and the choice of words used will depend on the style and personality of the person doing the preparation. Regardless of the style or approach, it is important for that person to be familiar with every procedure described, as well as with the techniques of each physician and anesthesiologist. Information given the child should, of course, be accurate, honest, brief, and reassuring. Too many details at one time will overwhelm the child. Moreover, for information to be assimilated, it must be repeated a number of times under varying circumstances.

A child's mental preparation begins when he is first informed of the necessity for hospitalization. At the time of the preadmission visit a new dimension is added. His mental working-through continues after the visit, which hopefully opens the way for continuing discussion with family members.

It is helpful to the person doing the orientation to know what the child's concerns are, but children are often reticent about expressing themselves and sometimes do not get the information they need the first time they have the opportunity to ask. A mother's questionnaire comment points this out:

There was still concern about where and what was going to happen to his tonsils.

The benefit of ongoing preparation is shown in the example of another child who had been provided a brief span of time between preparation opportunities during which he thought about his surgery, formulated questions, and worked up enough courage to enable him to ask them.

Robert (8 years old) came for his preadmission visit knowing that his hernia was a "lump" that his doctor was going to "get rid of." He also knew that he was going to be put to sleep during surgery. Robert's physician had talked to him about it a week before his visit. After having thought about it for a week but refusing to talk about it (according to his mother), he came for the visit wanting a great deal of specific information but was extremely hesitant about asking.

Obviously intelligent, Robert was nervous, hyperactive, and seemingly anxious at the time of the visit. He was inquisitive about and interested in everything he saw. He asked about the oxygen tent and the inhalation equipment. He read a poster in the lobby soliciting donors for the blood bank and wanted to know if blood would be given to him. Early in the visit, when he was asked if he knew why he was coming to the hospital, he said that he did not want to talk about it. After the tour, when given an opportunity to ask questions, he was hesitant. His first questions had to be relayed by his mother, since the only way he

could express them was to whisper them to her. How would the doctor get rid of his hernia? How would they know that he was *really* asleep before they operated? Before the conference was over, Robert had verbalized the fear that they would operate while he was still awake and that once asleep, he would not wake up. He ended the discussion by asking about less "emotionally loaded" topics, such as the food and whether his stitches would hurt.

Robert's questions were answered simply and honestly, and an additional measure of reassurance was added when, on the way out, he was taken back to the ward to be introduced to three boys who were awake and in good spirits after having had surgery earlier in the day. One of the boys had had a hernia repair. Robert's mother subsequently reported that he relaxed considerably after the visit. His hospital course was "uneventful" in the sense of the usual medical jargon but obviously eventful as an experience in mastery of a feared event.

The case of Robert also points out some usual fears of children in that age group. Although each child's fears are unique, some fears are common to most children and vary with different ages. Separation from home and exposure to strange hospital surroundings are the greatest fears in children under 5 years of age. For the very young child, the agony of separation is immense and, in reality, a threat if his well-being. In children between 5 and 8 years of age, fear shifts to the operation and anesthesia. Many are afraid of being put to sleep because they think that they might not wake up. They also fear the operation itself, as well as being injected with needles. In children over 8 years of age, fear of loss of control during anesthesia is a major concern. Some fear inability to control their own impulses; others fear losing control over the environment.[10]

Our initial apprehension about the possible traumatic impact of the visits was unfounded. Only one parent wrote that her child had seen something upsetting.

As we arrived for the previsit, there was a little boy at the entrance crying and crying for his mommie. This did upset Michelle and worried her. Perhaps the visits should be made when the younger children are napping and the older children in the craft room.

Although some anxiety was apparent in most of the children, many of them defended against too much anxiety by the liberal use of denial. Time and again, in the presence of something that could have been upsetting (from the adult's viewpoint), children found the fire hose, furniture, or some other commonplace, nonthreatening object a subject for examination and exploration. During the conferences after the visits, children were given an opportunity to talk about what hospitalization would be like. Many of them changed the subject and looked out the window to point to or talk about something outside. This happened too often to be a coincidence. One 5-year-old girl denied that she was still in the hospital, saying that she was in New York City, which was probably the most faraway place that she knew about.

Most of the children's questions were about safe subjects such as what kind of food they would have or whether they could have a television set. A few children wanted to know where their tonsils or adenoids were. One little girl wanted to know what "they" would do if she woke up in the middle of the operation. Other children were more interested in the practical aspects of the hospital. One child wanted to know how she could find her room if she left it to go to the playroom. Another wanted to know what to do if the bathroom was occupied when she had to use it.

Helping parents

Parents, as well as children, have fears, and they also benefit from this type of preparation. If a mother, for example, is helped to make positive use of her anxiety, the child is also benefited. If she is anxious and fearful about the welfare of her child, her feeling state may be communicated to and increase the stress on him. The communication of emotions between a mother and child may take place by nonverbal as well as verbal means and on conscious as well as unconscious levels.[6] Moreover, anxiety often decreases the mother's ability to help and support her child, and it is usually she who has the greatest potential for meeting his emotional needs, as the one to whom the child is most likely to turn. A previous study of nursing care demonstrated that mothers' anxiety can be decreased and their children's postoperative course improved by the provision of sensi-tive, personalized nursing intervention with the mothers at the time of their children's hospital admissions.[11,21]

Although the major portion of the preparation is directed to the child, during the course of the visit his mother will become familiar with the setting and hospital regulations. She, like her child, will benefit if warned in advance of possible disquieting events. It will help her to know that her child may be angry with her when he returns from surgery and that he may be cross, demanding, and irritable for the first day or two. It will also be helpful to her to learn that her child may have some blood on his face or gown if he has had a tonsillectomy. She should also expect that his behavior afterward at home may be different and that he may be clinging and fearful, have sleep disturbances, or revert to earlier forms of behavior such as wetting and soiling, depending on his age. On one of the preadmission visits, for example, a child with bright red sclera, resulting from eye surgery, was brought to the attention of a mother whose own child was scheduled for the same surgical procedure. She said that she was glad to have seen, in advance, how her child's eyes might appear, since she would be "terrified" if she were to see it without warning. Such subjects should be discussed when the child is not present or while he is busy on the other side of the playroom, perhaps, out of hearing.

A child's mother, during the visit, can be advised to be present before he goes to the operating room and when he returns. She can be told how to determine the scheduled time of surgery and how long he might be expected to remain in the recovery room. Many mothers need to be reminded, even urged, to approach nurses for help if they need it, even if the nurses are busy. This might be an appropriate time to discuss with the mother the feasibility of rooming-in, taking into account the needs of children at home. It is important to include fathers in the preparation as much as possible, since they too will have fears for the child, and they too can be enormously supportive.

The kinds of information that parents are given at the time of the visit will depend on the routines and procedures in a given hospital and on each family's particular needs. It is not always possible to know in advance exactly what will be done to a child. If parents ask for information that cannot be supplied at that time, very effort should be made to get it for them or to assist them in getting it from another source.

Five-year-old Juliet was brought for her preadmission visit a few days before she entered the hospital for diagnostic tests for diabetes insipidus. She was accompanied by both parents and a younger sister. Juliet was interested in everything, particularly the playroom. She did not show any recognizable anxiety; in fact, she did not want to go home but to stay and play for a while. When the option to room in was mentioned, her mother was hesitant and subsequently decided that it would not be necessary. Juliet's father seemed somewhat anxious and asked many questions about the tests that would be done. The nurse who conducted the visit did not have that information. She referred the parents back to the admitting physician, but the pressure of his busy schedule prevented him from seeing them before admission.

Juliet's admission to the hospital two days later went well. Her father commended the preadmission visit, saying that the whole family had enjoyed it and there had been no adverse reaction by either child. However, when hospitalization continued beyond their expectations and as more and more tests were introduced, Juliet became despondent, tearful, and angry and demanded to be taken home. Her father decided to room in with her to provide the support that she needed. He reflected that the rosy glow of the first contact with the hospital had worn off and that, as nice as the hospital was, perhaps Juliet should have been told that she would be subjected to an eighteen-hour fast and an intravenous pyelogram.

Juliet's preparation had been chiefly in the area of the pleasant aspects of hospitalization, and she was not sufficiently prepared for the unpleasant. In addition, her father's anxiety had not been relieved by supplying him with the information that he needed and wanted. Juliet's distress and her family's dissatisfaction might have been prevented, had her preparation included more direct and specific information about the tests. It is not always possible to foresee and predict all eventualities, of course, but every effort should be made to be as honest and specific as possible.

EVALUATION OF THE PROGRAM

Although not every visit was successful, we thought that almost all the children and parents who made the visits benefited. This conclusion is based on observations during the visits and discussion afterward and on written and verbal comments of parents and hospital staff. Several parents attributed a smooth, uneventful course of hospitalization directly to the preadmission visit. Pediatricians and other staff members made laudatory comments, and several pediatricians took the initiative in recommending the visits to their patients. The social worker who conducted discussion groups for mothers during hospitalization of their children reported that mothers often talked favorably of the visits in their group meetings and also seemed to be more comfortable during their children's hospitalization than were many mothers who had not made the visit.

The father of one child was a psychologist who wrote his doctoral dissertation on the emotional reactions of children to tonsillectomy. He reported that his 5-year-old son, who had been anxious and wakeful at night after hearing about his impending surgery, relaxed and was able to sleep after his visit to the hospital. Many other parents made similar comments, such as that the visit seemed to reassure and relax their children.

Several mothers wrote letters to the hospital administrator commending the visits. Although not all parents returned the questionnaires asking for their evaluation of the visits, all who did made positive comments to a question that asked whether they would elect to make the visit again if a child were to be hospitalized. All answers were affirmative, with numerous comments such as the following: "Very definitely," "Definitely," "Most definitely," "Oh, yes!" and "Yes, it helped considerably."

The following comments from parents are cited not as evidence of the benefit of these visits, since we are convinced from many years of experience of the importance of such a preparation, but as added substance for the reader.

[After hospitalization]. . . he showed no signs of being upset. He seemed to forget the discomforts very rapidly, and he seems to remember the visit with pleasure. He seemed to gain maturity and self-confidence. I was very pleased with the way everything was handled.

Roger (and his sister) enjoyed their visit and were very interested in everything, especially the school and craft rooms. They discussed it afterward, and Mary Anne insisted that now they play hospital with *her* as the doctor and Roger as the patient, since this was the way things would be.

John was very pleased to have been invited and told all his friends he was going, afterwards told everyone he had been, and all about it.

I was impressed and reassured by our visit and felt quite grateful that the hospital provided such a service.

One 7-year-old child came for a visit from a residential treatment center for emotionally disturbed children. He was brought by a social worker who had worked in the center for many years. She responded to the questionnaire as follows:

David's past experiences were such that he was most fearful of going to the hospital. It helped him tremendously to have the 'preplacement' visit. He was free to ask any questions he wished and to see for himself just exactly what the place he was going to was like . . . . I knew you had some very sick children on the floor to which David was going, and I was very fearful of what it would do to him to see them. Apparently he was so wrapped up in himself that they did not bother him. Either that, or he accepted the fact that they were there to be helped as he would be when he went. . . . My chief reaction to the visit was to wish this type of program had been inaugurated at least twenty-five years ago. I have been taking children to the hospital for a long, long time and have had to do all the preparation without their really seeing what I was talking about. They have had to take my word for what the place was really like and what would happen to them when they were admitted.

The parents who elected to make the visits were a rather select group. Most of them seemed to have above-average education. All were knowledgeable about the benefits of preparation. Every child who visited had been given some preparation at home. Even the youngest children knew why they were going to the hospital.

In several instances the visits were family undertakings: children were accompanied by parents, grandparents, siblings, and, on two occasions, by playmates. One father explained the inclusion of two older siblings by saying, "Tommy's hospitalization affects them too." A mother of a 7-year-old girl brought along a younger sister who was feeling jealous of all the attention that was being paid to her sibling. Another family included an older brother who had been telling the younger boy frightening stories about hospitals, even though he had never seen one.

Many parents seem to be resistant or reluctant to accept this kind of preparation. Of the 464 families invited, only 105 responded by bringing their children to visit. Almost all the children who visited were private patients. Parents of clinic patients tended not to respond to the invitations. Possibly the children who did not visit were the ones who received less preparation at home and therefore needed the visit most.

In addition to benefiting parents and children, the experience of planning and implementing the program of taking families on preadmission visits was challenging and rewarding.

In many years of nursing experience, I, as the nurse who conducted the visits, had neither before nor have I since enjoyed the same type of spontaneous, instant, trusting, seeking-out relationships that were established with the visiting children. They remembered my name and looked for me at the time of admission. If I was not there, they asked for me. Typical of the children's reactions was that of an 8-year-old boy admitted on a day when I was not on duty. He looked for me, even though I had explained that I would not see him until the following day. His dismay at not seeing me on admission was considered worthy of mention by his mother on her returned questionnaire:

One very important thing to John was that you were going to stop in to see him. He talked a great deal about it, and although you had told him you would see him on Monday, not Sunday, I had to explain to him several times that you were entitled to Sunday off. . . . With John, this was a promise that had great meaning, even though his father or I was with him the whole time.

It seemed as though, in the eyes of the children, the nurse who had taken them on a safe and pleasant journey had some kind of "magical" protective power. The importance of my presence, which was enormous on the day of admission, diminished rapidly as the children stayed in the hospital and continued to meet other "safe," nonthreatening persons.

CONCLUSION

The purpose of a personalized preadmission visit is to acquaint the child and his parents with the hospital and, according to their unique circumstances and needs, give them information about what they may expect during the first twenty-four hours of hospitalization. It also provides an opportunity for them to seek information, clarify misconceptions, and communicate their feelings about the experience. The fact that the hospital staff and the person doing the preparation are concerned enough about them to make such a visit possible increases their feelings of being supported over a difficult period.

This differs from preparation for specific procedures faced throughout the course of hospitalization. Ideally, preparation should be an ongoing process with additional exploration and explanation offered as situations arise. To be optimally effective, it requires the coordinated efforts of the child's parents, the admitting physician, and the hospital staff. In this effort, the nurse is a centrally important figure.

Children who are prepared for stressful events and supported through them will have anxiety, of course, but no trauma or greatly lessened trauma, and that is what we want to achieve. Moreover, if conditions are optimal, a child can experience hospitalization as a challenge to be met and mastered, and, if he copes with it successfully, it can be a maturing experience.

References

1. Blake, F.: In quest of hope and autonomy, Nurs. Forum 1:9, Winter, 1961-1962.
2. Caplan, G.: An approach to community mental health, New York, 1961, Grune & Stratton, Inc., pp. 46-47.
3. Chase, S.: A visit to the hospital, New York, 1958, Wonder Books.
4. Clark, B.: Pop-up going to the hospital, New York, 1970, Random House, Inc.
5. Clark, J.: Danny goes to the hospital, New York, 1970, W. W. Norton & Co., Inc.
6. Escalona, S.: Emotional development in the first year of life. In Senn, M. J., editor: Problems of infancy and childhood, Packanack Lake, N. J., 1953, Foundation Press, p. 11.
7. Freud, A.: The role of bodily illness in the mental life of children. In Psychoanalytic study of the child, vol. VII, New York, 1952, International Universities Press, Inc., p. 75.
8. Haller, J. A., editor: The hospitalized child and his family, Baltimore, Md., 1967, The Johns Hopkins Press, pp. 79-117.
9. Hartman, H.: Ego psychology and the problem of adaptation, New York, 1958, International Universities Press, Inc., p. 18.
10. Jessner, L., Bloom, G. E., and Waldfogel, S.: Emotional implications of tonsillectomy and adenoidectomy on children. In Psychoanalytic study of the child, New York, 1952, International Universities Press, Inc., p. 141.
11. Mahaffy, P. R., Jr.: Effects of hospitalization on children admitted for tonsillectomy and adenoidectomy, Nurs. Res. 14:12, 1965.
12. Jimmy and Susie at the hospital (Wonder Book No. 686), New York, 1969, Media Medica, Inc.
13. Murphy, L. B.: Preventive implications of development in the pre-school years. In Caplan, G., editor: Prevention of mental disorders in children, New York, 1961, Basic Books, Inc., Publishers, pp. 218-248.
14. Murphy, L. B.: The problem of defense and the concept of coping. In Anthony, E. J., and Koupernik, C., editors: The child in his family, New York, 1970, Interscience Publishers, Inc., pp. 65-86.
15. Petrillo, M., and Sanger, S.: Emotional care of hospitalized children, Philadelphia, 1972, J. B. Lippincott Co.
16. Plank, E.: Working with children in hospitals; a guide for the professional team, Cleveland, 1971, The Press of Case Western Reserve University.
17. Plank, E.: Working with children in hospitals, ed. 2, Chicago, 1971, Year Book Medical Publishers, Inc.
18. Ray, A., and Ray, H. A.: Curious George goes to the hospital, New York, 1966, Houghton Mifflin Co.
19. Sever, J. A.: Johnny goes to the hospital, Boston, 1953, Houghton Mifflin Co.
20. Shay, A.: What happens when you go to the hospital, Chicago, 1969, The Reilly & Lee Co.
21. Skipper, J. K., Leonard, R. C., and Rhymes, J: Child hospitalization and social interaction; an experimental study of mothers' feelings of stress, adaptation, and satisfaction, Med. Care 6:496, 1968.
22. Solnit, H. J.: Hospitalization, an aid to physical and psychological health in childhood, A.M.A. J. Dis. Child. 99:155, 1960.
23. Vernon, D. T. A., Foley, J. M., Sipowicz, M. H., and Schulman, J. L.: The psychological responses of children to hospitalization and illness; a review of the literature, Springfield, Ill., 1965, Charles C Thomas, Publisher, pp. 9-24.
24. Weber, A.: Elizabeth gets well, New York, 1970, Thomas Y. Crowell Co.

Maternity nursing

with an introduction by
Edith H. Anderson

Maternity nursing preserves and fosters optimal health of mothers, infants, and families during the period of childbearing. In this section authors present a wide range of topics in maternity nursing that have implications for all phases of the life cycle.

Raising the level of conscious awareness is the approach Tanner advocates to human sexuality as a means of developing understanding of self and others. She explores how nursing can help people reach the full potential of the human personality through counseling.

Caring is the key to Buten's philosophy of nursing directed toward quality nursing of women during labor and delivery. Affonso uses a model of pain to develop a guide to assess pain during labor and to plan nursing intervention based on individual needs.

Monitoring labor contractions and fetal heart tones is now widely used. Luckner views monitoring as a tool to assess and to predict the outcome of labor, thus reducing fetal mortality. She underscores the significance of the nurse as a facilitator in managing labor with a new degree of precision afforded by monitoring.

A maternity nurse clinical specialist writes about the development of her role as a counselor, teacher, and consultant to staff. Fowler's sensitivity as a practitioner comes through as she gives illustrations of her work with families.

Starting with the premise that the mother is the environment of the fetus, Strickland describes the state of knowledge of fetal environmental hazards and its application in the prevention of fetal defects.

In a clinical study, Walker identifies the concerns, conflicts, and strengths of mothers during the postpartum period. Not content to allow her findings to remain on a shelf, Walker describes how she presented her findings to a maternity nursing service and gained acceptance in initiating a teaching program based on individual family needs.

Changing the system is no easy task. Lytle describes how planned change was introduced into a maternity hospital. Her strategies and analyses should give inspiration to all caught in an unresponsive hospital system. Change can be brought about by intelligent, diligent professional nurses whose aim is to improve the nursing of mothers, infants, and families.

The academic discipline of religion can assist the nursing profession in resolving conflicts between the professional role and an individual's religious convictions. Accordingly, Milhaven, a Christian ethicist, and his wife, a nursing service administrator, respond to the conflict of nurses who believe that abortion is murder.

18

The maternity nurse as counselor in human sexuality

Leonide M. Tanner

In a time of expanding horizons in nursing the role of the maternity nurse is also reaching out into new dimensions. No longer exclusively focused on care of the pregnant and postpartum woman, maternity nursing in recent years has developed a broader concern for the family unit during the reproductive experience. This movement first encompassed the role of the husband, soon included the adaptation of the family unit to its new member, and recently involved variations on the theme such as contraceptive counseling and care of the abortion patient. Concern for increasing the quality and the personal meaning of the childbearing experience has also characterized the new dimensions of maternity nursing. This is illustrated by the growth of prepared childbirth classes, husband participation in labor and delivery, and mother-baby couple care (a revised method of rooming-in) on the postpartum unit. Recently the most noted extension of the role is that of the emerging maternity nurse practitioner, who provides physical assessment, diagnosis, and screening, as well as teaching and counseling for low-risk pregnant patients.

Moving into the field of human sexuality seems another natural expansion of the maternity nurse's role. Maternity nurses are already vitally involved in all aspects of the reproductive experience, which is one particular expression of sexuality. They now consider family planning an integral part of their role, and although contraception permits a family to limit its size, it is also undeniably a potentiator of the sexual experience. In fact, sex is so central to our specialty field it is a wonder recognition has been so slow in coming. Being informed about human sexual functioning

and understanding its complex relationship to family interaction and reproductive problems seems an increasing necessity for good practice of maternity nursing.

There are numerous ways in which sexual concerns of the patient come to the attention of the maternity nurses. Probably the most frequent source is the family planning clinic, where confusion and misconceptions about both sex and contraception are discovered in the course of counseling about use, advantages, and disadvantages of various methods. Prenatal and postpartal clinics are also areas where sexual myths and fallacies can be uncovered, especially in relation to the effects on the baby and the "safe" period while breast-feeding. Even in the labor room, important cues of how a woman feels about herself as a sexual person are available to the perceptive nurse. Does the patient give herself cooperatively to the natural rhythms of labor, or does she fight them with fear, tension, withdrawal, and aversion? On the postpartum unit, a surprising number of sexual concerns can be brought to light with the right atmosphere. In routine postpartal contraceptive counseling one woman made the amazing statement: "I've just had my third baby after five years of marriage, and I've never had an orgasm." Obviously, many problems related to sex surface in youth or free clinics, specifically during venereal disease diagnosis and treatment, pregnancy testing, and abortion counseling.

The need for maternity nursing to extend into the area of sexual counseling is immense. The question to be answered is how? At least initially, the nurse's contribution could probably be twofold: First, the nurse could be a major source of education and information about sexuality. If possessing broad and accurate knowledge, the maternity nurse in numerous points of contact with patients could help dispel sexual myths, fallacies, and misconceptions that have negative influence on sexual experiences. Second, the nurse could function as an important screening agent in the recognition of more serious sexual problems. Identification of sexual inadequacies and helping the couple recognize and accept their need for help would be a great service to these distressed individuals. The nurse would need to be informed about sources of referral for therapy for such sexual problems.

The maternity nurse can perform another frontline service in a more informal way. Many times friends, students, and colleagues seek sex-related advice from maternity nurses because they are perceived to be in a key position to understand problems in sexuality and femininity. As a sympathetic source of accurate information, the nurse could do much in helping individuals grow in both their personal adjustment and professional expertise.

Unfortunately, few nursing curricula include courses in human sexuality. Even information on contraception is a recent and by no means universal addition. Maternity nurses do have a solid foundation in reproductive anatomy and physiology, including full understanding of the processes of menstruation, fertilization, pregnancy, labor and delivery, and involution. From this base line, what are the needs of the nurse who wants to become a skilled counselor in human sexuality?

THE NEED FOR INFORMATION

The nurse's first need is to seek information about human sexuality from books, articles, regular or extension university courses, workshops, and symposia. Most of these have mushroomed recently, and the nurse might be surprised by the extent of the literature and the numerous educational opportunities available. Questions about quality and reliability inevitably arise.

Workshops, symposia, and courses offered by reputable organizations and by colleges and universities can usually be re-

lied on to be accurate and professional. Some such sponsoring organizations are university medical, social science, psychology, or nursing extension departments; the state medical or nursing associations; Planned Parenthood–World Population; and the Sex Information and Education Council of the United States (SIECUS). A number of professional periodicals such as the following contain varying amounts of information related to sexuality and sexual problems:

> *Medical Aspects of Human Sexuality*
> *Journal of Marriage and the Family*
> *The Journal of Social Issues*
> *Journal of the American Psychoanalytic Society*
> *Journal of Nervous and Mental Disease*
> *Social Problems*
> *Psychology Today* (semiprofessional)

In the quest for information a large number of topics should be included. Of primary importance is attaining full knowledge and understanding of the anatomy and physiology of human sexual response, including the excitement, plateau, orgasmic, and resolution phases as documented by Masters and Johnson.[3] The functions of the organs involved, such as skin, breasts, clitoris, vagina, uterus, penis, scrotum, and testes, also have to be understood. The role of fantasy and other psychological factors affecting sexual response such as guilt, fear of inadequacy, negative associations, inhibitions, distractions, and fear of discovery are important in understanding variations in sexual response.

Early sexual experiences, including masturbation, nocturnal emissions, and menstruation, play a key role in shaping sexual response. The first experience(s) of intercourse may have profound effects on later sexual functioning. The nurse requires an understanding of the techniques of sexual arousal, positions of sexual intercourse, and their various advantages and uses. Sex during pregnancy and postpartum is of special concern, primarily regarding the best practices for mother and baby. Sexual response in the later years is another area full of prejudices and misunderstanding, and the nurse needs to appreciate the normality and significance of sex, as well as sexual problems, among the aged.

Understanding homosexuality is threatening to many nurses, and some feel uncomfortable or are unable to take care of homosexual patients. Currently there is much dissent regarding the abnormality of homosexuality: whether it is truly a pathological sexual adaptation, and whether it is biochemical or psychogenic in origin. The frequency of homosexual contact among both men and women at some point in their lives and Kinsey's continuum of sexuality ranging from exclusively heterosexual to exclusively homosexual, with many gradations of bisexuality in between, lead some to perceive homosexuality as a variation within a broad range of normal choices of sexual objects. Others believe homosexuality to be an abnormal variation of sexual object choice, largely on the basis of the psychopathology of family relationships in the child's developmental years. The homosexual's psychosexual development is thought to be arrested at an immature level without progression to full, mature sexual expression.[6] The frequency of personal maladaptation and neurosis with accompanying symptoms of distress contributes to the idea of homosexuality as abnormal. However, the effects of social disapproval and discrimination must not be overlooked as a source of maladaptation. The nurse should become familiar with the controversy surrounding homosexuality and recognize the social movement presently underway for acknowledging the rights of homosexual persons. When there are signs of personal conflict or distress on the part of the homosexual, the nurse should be ready to respond to the need for therapy.

It is helpful for the nurse to be informed about unusual sexual practices, although what is considered abnormal is often a matter of interpretation. Some of the practices most commonly labeled "aberrations" include sadism, masochism, exhibitionism, transvestism, transsexualism, pedophilia, and fetishism. There are many more rare and exotic sexual practices that are infrequently seen. These and the more common practices just listed are frequently associated with psychopathology and are within the province of the psychiatrist.

Developing an appreciation of the importance of sexuality in human relationships should be a basic outgrowth of the nurse's pursuit of knowledge. Sexuality plays a major role in masculine and feminine identity, contributes to full self-realization as a mature man or woman, and shapes the individual's mode of interaction. Through the process of giving and receiving, which is the foundation of sexual interaction, there is an enhancement of love and affection between the partners and a mutual gratification growing out of a reciprocal interpersonal relationship. The greatest intimacy between persons comes in a relationship in which all aspects of the personality are involved and shared, including the sexual.

One other important area of knowledge concerns sexual misinformation. The nurse needs knowledge to dispel the myths and fallacies so predominant in popular thinking, which interfere with sexual fulfillment or contribute to destructive or unhappy sexual relationships. There are a multitude of such myths; but it is not the purpose of this chapter to discuss them in detail. However, here are some common fallacies the nurse should have the knowledge to refute:

"Nice" women do not enjoy sex.

Sex is only justified for procreation.

There are only so many sexual experiences in a lifetime, and when they are used up, sexual activity is over.

Sexual intercourse should be avoided during pregnancy.

Oral-genital sex between a man and a woman indicates homosexual tendencies.

Virginity of the woman is an important factor in the success of a marriage.

There is a difference between vaginal and clitoral orgasms.

A large penis is important to a woman's sexual gratification.

Simultaneous orgasms are more satisfying than those experienced separately.

Menopause or hysterectomy terminates a woman's sex life.

It is dangerous to have intercourse during menstruation.

Sex desire and ability decrease markedly after 40 to 50 years of age.[5]

Books present a formidable challenge to the nurse wishing to become knowledgeable about sexuality. The challenge comes from sheer numbers alone and from the necessity to screen out unreliable, commercial, and outright pornographic material. Sexuality is an area that is extremely vulnerable to exploitation, as a large number of enterprising authors have found. Reliable professional sources provide books of quality and accuracy, such as those published by university presses, reputable professional publishing houses, PPWP, SIECUS, and the Association for the Study of Abortion. The popular books now flooding the market are of variable quality; probably their content should be checked against the professional sources.

Absolutely essential reading for any nurse who is increasing her knowledge of human sexuality are the two books by Masters and Johnson,[3,4] *Human Sexual Response* and *Human Sexual Inadequacy;* they stand out as the classic biological research in the field. Much of what is known scientifically about the biophysiology of human sexuality is contained in these books. Although technical, the books are not difficult reading for those with a background in the health profession. They are worthy additions to the libraries of nurses who work with couples and families.

Two other reliable professional books that cover a broad range of material related to sexuality and sexual problems are SIECUS's *Sexuality and Man,* and McCary's *Human Sexuality.*[5] Both of these books are written in language that lay persons can readily understand and could serve as a basic introduction to the field.

Reading popular books is recommended for several reasons. The informed nurse should be aware of what material the public is reading and what ideas and misperceptions might result from this. Some popular literature is informative, going into detail about sexual techniques, which professional sources usually avoid. Some are entertaining, combining humor, information, and advice in an uproarious fashion. These can also serve to desensitize the nurse to highly-charged sexual material and help her feel more comfortable thinking and talking about sex. There are real dangers in popular books, however, especially when they contain inaccurate, prejudicial, or "half-truth" types of information. Often written tongue in cheek, such books may only increase sexual inadequacies or dysfunctions if taken literally or too seriously. There

are always those popular books that are truly pornographic in the worst sense of the word, which in their vulgar approach manage to make sex as "dirty and bad" as puritan admonitions would have it.

Berne has a delightful "last word" on the subject of pornography, which he says comes in three variations:

(1) Literary realism (Joyce's *Ulysses,* Roth's *Portnoy's Complaint*). This includes books worth reading for themselves, which happen to contain sexual scenes.
(2) Erotica (found nowadays in reputable bookstores). These come as paperbacks with well-designed jackets and evocative titles. Their purpose is erotic stimulation of a reasonably healthy variety, buried with at least a pretence of style in some sort of plausible plot. *Evergreen* magazine belongs about halfway between (1) and (2).
(3) Filth (found in cigar stores that sell racing forms). This comes in paperbacks with plain covers and titles that are either common street slang or low-grade puns. They are often proctoscopic and are usually bummers.*

A brief review of some of the better professional and best-selling popular books is included at the end of this chapter.

THE NEED FOR SELF-AWARENESS

To be effective counselors, nurses must first be comfortable with themselves as sexual persons, with their feelings about sexuality and about discussing this emotional subject. They should become aware of their own attitudes toward sexuality—blind spots, prejudices, hang-ups, misconceptions—as well as their positive and healthy feelings. This is no easy task for most nurses, with the influence of their nursing education compounding their middle-class morality. All societies and every culture have in some way attempted to control sexual expression. As a result, no sex is truly natural and unhampered among humans. In our society the Judeo-Christian ethic and puritanical influences have led to repressive and negative attitudes toward sex: that it is "dirty" because it is closely associated with excretive areas of the body, that it is "bad" and "sinful" except under certain carefully spelled-out conditions, and that it is "abnormal" unless prescribed practices are followed between persons in certain relation-

---

*From Berne, E.: Sex in human loving, New York, 1971, Pocket Books, Simon & Schuster, Inc., p. 226.

ships. Such attitudes have led to a high degree (in up to 50% of all marriages, according to Masters and Johnson[4]) of sexual dysfunction in this country.

Basically, the nurse must come to grips with the idea that *sex is good.* The human personality develops along lines of sexuality, as illustrated by Freud's psychosexual theory of personality and Erikson's psychosocial theory, which describes how sexuality fits into the sense of identity and the eight stages of psychological development in man. Sex is not only good but also good for you. A large number of physical complaints have been shown to result from channeled sexual frustration. Cardiologists now believe that heart attacks are less frequent among those with regular sexual expression. Certainly marriages with full and satisfying sexual relationships are happier, for it is difficult for a couple to be truly compatible if one or both are sexually frustrated or unfulfilled. The sexual system is as much a part of the person as the digestive, respiratory, and cardiovascular systems, but it has more pervasive effects because it is pivotal in personality development and is a key to psychological condition.

Sexual drives are present in all of us; they are an integral part of our being and a source of identity, self-esteem, and pleasure. Except for the few who sublimate these drives in the service of an ideology, people strive throughout their lives with varying degrees of success to satisfy their sexual needs. Everyone has "conditions" attached to sexual fulfillment, but as professionals, nurses should not impose their "conditions" on others.

What of sexual abnormalities? Or sexual deviations? Most of what we think of today as aberrations is the result of legal and moral definitions growing out of the Judeo-Christian ethic. All types of practices have been considered normal in other societies, from the Eskimo's sharing of his wife with his guest as a sign of hospitality to the islander's practice of the father initiating his daughter into intercourse as a preparation for marriage. A broad definition of normal sexual expression is necessary. Such a humanistic definition would require only that:

(1) The participants are free agents, (2) that sex is an act of personal communion, and (3) that it must not damage the flesh beyond the perforation of the hymen. Then any sequence based on free, mutual, informed consent, which terminates in bodily contact and does not damage the tissues of either party is not a perversion.*

Although many states legislate sexual behavior, these laws are largely unenforceable and of questionable constitutionality in view of recent concerns about invasion of privacy. There seems some consensus among researchers of sex laws that in only three instances does society have reason to bring legal sanctions to bear on sexual behavior:

1. When force or duress is involved
2. When there is sexual contact between children and adults
3. When sexual behavior constitutes public nuisance[2]

The maternity nurse who wishes to become a sexual counselor must develop tolerant attitudes toward varieties of sexual practices. The question to ask is whether these practices bring pleasure and fulfillment to both partners, without inflicting bodily or psychic harm. If the answer is yes, then for these people the practice is normal. Developing attitudes of acceptance is a process the nurse can deliberately embark upon. Knowledge is the first step, which can be acquired in the several ways already mentioned. Seeking perspective on societal attitudes toward certain practices, such as oral-genital contact or homosexuality, provides insight into the negative values associated with these. By constantly questioning, "Why is this considered bad? Why does society disapprove of this?" perhaps the nurse can require more substantial reasons before accepting such values.

In addition to questioning values, the nurse needs desensitization through confronting herself with her reactions to controversial areas. This can be done by attending workshops and lectures on homosexuality, group sex, changing sexual mores, abortion, sex education in the schools, etc. Make a real attempt to truly understand both sides of the controversy, especially the "opposite" side. These opportunities are

---

*From Berne, E.: Sex in human loving, New York, 1971, Pocket Books, Simon & Schuster, Inc., p. 75.

plentiful in most metropolitan and university communities. Another way is to engage in informal discussion with friends and colleagues, testing ideas and gauging reactions, especially one's own. These exposures and discussions will usually result in the nurse becoming more comfortable in dealing with sexuality.

THE NEED FOR COUNSELING PRACTICE

When entering a new clinical area, a period of time is necessarily spent gaining experience before clinical expertise can be achieved. In sexual counseling this is also true. However, the beginning counselor can enter the situation armed with as much knowledge and self-awareness as possible. Another essential asset is good interviewing technique, which also includes good interpersonal skills. Usually acquired during basic nursing education, these skills can be combined with a specific approach in taking sexual histories. The sexual history can be integrated into the more general health history or used separately in especially conducive settings, such as the family clinic or VD clinic.

The techniques and principles in taking sexual histories have been well described by Wahl[7] in *Sexual Problems: Diagnosis and Treatment in Medical Practice*. Recommending that the sexual history be left until the end of the interview so that an attitude of candor, confidence, and trust can be established, Wahl describes general principles for sexual history-taking:

1. Progress from topics easier to discuss to those more difficult to discuss. For instance, the interview should move from information about birth and sexual reproduction to masturbation to intercourse and lastly to homosexuality and other different sexual practices.

2. Ask the patient first how he acquired sexual information before he is asked about sexual experiences. For instance, ask how old he was when he first learned about masturbation, any frightening or worrisome things he heard when young, then how old he was when he first began to masturbate and feelings associated with this.

3. When appropriate, questions are preceded by informational statements on the generality of the experience (ubiquity statements). These reassure the patient as well as supply information; they significantly reduce his shame, anxiety, and evasiveness. For example: Many people have had the experience of being approached by a homosexual person during the time they were growing up. This sometimes happens at movies, in public restrooms, at parties, or on the street corner. When you were very young, did this ever happen to you? Frequently this experience is very disturbing. How did you feel about it?

In taking a sexual history, it is important that the nurse be warm, be objective, show respect for the patient as a person, and provide an atmosphere of understanding and acceptance. Confidentiality should be assured and note-taking kept at a minimum or postponed until later. The patient also deserves recognition for sharing this intimate information about his personal life frankly and honestly. Usually the process of a history-taking interview is valuable to the patient in itself. He may gain increased self-respect and a feeling of hope through the communication process with a nonjudgmental, relaxed professional. Even if there seems no immediate solution for the sexual problem, almost all patients see the opportunity to unburden themselves as a great advantage. According to Wahl:

> Experience reinforces the conviction that a well-taken history is of benefit to the patient even in itself. Most patients welcome the chance to discuss difficulties that all the forces of previous habit, custom, and convention have conspired to keep hidden and suppressed.*

Of course, it is preferable for the nurse to take some action on the sexual problems identified through history-taking. Many problems are the result of ignorance and misinformation, which can be corrected by educating the patient in human sexuality. Sometimes reassurance and reinforcement is what the patient needs, especially regarding the normality and acceptability of his sexual practices or feelings. The health professional can often act *in loco parentis* to

---

*From Wahl, C.: Psychiatric techniques in the taking of a sexual history. In Sexual problems: diagnosis and treatment in medical practice, New York, 1967, The Free Press, p. 20.

give the permission needed for the patient to relax and enjoy his sexuality. When more serious sexual problems such as premature ejaculation, impotence, and orgasmic dysfunction are identified, the nurse needs to judge whether her own abilities are adequate for treating the problem or if a referral is necessary. Long-standing sexual problems or those in which psychopathology seems involved are best referred to psychiatry. Since Masters and Johnson pioneered their effective techniques for treating these problems, other psychiatrists have been using and modifying them in outpatient practice. The local office of the psychiatric association should have listings of psychiatrists who offer therapy for sexual problems. Some social workers and marriage counselors may also have these skills and could be available as consultants or referral sources for the nurse.

Maternity nurses, from their special closeness to human reproduction, can offer critical services to their patients with problems or concerns about sexuality. To provide this service, a consciousness-raising approach is required, involving knowledge, self-awareness, and skills. The resources for accomplishing this are available both within the nurse and in the surrounding professional community. The challenge is present; the opportunity exists; the nurse need only be motivated by concern for others. She can aspire to meet the goal of Spinoza:

I have, in my life, sedulously endeavored not to laugh at human actions, not to lament them, not to detest them, but to understand them.

The nurse can take this one step further—to help people find greater happiness and fulfillment in their human sexuality.

REVIEW OF SELECTED BOOKS ON HUMAN SEXUALITY

Masters, W. H., and Johnson, V. E.: Human sexual response, Boston, 1966, Little, Brown & Co.

A new era in sex research was initiated by the scientifically documented studies at the Reproductive Biology Research Foundation in St. Louis. The details of the complex physiological sexual responses of men and women are described with accompanying psychological responses. Orgasmic expressions of both sexes are covered extensively, dispelling finally many myths such as those concerning female orgasm and penis size.

The similarity in orgasmic response between men and women is emphasized. Sexual response cycles in the aging population, during pregnancy, and in relation to the cardiovascular system are also reported. In addition to the physiological facts, the accepting attitude toward sexuality that permeates the book is significant. Although recognizing societal barriers, the importance of sexuality as a normal and natural human function is constantly upheld. An enormous amount of complex data is contained in this book; although general understanding may be readily gained, much rereading is necessary for full comprehension.

Masters, W. H., and Johnson, V. E.: Human sexual inadequacy, Boston, 1970, Little, Brown & Co.

A therapy format for treatment of sexual dysfunctions, including premature ejaculation, impotence, ejaculatory impotence, orgasmic dysfunction in women, vaginismus, and dyspareunia, is presented. The basic premise of this approach holds attitudes and ignorance responsible for most sexual problems. Mental or physical illness affects only a small number of patients. Treatment is aimed at unraveling the development of sexual dysfunctions, seeking understanding of how current behaviors perpetuate the problem, improving communication, and educating the couple in the psychophysiological aspects of sexual response. Physical examinations, therapy sessions with male and female co-therapists, and specific sexual techniques to be practiced in private are included. The overall success rate for all cases treated is 80%. The marital relationship itself rather than particular partners is considered the patient. With a sexual problem neither partner is uninvolved, thus both are treated, although one may not appear dysfunctional. Case studies are used to illustrate various sexual dysfunctions. The principles and techniques for intervening in sexual problems are invaluable information for those concerned with human sexuality.

McCary, J. L.: Human sexuality, Princeton, N. J., 1967, Van Nostrand Co., Inc.

As a comprehensive resource that encompasses a broad range of information in many areas of sexuality, this book stands out. Included are attitudes, factual data, and sexual myths and fallacies. Content covers the development and physiology of male and female reproductive systems, contraception, techniques of sexual arousal, orgasmic response (based on Masters and Johnson), sexual behavior and attitudes, sexual diseases and disorders, dispelling sexual myths, and legal aspects of sex. The author, a professor of psychology at the University of Houston, based the book on a course in human sexuality that he pioneered. His goal was to explore the physiological, sociological, and psychological components of human sexuality in a readable and sufficiently detailed manner to dispel mystery and confusion. This goal is certainly accomplished in this well-documented book. Written primarily for college students, this book is useful for both lay and professional readers.

SIECUS: Sexuality and man, introduction by Mary S. Calderone, New York, 1970, Charles Scribner's Sons.

SIECUS is a voluntary, nonprofit health organization dedicated to providing information and education about human sexual behavior. This book, a compilation of study guides, presents facts concerning male and female sexual responses (based on Masters and Johnson), sexual relations during pregnancy and postpartum, and sexual life during childhood, adolescence, adulthood, and in the later years. Information is provided and attitudes explored related to premarital sexual standards, masturbation, sex education, homosexuality, and sexual encounters between adults and children. Nontechnical language appropriate for the late adolescent and adult population contributes to readability. A calm, matter-of-fact approach covers sensitive material in a nonthreatening way. An appendix of film resources for sex education for various grade levels is useful to educators. This book is a good introduction and primer in human sexuality.

Wahl, C. W.: Sexual problems: diagnosis and treatment in medical practice, New York, 1967, The Free Press.

Medical education has until recently been as remiss as nursing in providing courses in human sexuality. This book is an attempt to fill the gap; it is based on a course at the UCLA Medical Center, which brought together authorities in several areas of sexuality that are frequently problematic. Twenty-two papers are included, many written by pioneers and leading authorities in different aspects of human sexuality. Some of the topics dealt with are masculine and feminine identity, variety in sexual behavior, conception control, abortion, problems in sexual identity, sexual problems in children, homosexuality, sexual promiscuity, transsexualism, and psychosexual implications in multiple surgery. Although written for the nonpsychiatrically trained physician, nurses will find much of value in this book. Frequently the nurse can utilize management or treatment techniques suggested. The chapter written by Wahl on techniques of taking a sexual history is excellent and could readily be adopted by nurses. Valuable insight into the recognition and psychodynamics of sexual problems is helpful to the nurse in screening and referral.

Berne, E.: Sex in human loving, New York, 1971, Simon & Schuster, Inc. (Pocket Books).

Berne, famous for developing the transactional analysis approach to psychotherapy, is witty, irreverent, and provocative when dealing with sexual foibles. He is much more concerned with the quality of the relationship than with sexual information and techniques. Sexuality is seen as an important part of the whole human personality with which we relate. Observations about our relationships are based on Berne's concept of personality, the three ego states of parent-adult-child. Human interactions are seen as transactions between these ego states. A good portion of the book is devoted to explaining these concepts. The approach to sex is oblique rather than direct, with Berne using poetic exuberance interspersed with folksy idioms. Those seeking information about sex can eventually learn an array of facts, some rather far removed. These are well camouflaged in humor and philosophy. The author also has a preoccupation with conception and babies as the ultimate and loftiest purpose of sex, for example, "The orgasm is her [nature's] reward for making a new baby." Occasionally Berne seems opinionated, and more scientific support of his views seems needed. Particularly questionable is the section on physical ailments that sex can cure or prevent, ranging from back pain to hemorrhoids.

Fromm, E.: The art of loving, New York, 1956, Harper & Row, Publishers, Inc.

Fromm, a psychoanalyst, has written one of the all-time best-selling books about sex and love. It does not contain facts and information about sexuality but expounds a philosophy of love and human relationships. If you are secure in yourself as a sexual person, reading Fromm is an interesting trip into convoluted semanticism. If you have doubts or problems related to sex, you will probably find neither help nor answers. You will get the feeling that your problems are due to your inability to really love, an ego-defeating conclusion hardly helpful when trying to cope with problems of sexual inadequacy. Fromm negates all concern for learning techniques of sexual arousal. He believes the current emphasis on techniques comes from an industrialized mentality that believes all problems can have mechanical solutions. This, to Fromm, is the wrong approach because "Love is not the result of adequate sexual satisfaction, but sexual happiness—even the knowledge of the so-called sexual technique—is the result of love." Thus the premise is that if partners really love each other, sexual satisfaction necessarily flows without specific knowledge of techniques. If a couple is having sexual problems, they must therefore not really love each other. The fallacy of such a premise is seen repeatedly in couples whose love has gradually eroded because sexual ignorance or dysfunction leaves one or both chronically frustrated sexually. In negating the value of knowledge and skill, Fromm consigns people to the mists of the romantic ideal, there to stumble on in ignorance, having no right to ask. Romanticism may be nice as a philosophical ideal, but it has little to do with everyday human problems.

Reuben, D.: Everything you always wanted to know about sex, New York, 1969, David McKay Co., Inc.

A best seller that catapulted sex manuals onto the national popular market, Reuben's book is written in a catchy, popular style. It contains a broad range of information, much of which is accurate, but frequently he resorts to generalizations and stretching of facts, which come dangerously close to misinformation. Partly this results from the "cuteness" and attempts at humor that make the reader uncertain as to whether statements are meant seriously. Particularly misleading are statements such as those on direct stimulation of the clitoris, intercourse via urethra, and the morning-after pill. Reuben appears opinionated or even prejudiced on certain topics. The chapter on homosexuality is especially objectionable, with disparaging statements revealing a disdainful, rejecting attitude. In painting the picture of the menopausal woman as desexualized, Reuben seems to offer hormone supplementation as a panacea for the problems of aging. The man is seen as a similar, although less severe, case. Another characteristic that decreases credibility involves his unidimensional case studies, which portray stereotypical people who all talk alike. Even more remarkable are his rapid and nearly universal "cures" of assorted sexual problems. If taken seriously by those who have no other sources of accurate sexual information, this book could be harmful. It may engender feelings of unnecessary inadequacy by setting unrealistic ideals (e.g., multiple orgasm, fantastic ecstasy). Its positive service is to encourage sex as good and perhaps stimulate those with problems to seek help.

Reuben, D.: Any woman can! New York, 1971, David McKay Co., Inc.

If the reader did not have a complex about being a woman before reading the first few chapters, she certainly will afterward. Overexaggerating to make a point, Reuben makes women look like patsies who appear maudlin in their oppression. It seems that every woman who is unmarried is unhappy and has a sexual problem (or is defending against these). A strong bias for marriage permeates the book. The section on contraceptives is a disaster. The pill and IUD are described in such frightening terms that uninformed women may panic and stop their use. Omitted is any comparison of risk of the pill versus risk of pregnancy or discussion of the actual incidence of complications. Ultimately Reuben seems to recommend foam and condom, and the "small risk of pregnancy" with these methods seems acceptable to him. His husband-hunting advice is mercenary: check him with the Credit Bureau, through comprehensive ex-FBI-men who run "reporting agencies," and by his auto registration tag. A woman still must define herself in terms of her relationship with a man, and career must always play second fiddle to family and husband. After careful reading, Reuben emerges as a traditional male who has provided some one-sided advice intended to help women be happier in their "proper" place in life. This book suffers from the same credibility gaps as the first, the same cute, popular gimmicks, and is much longer as well.

"J": The sensuous woman, New York, 1969, Lyle Stuart, Inc.

The first of the "sensuous books" presents, in cookbook style, recipes for women to develop their ability to experience and give sensual pleasure. Ranging from exercises to increase tactile awareness to specific techniques of oral-genital sex and intercourse, some suggestions can indeed increase sensate awareness. Others seem rather impractical, especially the whipped cream approach to fellatio. The book does not provide information about physiological sexual response but focuses mainly on attitudes and approaches. Women are told how to go about finding and selecting a man, with helpful hints on "his" and "hers" orgasms. The heterosexual relationship becomes mechanical and depersonalized, with stereotyped roles. One gets the impression that "J" is tongue in cheek in many of her comments, which leaves the problem of sorting out those that are more accurate and serious. The possibility that misinterpretation could be dangerous to the ill informed does exist. The general premise of the book—that women should become better acquainted with their bodies and develop their various senses—is a positive one. Setting up unrealistic ideals for the reader is a drawback.

"M": The sensuous man, New York, 1971, Lyle Stuart, Inc.

Written with humor and graphic language, this book gives explicit direction for sexual techniques to pleasure women. It contains some good information about what is erotically arousing to many women and what is inhibiting and detracting. The information on sexual response is reasonably accurate (based on Masters and Johnson), although suggestions for self-cure of impotence, premature ejaculation, and frigidity seem unrealistic. Although the theme that women deserve their sexual satisfaction is consistent throughout, the man still comes out as a hunter ever on the prowl for the ultimate target—sex and orgasm. Women seem to become depersonalized sexual objects, despite numerous author protestations to the contrary. "Love" is used loosely; transience, as well as limited involvement, seems to typify "M's" concept of man-woman relationships. The human need for deep, personal involvement seems less important than techniques for ecstatic sexual experiences. One danger is that techniques may be taken as panaceas for personal unhappiness. A completely literal interpretation by uninformed persons may lead to greater disappointment and confusion. Explanations are partial, and the reader needs the ability to screen out the implausible, recognize tongue in cheek statements, and supplement partial facts with fuller knowledge and understanding.

Chartham, R.: The sensuous couple, New York, 1971, Ballantine Books, Inc.

This book capitalizes on the two previous "sensuous books," adding little if anything. Although the author is billed as "Britain's leading sexologist," the book has little substance. Many of the suggestions given raise serious questions, and no attempt is made to validate "prescriptions." Much advice seems to be personally drawn conclusions and opinions; the reader certainly wants to know what research supports these. The book contains much questionable, if not outright erroneous, material. As with other popular books, it is a commercial venture intended more to stimulate and titillate than to inform.

References

1. Berne, E.: Sex in human loving, New York, 1971, Simon & Schuster, Inc. (Pocket Books).
2. Gebhard, P. H.: Human sex behavior research. In Diamond, M., editor: Perspectives in reproduction and sexual behavior, Bloomington, Ind., 1968, Indiana University Press, p. 396.
3. Masters, W. H., and Johnson, V. E.: Human sexual response, Boston, 1966, Little, Brown & Co., pp. 27-220.
4. Masters, W. H., and Johnson, V. E.: Human sexual inadequacy, Boston, 1970, Little, Brown & Co., p. 369.
5. McCary, J. L.: Human sexuality, Princeton, N. J., 1967, Van Nostrand Co., Inc., pp. 312-326.
6. Wahl, C. W.: The evaluation and treatment of the homosexual patient. In Sexual problems: Diagnosis and treatment in medical practice, New York, 1967, The Free Press, pp. 194-195.
7. Wahl, C. W.: Psychiatric techniques in the taking of a sexual history. In Sexual problems: Diagnosis and treatment in medical practice, New York, 1967, The Free Press, pp. 15-20.

19

A philosophy of labor and delivery nursing

Judith Ann Buten

Caring is the cornerstone of professional nursing.[1] Caring is an attitude of active concern for the patient's welfare, of understanding and accepting the patient as a worthy, respected human being. It is an attitude that is highly vulnerable to the pressures of a hospital bureaucracy; it is often destroyed by the very system it strives to serve. Caring is a singular attitude that manifests itself in a multitude of nursing actions. This chapter describes manifestations of caring in the labor and delivery suite of a large, busy university teaching hospital.

This hospital has a strong emphasis on research and technology and extensive teaching programs for residents, interns, medical and nursing students, and paramedics. The labor and delivery suite handles up to 250 deliveries a month. Maternity patients come from all levels of society and represent a great diversity of cultural backgrounds and native tongues. Obstetrically, patients are admitted at twenty weeks of gestation and over. The department estimates that 60% of these patients have complications such as diabetes mellitus, congestive heart failure, sickle-cell thalassemia, lupus erythematosus, psychotic disorders, hemorrhage, ruptured uterus, abnormal fetal presentations, and seizure disorders. Some 15% to 20% of the patients are cared for surgically in the suite by cesarean section, hysterotomy, bilateral tubal ligation, and cerclage.

TO CARE is to recognize, accept, and respect patients as human beings with needs, emotions, and responses and with strengths and weaknesses common to all persons. Nurses must recognize, accept, and respect their own state of humanness. They must be free to feel and to express joy and pleasure, anger and frustration, and worry and sorrow. Such freedom and self-understanding equip them to work with similar emotions and behaviors of the patients. To remain professional and therapeutic with them, they must know where and how to handle their own feelings and behaviors. Understanding the human side of all people is the undercurrent that permeates the entire atmosphere of this particular labor and delivery suite. To recognize, accept, and respect the human state of people is the nurse's springboard to caring.

TO CARE for patients undergoing parturition begins long before the first labor contraction and continues long after delivery is over. Given the reality of busy inpatient and outpatient maternity departments, labor-delivery nurses can participate in extradepartmental care on a limited basis only. Nurses do take part in the weekly tours of the maternity unit provided for expectant parents. They meet patients on a face-to-face basis, answer questions, and explain policies and procedures. As their confinement approaches, antepartum patients are encouraged to telephone the nurses and physicians in the labor delivery suite to have questions answered. The availability of a line of communication between patients and professional help—regardless of the hour—provides patients with answers, information, and instructions and can reduce the anxiety that accompanies waiting and wondering what to do.

Antepartum patients hospitalized on the maternity ward are discussed during team conferences at which plans of care are developed. Nurses meet and talk with these patients to assist them to become familiar with the labor-delivery staff and with what to expect in their approaching confinements. Antepartum clinic patients whose problems come to the attention of the nurses are cared for selectively as in the following example.

Mrs. S (gravida ii, para i at thirty-eight weeks' gestation) had arrived in the United States from England in the sixth month of pregnancy. She had practiced natural childbirth in delivering her first baby at home attended by a midwife. During a visit to the clinic, she voiced concern over the purpose of stirrups on the delivery table, how much medication she would have to receive, and the necessity of an episiotomy. The case was presented to the nurses, who discussed and created a plan of care. Accordingly Mrs. S later toured the suite, met the staff, and saw what stirrups were. Over tea she received further information, answers, and reassurance from the two English nurses on the staff. When Mrs. S was admitted in active labor, the nurses discussed with the physician the patient's concerns and the nurses' plan of care. Mrs S was followed through a rapid and natural labor by one of the English nurses and delivered a healthy baby without an episiotomy. Because the nurses set up and carried out an appropriate plan of care, Mrs. S found her hospital delivery to be "as satisfying" as her home delivery and her worries "quite ridiculous."

As to postpartum follow-up, nurses make individual ward rounds on patients that they cared for previously in the labor-delivery suite. This allows the nurse to assess the patient's progress, study family relationships, assist in teaching, answer questions, and update care plans. Patients often ask, "Was I bad in labor?" or "Did I scream a lot?" Once the experience is over, the patient can look back on it more objectively. She needs information to help her work through her feelings associated with parturition and to help her to establish her maternal role. Nurses deal with these questions honestly, but in a skilled, supportive, and constructive manner:

> Yes, you made some noise, but it couldn't be heard outside of your room. Working with pain is a very difficult thing to do. On the whole, you managed very well.

> Yes, you lost control near the end of labor. This often happens to mothers when the contractions become very strong and they feel pressure and begin to bear down. It is perfectly normal.

> You were a little apprehensive when you first came into the hospital. Most mothers are. Once we taught you how to breathe and work with contractions, you calmed down and did very well.

As discharge time approaches, the nurse terminates the relationship with the patient at a natural break-off point.

TO CARE is to take or make a few minutes to be present when the patient is wheeled through the doors, to know the patient's name beforehand, and to welcome her in a warm yet professional manner. A smile and a sincere greeting, "Hello, Mrs. Smith; I'm Miss Jones, your nurse; I'll be caring for you," is of immeasurable value in establishing an effective nurse-patient relationship. The nurse's interest and concern from the first moment enhances the patient's ability to handle the anxiety, fear, and pain of labor. The husband accompanying the patient is likewise welcomed and directed to the waiting room as his wife undergoes the admission procedures.

TO CARE is to take the time to carry out the admission procedures slowly, while structuring a solid trust relationship with the patient. Basic to this relationship is the understanding that the patient as a person is of greater importance than the admission tasks to be done. The nurse can demonstrate in several ways the importance of the patient as an individual. First, the nurse respects the patient's need for privacy as she is escorted to her individual labor room, asked to change into a hospital gown, and has the curtain pulled about her before she undresses. Second, a relationship must be given room to root firmly before it can grow. Therefore the nurse directs other health personnel to wait their turn to care for the patient. The admission period is a necessary time to establish a good relationship. Third, the nurse must be skilled at intertwining questions, statements, and instructions into a seemingly casual but goal-directed conversation with the patient. The nurse outlines the stages of progress and the expected plan of care. The patient is instructed how to breathe with contractions to reduce her discomfort and is invited to reciprocate with questions and statements of her own, so that a give-and-take attitude is created. Simultaneously, the nurse carries out actual tasks in an organized, confident, and unobtrusive manner, always remembering to prepare the patient before each procedure. Fourth, the nurse knows and utilizes the value of face-to-face contact. Persons of importance are persons to be looked at. Look at the patient! Pause and listen attentively to the patient. When the admission equipment is readied before the patient arrives, the nurse can center attention on the patient rather than on the prep kit, enema can, and pen and paper. Fifth, nothing is gained by hurrying the patient. When the patient is having a contraction is the wrong time to ask her to change position, sign a consent, or even answer a question. Working with the contraction taxes all the patient's efforts without adding effort to accommodate the nurse's needs. To insist that the patient do something during a contraction simply adds to her pain; a natural defense against additional pain is to resist. Resistance by the patient and insistance by the nurse create ill feelings, with each person working against the other. It is better to wait for the contraction to ebb. Waiting demonstrates to the patient that the nurse is willing to work with contractions—something the nurse expects the patient to do. After the contraction, the nurse can give instructions and help the patient do as requested. If necessary, the nurse can instruct during the contraction as long as the explanation is added that "I don't expect you to answer or move while you contract." Sixth, the nurse should keep all movements slow, minimal, and organized. Avoiding hustle and bustle gives the patient confidence in her nurse; it calms the patient and puts her more at ease and in control of her situation.

TO CARE is to handle the patient's possessions in a concerned manner, for possessions are simply extensions of the person. How the nurse treats possessions indicates to the patient how she herself will be cared for. With this thought in mind, the nurse folds and stores clothing, rinses out bloody garments, and labels suitcases—be it a Samsonite case or a cardboard box tied with twine. Personal belongings such as rings, watches, rosaries, necklaces, and hair ribbons can be left on the patient. These things help the patient to maintain her sense of identity and to reduce the feeling of depersonalization that most patients experience when hospitalized. Because these possessions are important, the caring nurse assumes the responsibility of looking after them.

TO CARE is to conclude the admission procedure by making sure that the patient is "at home" in her surroundings and that she knows where her possessions and call bell are, how to raise the head of the bed, what the restrictions on walking about, eating, and smoking are, when to expect the physician, and the general outline of care to follow. Her husband is accompanied to the labor room and likewise made "at home."

The outcome of such an admission procedure is the establishment of a solid nurse-patient relationship. The patient knows that she has a professional nurse in whom she may have confidence, she has information and answers to ease her fears and anxieties, and she has concrete instructions on how to breathe with contractions to reduce her discomfort. She is free to question, to know her stage of labor, to know what will happen before it happens, and to help to make some of the decisions about her care. Instead of being a passive outsider to whom things are done, she becomes actively involved in this experience. She feels that her nurse is likewise actively involved and interested in her and her welfare. It is this sense of involvement and comradeship between herself and a caring nurse that gives her the impetus and strength to put forth efforts that she never thought possible in handling the pain, fear, and self-doubt of labor.

The nurse has gained a wealth of information about the patient and her feelings toward pregnancy, about her family relationships, and about her medical condition. Such information is the basis for the plan of care. Not only have the admission procedures been completed, but also the patient is now prepared, cooperative, and willing.

TO CARE is to be at the bedside with the patient in labor. Appropriately, two chairs are at each bedside: one for the husband and one for the nurse. The nurse provides the patient with information. Using *simplicity* as a rule of thumb, the nurse explains policies and procedures, mechanisms of labor and delivery, and steps of progress; outlines the general plan of medical and nursing care; instructs as to breathing exercises to be used with contractions; and clarifies the physician's statements. Unlike medical and surgical patients, obstetrical patients have had nine months to anticipate labor and delivery—nine months of seeking information (often misinformation), listening to other women describe labor, reading books and attending classes, raising questions, and developing fears and anxieties. The professional nurse has a refined skill and finesse in talking with patients so as to rectify misinformation, answer questions, and give explanations without further alarming the patient. The nurse must draw on a solid background in the psychology of labor and delivery to help the patient work with her fears and anxieties about childbirth. By virtue of a knowledge and understanding of both parturition and human nature, refined communication skills, and a full-time position at the bedside, the professional nurse becomes an adept judge of what and how information should be given to the patient and by whom. The patient's comprehension ability, the impact of the data on her, and the need for further information are assessed. Patients in labor, both lay persons and health professionals themselves, need explanations and instructions. To the health professional in labor, the nurse can preface the first explanation or instruction by saying the following:

> I know you are a doctor [or nurse], but I will not assume you know everything that is going on. You are a mother-to-be now, and I'll explain things to you as I do to other patients.

The difference between the handling of health professionals and of lay persons rests in the choice of vocabulary, not in the presence or absence of the actual instruction or explanation. For example, in setting up an infusion pump for an oxytocin induction of labor by the intravenous piggyback method, the nurse can say to the health professional, "This infusion pump provides a more regulated flow of I.V. fluid." For the lay person, the nurse can point to the drip chamber of the existing intravenous fluid and say, "This machine counts more accurately the number of drops of fluid you receive."

Keeping the patient in control of herself and her situation during labor assumes a major part of the nurse's time. A rather alert and responsive patient must be carried through labor by the professional nurse, since patients in this labor-delivery suite receive limited doses of medication.

Sodium pentobarbital (Nembutal) is given in prodromal labor. Meperidine hydrochloride (Demerol) and diazepam (Valium) or promethazine hydrochloride (Phenergan) or all three are often given when the cervix is 4 to 5 cm. dilated and repeated in a lesser dose around 7 or 8 cm. dilatation. Occasional paracervical blocks are administered late in the first stage of labor as is the epidural block. For delivery, saddle blocks are given predominately to primigravidas and pudendal blocks, to multigravidas.

The nurse can use various techniques to keep the patient in control. First, patients respond well when they are given something concrete with which to work. Therefore each nurse has a good knowledge of natural childbirth practices on which to draw to instruct and help patients to breathe and relax with contractions. Whether or not the patient is practicing natural childbirth, the patient who works with contractions as directed often finds her discomfort lessened and her progress steady if not rapid—two incentives to make her work even harder with contractions. The patient can concentrate on her breathing when instructed to keep her "eyes open, pick out a spot, and stare at it," during the contraction. One of the most effective "spots" is the husband's or the nurse's eyes. Use of the human face instead of an inanimate object reconfirms for the patient that she is not alone and that some other human being is involved with her and her labor. She also stays in touch with the reality of labor when she keeps her eyes open. Closing her eyes and wishing "to go to sleep" or to "be knocked out" are often the first steps in attempting to escape reality, with a resultant loss of control.

Second, a patient can handle her labor more effectively when she understands what is expected and receives positive reinforcement for her efforts. When the patient responds readily to directions and works with her labor, the nurse simply tells the patient how well she is doing. For the laboring mother with a more tenuous grip on self-control, the nurse must be patient and accepting and gentle but firm. The most effective way to get the patient under control is for one person only to assume the task of coaching the patient. The nurse leans close to the patient, places one hand on each side of the patient's face, and calmly gives a simple instruction, "Jane, open your eyes and look at me." The nurse repeats the instruction until the patient responds correctly. Using the patient's first name, as well as face-to-face contact, is often a rapid way of getting the patient's attention. The nurse gives positive reinforcement, restates the first expectation, and adds a second instruction, "That is very good. Now, again, stare into my eyes. This time take a slow, deep breath with the contraction." As the patient responds correctly, the nurse gives further encouragement, clarification of expectations, and directions. In this slow, minute-by-minute process, the nurse helps the patient to gain a greater degree of self-control.

Third, the nurse is totally accepting of the patient as a person, although her *behavior* may have to be reprimanded and limited. For example, the nurse may say the following:

> Bearing down now will not help your labor. Bearing down will make the cervix swell and tear.
>
> I cannot understand whining.
>
> Thrashing about the bed will cause you to hurt yourself.

The behavior—bearing down, whining, thrashing about—and not the patient is being criticized. Behavior that is detrimental to progress or safety must not be accepted. The nurse demonstrates acceptance of the patient by constantly remaining at the bedside, even though limiting and correcting patient behavior.

The nurse at the bedside evaluates the patient's progress and provides her with good physical care. Patients are kept clean, dry, and comfortable with close attention to the perineum, skin, and mouth. Sponge baths, linen changes, and hair care are provided at least once a shift or more often, if the patient's condition warrants. Positioning the patient on her side when she complains of the "back labor" associated with the occipitoposterior lie of the fetal head can ease her discomfort. Rubbing the patient's lower back does likewise. Using Sim's

position when bearing down is often more comfortable for this particular patient than lying on her back. The nurse maintains close surveillance of intake and output. The patient must void a sufficient quantity each shift or be catheterized, particularly for a distended bladder. An intake of 800 to 1,000 ml. per shift is maintained. Blood pressure and TPR are recorded on a two- to four-hour basis—more often at the discretion of the nurse or as ordered by the physician. The nurse evaluates the pattern of fetal heart tones and records them at least every thirty minutes. The contractions are evaluated as to occurrence, strength, and duration. The relationship of the fetal heart tone and the contraction patterns are assessed, as well as the patient's progress and her need for medication and vaginal examination.

TO CARE for patients in labor is to manage machines and equipment and monitors without losing sight of the patient as a person. Nurses in this labor-delivery suite use a small, portable, external, ultrasonic fetal heart monitor on each patient in labor, in place of a fetoscope. This monitor provides an audible, continuous report of the fetal heart tones. The patient readily accepts this monitor when the tiny transducer is taped to her abdomen and she herself can hear the fetal heart tones. She is told that, if the mother or fetus changes position, the heart tones may not be heard, unless the transducer is moved somewhat. This monitor allows the nurse to evaluate fetal heart tones by a turn of a knob and not to disturb a sleeping patient.

When more complicated equipment is required, the physician explains to the patient and her husband just what her condition is. He explains why and how the equipment will help in managing her labor. The nurse is present to provide support, clarification of medical statements, and additional information. The nurse is knowledgeable and adept in handling the equipment and assisting the physician to use it. Patients are often monitored by using complex fetal monitoring systems complete with intrauterine pressure catheters and internal fetal ECG electrodes. The contraction and fetal heart patterns are continuously recorded on graph paper for a permanent record. Nurses in this labor-delivery suite have found that the fetal heart tone recorder on this machine stops momentarily, every little while. Unless the patient is prepared by being told of this fact, she often panics, thinking that the "baby has suddenly died." Patients have accepted this monitor readily when they discover it does not replace either the nurse or the physician at the bedside. Second, this monitor adds to the patient's comfort because the nurse does not have to palpate the patient's abdomen to evaluate contractions: the monitor does it instead. Third, the patient accepts this machine when she understands that it provides the nurse and physician with a highly refined tool for better care of herself and her baby. Finally, the patient, not the machine, is still the nurse's focus of attention.

TO CARE is to incorporate the participation of the father-to-be (in his absence, a friend or relative) into the labor process. The nurse accepts the husband's degree of participation without passing judgment. Some of them sit quietly at the bedside holding the patient's hand; others pace between waiting room and bedside; others never appear in the labor room. When invited, some husbands become actively involved in their wives' labor. The nurse assesses the husband's reactions to labor, sets examples for him to follow, issues an invitation to participate, evaluates his responses and actions, and gives him feedback on his effectiveness. Even without natural childbirth training, many husbands become interested and successful labor coaches: all they need is encouragement and examples to follow. The husband can encourage the patient in breathing, panting, or pushing with the contractions, help to position her, time contractions, rub her back, supply her with cool, wet washcloths for her face, and provide support and encouragement—all with examples set by the nurse. Couples with training in natural childbirth often need the nurse there to assess their effectiveness, to intervene if they lose control, to redirect their energies, and to give encouragement. Having a husband-labor coach present does not excuse the nurse from the bedside. The nurse does respect the wishes of natural childbirth

couples who are doing well and wish to be alone but remains readily available and observant, provides physical care, and evaluates progress—all in a quiet and unobtrusive manner.

The nurse who cares does not neglect the needs of the husband in evaluating how well he handles the stress of labor, his level of fatigue, and his need for food and to escape the situation momentarily. The nurse prepares the couple early for the husband's need to take occasional "coffee breaks." The couple readily cooperate when they understand that the husband will be of more support to his wife with such breaks. And when she is in active labor, the patient finds that she can use these separations as a time to let down her guard or brave facade and cry tears that she does not want her husband to see. Such an emotional release allows her to regain her energy to continue working with her labor. The husband who hesitates to leave often does so when the nurse suggests that he "telephone the relatives at home who must be concerned" or suggests that he take a break while the physician is with the patient administering an analgesic or doing an examination.

The caring nurse involves family members in the process of labor insofar as is possible and serves as a communication link between patient and relatives. The nurse telephones the family at home and reports on the patient's condition. When relatives accompany the patient to the hospital, they are often left out of the situation. They may arrive at the delivery-suite doors distraught and angry, demanding to see the patient or physician or threatening to report their treatment to the administration or both. The nurse meets these relatives on a face-to-face basis. Taking her cues from what they say, she allows them to express their feelings:

Relative: This is sure some place! We've been sitting down there—just waiting! No one bothered to tell us our daughter had been admitted!
Nurse: Yes—the waiting and not knowing can be very hard on you. I'm sorry it happened.

Once they have vented their emotions to an accepting and supportive nurse, the family needs information about the patient's condition. Hearing of progress, they usually calm down. The caring nurse asks if they would like to speak to the physician, offers them a cup of coffee, and directs them to the waiting room where they can be telephoned about the patient's progress. They are told that, should they begin to worry and to "feel left out," they are free to return to the delivery-suite doors and talk with the nurse again. By this time even the most distraught relatives usually relax, cooperate, and state their appreciation for the nurse's assistance.

TO CARE is to be at the patient's side in the delivery room. The nurse who follows the patient through labor also follows her through delivery. While the nurse is assisting the patient to the delivery table, positioning her for anesthesia and the perineal prep, a second nurse enters the delivery room long enough to set up the baby's resuscitation crib and the physician's instrument table and splash basins. The nurse beside the table times contractions, encourages the patient to bear down or to pant, cools her face with a wet, cool washcloth, monitors fetal heart tones using the portable, audible ultrasonic monitor, takes blood pressures, adjusts the mirror so that the patient can observe the delivery, and gives support and encouragement.

After delivery of the newborn, the nurse assists with needed resuscitation and the Apgar scores. He is weighed and measured and provided with eye care and identification bands. He is shown to the mother and transferred to a warm incubator near the head of the delivery table: the mother can watch her newborn while the episiotomy is being repaired. When the newborn requires extensive resuscitation, the nurse reports on the baby's condition:

Let the doctor clear the fluid out of the baby's nose and mouth so he can cry. It will take a minute or so.

The baby had a difficult time. The doctors are helping him to breathe for a few minutes. He is nice and pink.

After completion of the third stage of labor, administration of medications, monitoring of vital signs, and checking on the patient's warmth and comfort, the nurse then turns to her paper work. After the episiotomy is repaired, the mother and baby are put to bed together and wheeled to the recovery room to see the waiting father.

TO CARE is to extend to the mother the privilege of announcing to her husband the sex and statistics of the newborn. In the recovery room, it is a delight when father and mother and baby come together and share in privacy, often with happy tears, their first few minutes as a newborn family. In the recovery room the baby is held and cuddled and unwrapped and checked by the parents for abnormalities and for the correctness of the identification bands. Shortly thereafter, the baby is transferred to the nursery. In the recovery room the mother is checked closely for vital signs, for the condition of the fundus, lochia, and urinary bladder, and for general comfort. She is given an overall outline of the nursing care to be expected. When stable, whether in one hour or thirty-six, the patient is transferred to the postpartum ward.

TO CARE is to practice continuity in caring. Insofar as is possible considering the limitations of an eight-hour shift, the nurse who admits the patient also follows her through labor, delivery, recovery, and transfer to the postpartum ward. In this manner, the patient has to establish only one relationship (or possibly two) with a nurse at this stressful period in her life, and this one relationship is of a deeper, stronger, and more binding quality than several would be. After establishing this relationship, the patient can direct her energy to working with her labor.

TO CARE is to intervene when other personnel responsible for looking after the patient do not measure up to the high standard of caring. This hospital has an emphasis on teaching and research, as well as patient care. People must learn, and research must be done—but not at the expense of the patient. Because of this learning atmosphere, not all personnel have the finesse, skill, and ability of the private staff physician or the experienced professional nurse. Therefore the nurse must intervene, for example, to introduce the intern who forgot to introduce himself; to remind the research resident to obtain the patient's permission before using her in his research; to follow through on getting medications for patients when the promised anesthetic failed in the hands of the beginner; to limit the number of attempts (only two permissible) by medical students in starting an intravenous drip. Such interventions do not interfere with the goal of teaching; they demonstrate the principle of caring for the patient as a human being—the most important lesson any beginning health professional can ever learn.

TO CARE is to be honest with patients, to respect the right of the patient and her husband to know what is happening. To be honest in this labor-delivery suite is difficult because patients are awake through labor and delivery; they ask questions pertinent to a life-and-death situation; they can see and hear problems, thanks to modern fetal monitors. "Is my baby normal?" "Why does the baby's heart speed up and slow down?" "Why are you shaving my abdomen?" Honesty is knowing that patients understand that something is wrong, when there is a sudden tension or quietness in the room or an artificial cheerfulness or reassurance. To be honest involves time: first, the physician must explain the problem or situation to the patient and her husband. The nurse is there to provide support and further explanation. To be honest involves courage: the nurse must not try to avoid or escape the unpleasant situation but must realize that patients can handle even the worst of news when they are given simple but honest answers by a supportive and understanding staff. A sincere "I'm sorry" or "I have no words to help you" shows concern when the patient has been given bad news such as that her baby is abnormal or stillborn. Words are often a too sophisticated level of communication in dealing with problems of such emotional depth. Nurses can effectively show nonverbally that they care by fluffing the pillow, patting the hand, giving someone coffee, sitting with the patient, and encouraging and accepting the patient's emotional response. It is surprising how much built-in courage can be drawn on to tide a person over a difficult period of living—and dying.

TO CARE is to dare to give of oneself and to become professionally involved in the welfare of the patient, the family, and even one's fellow team members, for caring knows no boundaries. It means daring to assume a burden of additional responsibility; as the nurse's concern and involvement increase, so does the level of responsibility. Caring is daring to stand up for an ideal in the face both of bureaucratic obstacles and criticisms from those who fail to understand what caring is. It is refusing to settle for second best. To care is to dare to know oneself both as a person and as a professional nurse.

In summary, caring is an attitude of active involvement with the welfare of the patient. This attitude manifests itself through many activities of the nurse. This chapter has described a multitude of nursing behaviors in a labor-delivery suite—behaviors that I believe to be manifestations of caring.

References

1. A position paper; educational preparation for nurse practitioners and assistants to nurses, New York, 1965, American Nurses Association.
2. Taylor, C. D.: Sociological sheepshearing, Nurs. Forum 1:75, 1962.

20

Assessment of pain during labor

Dyanne Affonso

Labor and birth is a time of stress and crises.[2,3,8] The most intense stimulus during labor is pain. Pain has been identified in the literature as a main source of anxiety and fear associated with childbirth.[5-7] The impact of the pain is expressed by women in labor with comments such as the following:

Another one. I'm having another pain.

How much longer will this pain last?

Can't you do anything? Please make the pain go away.

Nursing approaches to patients in labor do not demonstrate that management of pain is a goal; following are comments frequently made by nurses:

You're just having a baby. There's no need for all this reacting.

Relax. It's *just* a contraction.

You're making too much noise. Quiet down or you'll disturb the other patients.

Are you having a pain? Tell me when you have a pain.

In one large hospital I know of, nurses who are excellent practitioners during the delivery process seem to avoid interaction with the patient during the first stage of labor. Asked about this, nurses said:

I can't do much for her. You can't make the pain go away unless the doctor orders medications.

I get upset when they scream and become restless. It makes it harder for me to give care.

The pace is too slow. It's a long process with slow progress. At least in the delivery room I'm doing something, and things get done.

I don't know what to say. How can I answer her questions about how much longer?

Student nurses in the baccalaureate program affiliated with the hospital expressed similar attitudes:

The labor patient creates a lot of disorganization. She is restless and makes it hard for you to do your work.

They always ask if you can do something to take the pain away. I feel helpless, especially when it's too early for medications.

I think of how I cope when I'm in pain. I go away and want to be left alone. I tend to want to do that with the patient and find it difficult to assert myself on her.

The worst thing is to hear the patient screaming from the hallway. You just dread going into the room.

One difficulty nurses have in working with patients in labor is the management of pain. Failure to recognize and accept pain as a legitimate part of the labor experience interferes with the ability of the nurse to give care. The discontinuity between the patient's pain experience and the nurse's recognition and acceptance of it leads to ineffective nursing approaches. Difficulty in identifying, organizing, and implementing actions to effectively deal with the pain of labor is a clinical nursing problem.

The purpose of this chapter is to use a conceptual framework for understanding the pain and to illustrate its application to the patient in labor. The goal of this chapter is to present a systematic approach to guide nursing actions in the management of pain during labor. The conceptual model is presented in Fig. 20-1.

How does the experience of labor fit this conceptual model of pain? The pain source in labor is uterine contractions. Mechanical stimulation to receptors occurs as follows:
1. Myometrial anoxia, creating an ischemic state during contractions
2. Stretching of the cervix
3. Pressure on nerves
4. Traction on tubes, ovaries, peritoneum, and supporting ligaments

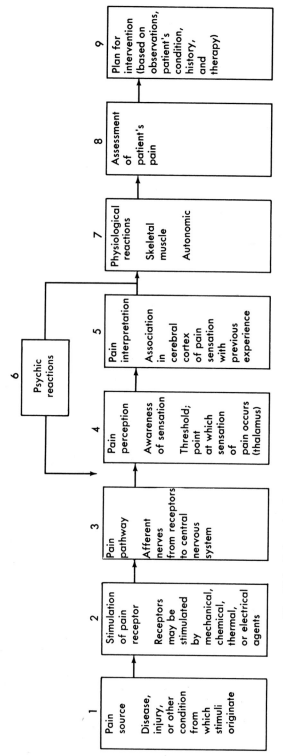

Fig. 20-1. Pain stimulus-response sequence. (From Am. J. Nurs. **66:**1085, 1345, 1966.)

5. Pressure on urethra, bladder, and rectum
6. Distention of muscles of pelvic floor and peritoneum[7]

The pain pathway of labor has been established.[4] Pain perception threshold is decreased by the mechanical stimulators just mentioned, as well as maternal fatigue, lack of sleep, decreased nutritional intake, anxiety, and fears. An important variable in the pain perception threshold is the frequency, intensity, and duration of the labor contractions. When labor patterns are established, the pain perception threshold can decrease. Following is an illustration:

A 19-year-old primipara is admitted in labor, 3 cm. dilated, 0 station, membranes intact, and contractions every 6 minutes. She is tossing and turning, crying, "I can't take this any longer. Please take it out." She refuses to accept the limitations of NPO orders and intravenous therapy. She reveals that she has not slept well for two days because of Braxton-Hicks contractions; she has not eaten a full meal since that time. She shares her fears of labor from the "stories" heard from friends; finally she states that she was doing fine until the "pains" kept coming and coming regularly.

From these data, it is evident that the patient perceives pain intensely, although the physiological effects of the contractions are minimal in terms of dilatation.

Pain interpretation occurs from experiences that are tangible to the patient in labor. She might compare the labor with past hospitalizations, injuries, or childhood pain experiences. She may refer to previous childbearing experiences and to cultural conditioning regarding expectations about pain and labor. For example:

A 22-year-old gravida ii, para i Mexican is 4 cm. dilated −1 station, membranes intact, with contractions every 5 minutes. She is screaming and attempts to climb over the bedrails. She has been reprimanded repeatedly by the physician and told that her screams are disrupting others and that she will hurt herself if she continues. Later the nurse's assessment revealed that her first labor was twenty hours long; she recalls the agony and pain of having to push the baby out. She also states that her mother and aunts have told her that an occasional scream or yell helps to bring the baby out.

It is evident that emotional or psychic reactions are elicited during a pain experience because of threats to the self. Kartchner[5] states that there are three classic threats or fears during the childbearing experience: fear for the self, fear for the baby, and fear of the unknown. Fear of the unknown relates to the strange environment, procedures, and bodily sensations and the ability to cope with the contractions for a duration of time.

A 22-year-old multipara described previously expressed fears of being injured by the baby during the second stage of labor. She also worried about the baby being injured as she was pushing and her physician's sudden command during the delivery "Don't push, or your baby will fall into the bucket!" She expressed concern about having her blood pressure and the baby's heartbeat checked so often. Her frequent question was "Is everything all right?"

The physiological reactions elicited during the pain experience are similar to autonomic reactions during stress. Patients in labor become diaphoretic; they hyperventilate; their lips become dry and cracked; their face and skin flush and become hot; they become restless and irritable; and they are unable to maintain a comfortable position for a period of time. These reactions impose discomfort on the already existing and uncontrollable pain source.

The key to nursing intervention in the management of the patient in labor is the assessment process. Assessment is the systematic collection of data about the physiological, psychological, and sociocultural behavior of the individual. The tools used in assessment are direct observation and interviewing. The significant factors to assess regarding pain in labor are as follows:

1. *The psychosexual development of the individual.* Childbirth is greatly affected by attitudes toward and adaptation to femininity and motherhood. Feelings about the genital organs may affect pain perception. For example:

A 25-year-old primipara was able to cope well during the latent phase of labor. She became anxious and uncontrollable as her labor progressed. She slowly revealed that she did not like anyone touching her vaginal area and found the vaginal exams brutal not because they hurt but because she was being touched. She was labeled by the staff as uncooperative because of her behavior during the vaginal exams.

2. *Threats to the self-system.* During labor threats to the self-concept and body image occur in the form of anxieties con-

cerning disfigurement, role loss, and inability to cope with the sensations of pain. In addition to the three classic fears, other stresses on the woman are strange faces, sounds, and equipment and restrictions on normal activities such as use of a bedpan, limited fluids, and inability to sleep. The patient is forced into a dependent role physically, and her decision-making abilities are called to a halt. She feels that she is losing control over the situation, especially as labor progresses. Fatigue overcomes her, and the energy needed to cope with the multitude of stresses is diminished. Sensations during the second stage of labor give rise to feelings of "being ripped apart"; at the same time the patient is forced to actively participate in the labor process by either pushing or controlling the urge to push. Threats to the self are associated with the fear of death that increases as labor progresses.

3. *Present and past pain experiences.* Nurses often learn that patients in labor have little knowledge about the childbirth process. The patient does not know how contractions assist the baby to be born, what is happening to her body during contractions, and why she feels certain bodily sensations during contractions. This mystery breeds fears and anxiety and intensifies pain impulses. Nursing assessment of the woman's antenatal course can be helpful, since the degree of discomforts, complications, satisfactions, and frustrations will either support or hinder the woman's ability to cope during labor. A simple question directed to the patient in labor such as, "What did you expect labor to be like?" can yield much information.

4. *The social and supportive environment during and previous to the pain experience.* Assessment of situational support from spouse, family, friends, and the environment is important. Who is the significant supportive person as identified by the patient? Is that person allowed to be present during labor? The patient in labor may find her environment restricted to persons defined by the hospital staff rather than by her decisions. The relationship established with nurses and physicians prenatally can give clues to reactions and the degree of trust or anxiety elicited by the

environment. Have the pregnant woman's dependency needs been met during her pregnancy? These data give clues about her ability to cope under the stress of labor.

5. *The meaning of the pain experience.* In times of great stress, suffering, pain, illness, and loneliness, the meaning or purpose one ascribes to the experience can be a means of support.[9] Thus the nurse must assess for this if she is to help the patient mobilize her resources to cope with the pain source. Assessment should include data about the woman's attitudes and values concerning the childbearing experience. Was the pregnancy desired, planned, wanted? Was adequate adaptation made during the prenatal course? What is the value of children? What are the attitudes toward parenthood? Is the pregnancy seen as an illness, a bothersome event, or a means of fulfilling other needs besides a desired child?

6. *Cultural implications of the labor process.* Culture is important because it influences attitudes and feelings about pain, acceptable reactions, and the measures utilized in coping. Culture dictates the expectations and acceptance of pain, values and expression of pain, rituals for relief behaviors, and norms for seeking assistance in coping with the pain. Rituals and relief behaviors may conflict with norms set by the staff. Verbal expression in the form of moans, chants, or screams may be a cultural necessity to the patient but be prohibited by the staff. The cultural meaning and significance of labor and its bodily sensations may breed fears and anxieties or promote coping during childbirth.

What is the purpose of nursing intervention during the pain experience? The conceptual model of nursing intervention is presented in Fig. 20-2. It is not always possible to alter each component of the pain experience during labor. The pain source—the uterine contractions—cannot be eliminated because it is essential to the process. Therefore nursing must identify the variables to which effort can be directed and in so doing, differentiate the profession from medicine in the management of pain.

The key to intervention is the nurse-patient interaction, which is based on the nurse's assessment of the pain source, perception, interpretation, and reactions. Use of observational and interviewing skills is a necessity in working with a patient in labor.

Following are examples of the use of observational skills. First, a description of poor use of observational skills is given:

A 24-year-old multipara was in labor for four hours, during which time she dilated from 3 to 8 cm. without anyone's knowledge of this progress. The nurse commented how "well the patient was doing" as she periodically looked in on her. Suddenly the patient, now 8 cm., screamed and thrashed in bed. She eventually had a precipitous delivery because she could not follow commands to pant and allow preparation for delivery. The staff was confused by the patient's change in behavior during the transitional and second stage.

Good use of observational skills would have revealed the following:

At 4 cm. dilatation the patient was diaphoretic and hyperventilating. At 5 cm. she was gripping the siderails, grimacing, and becoming restless. At 6 cm. she was still hyperventilating, her face flushed, tossing in bed, and clutching the sheets. At this time she had asked the nurse for something to ease the pain, to which the nurse responded, "When you're in active labor, we'll give you something. Not until then, or we'll stop your labor." Stopping the labor was the last thing the patient wanted, so she tried her best to continue on her own until she could no longer cope.

Interviewing skills are also necessary to obtain information. Following is a description of the poor use of interviewing skills:

Mrs. A, a 21-year-old primipara, is admitted in the latent phase of labor. The nurse notices her tenseness and rigid positioning while waiting for the admission examination. The following conversation occurs:

Nurse: You're scared?
Patient: Yes! It's my first baby.
Nurse: Oh, there's nothing to be frightened about. If you're dilated good, it'll go fast.
Patient: I guess I don't know what to expect, and it frightens me.
Nurse: Don't worry about it. When it's all over, you won't remember a thing.
Patient: I've heard so many stories about labor. Are they true?
Nurse: Now, you're going to get yourself all upset thinking about things like that. It won't be so bad.

In this case the nurse never gave the patient a chance to express her feelings and concerns. The nurse is talking instead of gathering information. Following are sug-

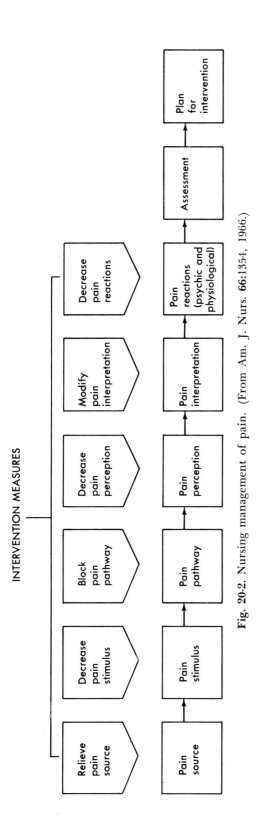

Fig. 20-2. Nursing management of pain. (From Am. J. Nurs. 66:1354, 1966.)

gested questions that the nurse might have asked to elicit valuable data:

What do you expect your labor to be like?

What have you heard or read about labor? How do you feel about it?

How have things been for you during your pregnancy?

How do you respond when you're uncomfortable or under stress? What helps you most during this time?

Do you understand what is happening to your body during labor and what you'll be feeling as you make progress?

What do you think would be helpful to you during your labor?

The nursing plan for intervention can be categorized into four main areas: (1) development of trust, (2) teaching, (3) role of advocate, and (4) support to the ego.

Essential in the management of pain is the *development of trust.* Trust lessens the opportunities for the patient to imagine or magnify the dangers in her situation.[1] Realistically, nurses cannot be present constantly when care is directed to groups of patients. However, the amount of time the nurse spends with the patient should increase as the patient's anxiety level rises during labor. The nurse's use of touch and a calm, reassuring voice can act as a distraction, thus increasing the pain perception threshold. The very presence of the nurse reduces the patient's fear of social isolation. Trust is also established by the nurse's anticipation of needs for physical care such as a clean perineum, oral hygiene, facial sponges, baths, and back rubs and by her acceptance of the patient's dependency as legitimate. The nurse attempts to meet the patient's demands for attention instead of retaliating with aggression.

Measures to ensure comfort and support include proper positioning, manipulation of environmental stressors, provision for rest and sleep through organized care, provision for presence of supportive persons, proper maternal-infant monitoring with data shared with the patient, and seeking of medical orders for pain relief instead of waiting for the physician to order it.

Teaching is essential to clarify the patient's misconceptions, prepare her for future phases of labor progress, and assist her to gain knowledge. In teaching the patient in labor, timing is essential. Certain content can best be presented during certain phases of labor. The patient's anxiety level and its effects on learning must be considered. Here is an example of presenting content at the optimum time during the labor process:

Latent phase (up to 4 cm.). This is the optimum time to teach about the mechanisms, stages, and bodily sensations occurring during labor. It is an excellent time for teaching because the patient is alert and her anxiety level does not interfere with learning. It is a good time to assess expectation and ability to cope and to explain breathing and other techniques to assist coping.

Active phase (4 to 7 cm.). This is the time to prepare the patient for expectations of the future phase of labor such as demands to push or pant. Give a rationale for limitations such as bed rest and NPO so that she can accept them. Reinforce previous teachings because she may forget or become confused as the pain source increases.

Transitional to delivery phase. This is a period of increased stress and anxiety. It is best not to introduce new content because the patient's perceptual field is narrowed and new learning is difficult. Speak in short phrases and reinforce teaching done during the active phase.

Content presented at time periods optimal for patients to participate in learning results in effective teaching during labor.

Pain affects the ability of a person to interact and cope by diminishing one's control of situations. The nurse strengthens this ability by assuming the *role of advocate.* The nurse can communicate the meaning of the patient's coping behaviors and protect her against prohibitions of behavior patterns dictated by her culture. To assume this role, the nurse must assess her own feelings about aggressive acts, moans, screams, and silence. The control the patient has of her situation increases when she is involved in decision making. Often patients are given a decision instead of a choice. How often is the patient allowed to say what positions offer comfort or what type of anesthetic or medicine she prefers for pain relief?

The nurse should give *positive support to the patient's ego.* Patients in pain are in a threatening situation in which all their resources have been mobilized in an attempt to cope. How often do they receive positive reinforcement for their efforts? Women frequently apologize for their coping during labor because the environment makes them feel their behaviors are inappropriate. Ego support appears simple enough, but some nurses have difficulty incorporating it into the care given. Positive reinforcement to a patient in labor is illustrated in the following process recording:

Mrs. D, a 23-year-old gravida iii, para ii, is 5 cm. dilated and in good labor for four hours.

Mrs. D.: They're getting harder. I'm so tired. How much longer?

Nurse: You've been working hard so many hours, and that's why you're exhausted. I can't tell you exactly how much longer, but the contractions are harder, which indicates progress. You're doing a good job handling these hard contractions.

At 6 cm. dilatation she becomes restless and gives out a scream during a contraction.

Mrs. D: I'm so sorry for being terrible. I didn't mean to yell. I couldn't help it.

Nurse: There's no need to apologize, and you were not terrible. You're in labor, and I don't expect you to be comfortable. Sometimes making noise helps to endure the discomforts.

Mrs. D: Yes. I always moan or make a sound when I'm in pain. It makes me feel better.

Mrs. D (at 7 cm.): Oh nurse, I can't go on. I've had it.

Nurse: Yes, you have a right to feel that way. You can go on. I'm here to help you do it. You're doing a good job tackling these contractions. That's one reason you've made good progress.

The nurse should give ego support during the labor and not wait till after the birth to shower the mother with praise. Patients need to be told that their efforts are not wasted, their behaviors are legitimate, and someone cares enough to see them through the pain experience.

In summary, this chapter presented a conceptual model of pain and applied it to pain of labor. The use of a conceptual model assists the nurse in a systematic way in problem solving and implementing nursing care. The goal of nursing in labor is to identify and to support the individual's adaptive behavior so that she can cope successfully with situations that she cannot alter or change herself. Labor fits the conceptual model of pain, and nursing assessment is the key to intervention in pain.

References

1. Beland, I.: Clinical nursing: Pathophysiological and psychosocial approaches, ed. 2, London, 1970, Macmillan International, Ltd.
2. Botella-Llusia, J.: Obstetrical endocrinology, Springfield, Ill., 1961, Charles C Thomas, Publisher.
3. Hays, J.: A labor and delivery—from the viewpoint of a psychiatric nurse, J. Psychiatr. Nurs. 2:157, March-April, 1964.
4. Javert, C., and Hardy, J.: Measurement of pain intensity in labor and its physiologic, neurologic, and pharmacologic implications, Am. J. Obstet. Gynecol. 60:552, 1950.
5. Kartchner, F.: A study of the emotional reactions during labor, Am. J. Obstet. Gynecol. 60: 19, July, 1950.
6. Klein, H., Potter, H., and Dyk, R.: Anxiety in pregnancy and childbirth, New York, 1950, Paul Hoeber, Inc.
7. Oxorn, H., and Foote, W.: Human labor and birth, New York, 1964, Appleton-Century-Crofts.
8. Shainess, N.: Psychologic experience of labor, N. Y. State J. Med. 63:2923, 1963.
9. Travelbee, J.: Intervention in psychiatric nursing: Process in the one to one relationship, Philadelphia, 1969, F. A. Davis Co.
10. Programmed instruction on pain, Parts I and II, Am. J. Nurs. 66:1085, 1345, 1966.

Bibliography

Allen, S.: Nurse attendance during labor, Am. J. Nurs. 64:70, July, 1964.

Crowley, D.: Pain and its alleviation, Los Angeles, 1962, Regents of the University of California.

Moss, F., and Meyer, B.: The effects of nursing interaction upon pain relief in patients, Nurs. Res. 15:303, Fall, 1966.

Reynolds, P.: Anxiety in pregnancy, Western J. Surgery 63:88, Feb., 1955.

Zabrowski, M.: Cultural components in response to pain. In Folta, J., and Deck, E., editors: Sociological framework for patient care, New York, 1966, John Wiley & Sons, Inc.

21

Fetal heart rate monitoring; the nurse's role as facilitator

Kleia Raubitschek Luckner

The purpose of continuous electronic fetal monitoring is to assess accurately the condition of the fetus by determining its response to labor. Circumstances of pregnancy affect development of the unborn and, consequently, its status during labor; it is therefore relevant to discuss pregnancy briefly. Medical or environmental factors may place the fetus in a hazardous position before labor begins. Determination of the degree of fetal risk has led to the development of the concept *high-risk pregnancy*.

HIGH-RISK PREGNANCY

Although maternal mortality rates have undergone dramatic and progressive reduction in the last three decades, perinatal mortality has failed to show the same decline. In spite of the fact that the quality and quantity of preconceptive, prenatal, and neonatal care has improved, approximately 40% of all perinatal deaths occur after thirty-seven weeks of gestation and after the fetus weighs 2,500 grams. Of these perinatal deaths, 40% occur immediately before birth. Gruenwald[5] has pointed out that deaths in perinates of this maturity and size are more readily preventable than with the premature. Further reduction in the incidence of reproductive failure has become one of the greatest challenges to modern medicine.

One practical approach to the problem is to identify and give special care to those patients who seem, for various reasons, to be particularly prone to reproductive failures. One tool that can be used during pregnancy is an objective screening system to aid clinical judgment in the initial identification of the high-risk patient.[8] This enables the practitioner immediately to recognize the patient as one who has a greater chance of having perinatal problems and to plan her care toward the reduction and, if possible, the prevention of the problems. Ideally, high-risk patients should be separated from routine antepartum patients and be treated in special high-risk clinics, staffed by a multidisciplinary team: obstetricians, neonatologists, internists, hematologists, nurses, social workers, nutritionists, and public health nurses. A team with such comprehensive skills can provide the high-risk patient with the best opportunity of having her needs met, with her care planned to reduce risks. Unexpected complications are infrequent in pregnant women who have had a thorough evaluation and careful medical observation; significant deviations can be treated during pregnancy and anticipated at delivery.[3]

With this problem in mind, the A.M.A. has taken an important stand. Their statement *Centralized Community and/or Regionalized Perinatal Intensive Care* described a perinatal care policy approved by the A.M.A. House of Delegates in June, 1971. This document encourages the establishment of programs that would enable the identification of a high-risk pregnancy in sufficient time to allow for delivery at those hospitals that are staffed, equipped, and organized for optimal perinatal care. It also describes the need for regionalized hospital-based newborn intensive care units.[1] This concept of regionalization is a practical solution, for a relatively small percentage of the obstetrical population gives rise to a disproportionately large percentage of perinatal casualties.[2]

The normal development of the fetus is threatened by many factors, both singly and in combination. Many are obstetrical in nature, in that maternal complications

194

play a threatening role. However, more factors are environmental, due to unfavorable social conditions, educational handicaps, or nutritional deficits.[3] Therefore the approach to these problems must be multifaceted: early identification of the high-risk pregnancy, with attention devoted to both medical and social conditions that contribute to the high-risk condition; the creation of a multidisciplinary team to handle the high-risk patient; and, finally, the development of regionalized high-risk neonatal centers to provide optimal care for those patients whose pregnancies are endangered.

Equal in importance to the medical problems that pregnancy may present to the fetus are the stresses of labor and their fetal effects. Healthy antenatal conditions may enable the fetus to respond favorably to the stresses of labor. However, the unborn infant, whose good health was established and maintained during pregnancy, may be put in jeopardy during labor. A means of evaluating fetal response during labor is crucial to fetal well-being.

PURPOSE OF FETAL MONITORING

In most cases, the fetus has the potential for survival at the start of labor. Often the only evaluation of the fetus during labor is an examination with a fetoscope to determine heart sounds. During labor and delivery, the fetus may become anoxic or depressed, which may cause the loss of a chance for normal development or death in utero because of failure to make a more strenuous attempt to assess its status.[9] Hospital emergency rooms and intensive care units are equipped with electronic devices that monitor every physical movement of the acutely ill patient. Until recently, scientific technology was not applied to labor and delivery. If childbirth is a natural physiological process, why is such equipment needed?

Ausculation of the fetal heart rate (FHR) with a fetoscope in pregnancy and labor is widely used to assess the fetal condition. Classically, the signs of fetal distress are the passage of meconium in a vertex presentation, hyperactivity, and fetal tachycardia or bradycardia. Information about FHR is critical in assessing fetal well-

being. The usual device for determining the FHR is the fetoscope. The use of this instrument is subject to three types of error: random error, error biased toward the norm when the heart rate is too fast or slow, and error based on the inability to determine FHR during a uterine contraction.[4] The sampling time is usually limited to the interval between contractions, when the fetus is under least stress. The fetoscope provides only periodic sampling of the FHR, and normal variability in rate is often obscured by averaging. Without continuous monitoring, a change in the FHR may be missed, leaving a fetus in unnoticed difficulty. Finally, the use of the fetoscope does not provide a permanent record that can be evaluated in terms of the early warning signs of fetal distress.

There are major limitations in the use of the classic clinical criteria for detecting fetal distress. Often these clinical signs are present when the fetus is well oxygenated. An emergency cesarean section for fetal distress could be performed under these conditions when the fetus is not really at risk.[7] Therefore the classic signs of fetal distress are unsatisfactory criteria. In addition, FHR changes in relation to uterine contractions are a significant index of fetal distress. It is difficult to detect FHR changes using the auscultation method. Fortunately, major advances have been made in this area, resolving these difficulties.

Two main groups of investigators are responsible for our present knowledge in this field and for the development of instrumentation that allows continuous monitoring of FHR and uterine contractions. These advances have allowed us to evaluate the unborn child directly and thus ascertain his status. Caldeyro-Barcia in Montevideo, Uruguay, devised, with Álvarez, a method for accurately recording the contractility of the uterus. His attention next focused on the effect of labor on a fetus and thus on the FHR pattern. Hon took up the challenge of interpreting FHR as a means of assessing fetal well-being and then correlated uterine contractility with the interpretation. Previously the clinical criteria used during labor to determine fetal distress were poorly defined and inadequately correlated with outcome. In contrast to the clinical indexes, continuous electronic surveillance of FHR and uterine contractions provides reliable, reproducible, and predictive information about the fetal condition during labor. Investigators have shown that FHR does not ordinarily drop during contractions and that decelerations in heart rate are not necessarily always ominous. However, certain specific FHR patterns appear to be indicative of fetal compromise.[10]

METHODS OF FETAL MONITORING
External monitoring

Monitoring may be external or internal, but in both methods the parameters of fetal heart rate and uterine contractions are noted and recorded on a permanent record. The external method of monitoring FHR may employ two different techniques: microphone and ultrasound. A crystal contact microphone is placed on the mother's abdomen over the area where fetal heart sounds are most clearly heard. The disk-shaped microphone is attached to a wire that is plugged into a bedside monitoring unit. The signal is audible, and a rate is computed by determining the frequency of the signals. The advantages are the following: the technique is noninvasive, it may be applied by a nurse, and the sound is similar to that heard with the fetoscope. The disadvantages are as follows: the disk-shaped microphone is difficult to keep in place over the fetal heart, transmission is lost in obese patients and patients with polyhydramnios, movement of the mother or fetus interferes with the signal, function in the lateral position is poor, and external noise interferes with the transmission of the signal.

The second method of externally monitoring the fetal heart rate employs ultrasound. A disk containing two receiving and transmitting crystals is used. Placed on the mothers abdomen, it is held in place by an elastic belt, which encircles the patient. The two transmitting crystals emit ultrasonic sound waves that are reflected back from bony structures and are modulated by the media through which they pass. If the media pulsates, as does blood through the major vessels, the reflected waves are modulated to reflect this pulsation. The modulation, or change, of the emitted sound wave, when compared to a reference time base, is used to indicate the FHR. Fig. 21-1, *A,* shows the external ultrasound bedside monitor. The advantages of this type of external monitoring are the following: the technique is noninvasive, it may be applied by a nurse, and the transmission is more reliable than the microphone technique. The disadvantages are as follows: the signal may be lost with excessive movement or in the lateral position, and the belt may be uncomfortable to the patient.

Uterine contractions are measured externally by the tocodynamometer. This instrument has a flat disk with a plunger in the center. It is fastened to the mothers abdomen by an elastic belt with the plunger pressing against the fundus. A uterine contraction produces a change in abdominal tension that is picked up by the plunger and converted to an electrical impulse that is recorded on the graph as a uterine contraction. Fig. 21-1, *B,* shows the tocodynamometer (upper belt) and ultrasonic disk (lower belt). The advantages are the following: the technique is noninvasive and can be used in early labor, it may be applied by a nurse, and it provides a continuous recording of the frequency of the contractions. The disadvantages are as follows: change in maternal position may alter the recordings, it is difficult to use in obese patients, and the amplitude of the contraction pattern is not quantitative. It provides information about the contraction's duration and some indication on the intensity of the contraction.

The advantages of external monitoring include the following: distress is minimal to the patient; the initiation of the procedure can be achieved immediately as part of routine nursing care; it can be used during an induction, when the cervix is closed and the membranes are intact; and finally, it is an ideal method with which to screen labor patients to determine the status of the fetus.

Internal monitoring

If the clinician needs more precise information about fetal status internal mon-

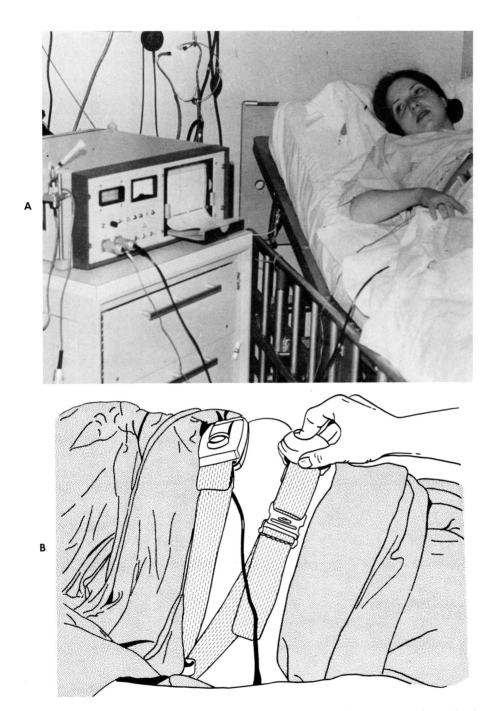

Fig. 21-1. A, External monitoring equipment: bedside unit. **B,** External monitoring equipment: tocodynamometer (upper belt) and ultrasound (lower belt). (**A** courtesy Thomas Blakowski, Director of Educational Services, The Toledo Hospital, Toledo, Ohio; **B** drawn by Carol Perkins, medical photographer, Institute of Medical Research, The Toledo Hospital.)

itoring is appropriate. The main prerequisite for the initiation of internal monitoring is rupture of membranes.

The internal method of measuring uterine contractions utilizes a fluid-filled catheter inserted into the lower uterine segment and connected to an external transducer. It is advisable to insert the catheter before applying the electrodes so that they will not become dislodged during catheter insertion. The polyethylene catheter is inserted through a transvaginal guide. If the presenting part is low (+1) station, placement of the catheter above the presenting part may be difficult.

As the pressure within the uterus increases during a uterine contraction, the fluid within the catheter also increases. The transducer converts this pressure change to an electrical signal that is then recorded on the graph as a uterine contraction. The advantages are that the data are quantitative because tonus (lowest pressure recorded between contractions) may be determined; amplitude, or intensity, is readily demonstrated; baseline values are useful in suspected abruptio placentae or during oxytocin (Pitocin) inductions; and obesity does not interfere with the recording of uterine contractions. Disadvantages are that the membranes must be ruptured; a trained operator is needed; and the catheter may become plugged or coiled, producing inaccurate recordings. Possible but infrequent complications include perforation of the lower uterine segment by the inappropriate use of the catheter guide (transducer) and infection attributed to poor aseptic technique.

Internal monitoring of the FHR may be done when the membranes are ruptured, the cervix is 2 to 3 cm. dilated, and the presenting part is −2 to −1 station. A scalp-clip electrode with silver-silver chloride barbs is pressed against the presenting part and closed. These barbs penetrate the skin and prevent the clip from being dislodged. In addition to the clip electrodes, there are hook, screw, and suction cup electrodes. My experience is with the Hon clip electrode.* Fig. 21-2, *B*, shows the scalp electrode forceps used to aid emplacement. The electrode is applied under aseptic conditions, with the patient in lithotomy position. The patient should be properly prepared for the procedure; a mild sedative may be necessary. Either the supine or lateral position is used. The electrode, held in place by a specifically designed forceps, is introduced into the vagina through a lighted endoscope or speculum. Occasionally the location of the presenting part may require the application of the electrode without an endoscope. Once the presenting part is located and visualized, slight pressure is applied to the forceps handles to allow the electrode to penetrate; then immediately pressure is carefully released, so as not to dislodge the electrode. The advantages of internal monitoring of the FHR are that there is little electrical interference from the patients movement, obesity is no problem, and the tracing most closely approximates the actual FHR. The disadvantages are that the membranes must be ruptured, the equipment must be applied by an especially trained person, the electrodes may become dislodged during a vaginal examination, and application is difficult when the cervix is posterior. Complications include hematomas of the vagina or cervix due to faulty application, as well as rare instances of fetal scalp hematomas or lacerations. Fig. 21-2, *A*, shows the equipment required for internal monitoring. Fig. 21-2, *B*, is a close-up of the Hon scalp-clip electrode; Fig. 21-2, *C*, shows the sagittal view of the pelvis with the internal monitor in place.

Occasionally the external and internal monitoring technique may be advantageously combined. If the cervix is minimally dilated (1 to 2 cm.), the presenting part is high (−3), making electrode application impossible, and the membranes are ruptured, the intrauterine catheter may be chosen to record uterine contractions and the ultrasound method, to record FHR. If the presenting part is a +2 station and placement of the intrauterine catheter presents difficulties, the external contraction belt may be used while the FHR is being recorded by the direct electrode technique. A combination of external and internal monitoring may be necessitated by the patient's condition and also by the functioning of either the operator or the machine.

---

*Manufactured by Corometrics.

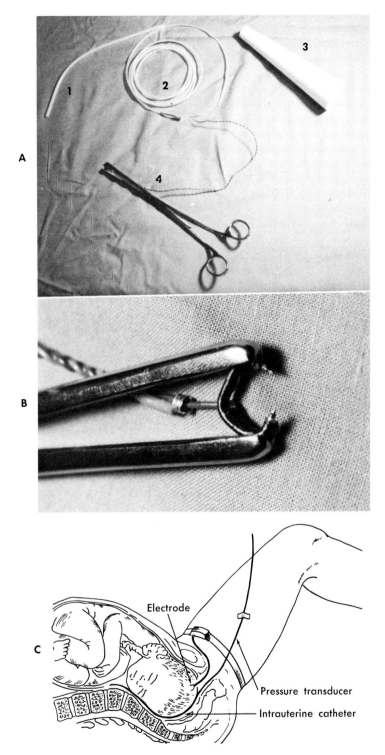

Fig. 21-2. A, Internal monitoring equipment: *1,* catheter guide; *2,* uterine catheter; *3,* endoscope; *4,* electrode forceps with fetal scalp electrode. **B,** Detail, fetal scalp electrode forceps. **C,** Internal monitor in place: sagittal view of pelvis. (**A** and **B** courtesy Thomas Blakowski; **C** drawn by Carol Perkins, medical photographer, Institute of Medical Research, The Toledo Hospital.)

The essential principle is that both parameters, FHR and uterine contractions, should be monitored simultaneously.

These are the major methods of fetal monitoring that currently are used in clinical practice. Other methods, such as transabdominal catheters and telemetry, are most often applicable in research settings. The type of monitoring used depends on many factors, such as the availability of trained and interested nursing and medical staff, financial resources, physical layout of the unit, availability of repair service from the manufacturer, characteristics of the patient population, the stage of labor, and patient cooperation. Regardless of the type of monitoring used, a primary advantage of fetal monitoring is the constant supervision and evaluation of the patient and the fetus by the medical and nursing staff.

TYPES OF FETAL HEART RATE PATTERNS AND THEIR SIGNIFICANCE

The FHR pattern represents the output of a physiological control system involving the interaction of cardioaccelerator and cardiodecelerator reflexes. An imbalance between these two opposing control mechanisms is reflected in an FHR acceleration or deceleration. The two major classifications of FHR changes are baseline and periodic changes, which are associated with uterine contractions. Periodic FHR changes are classified on the basis of the wave shape and on the time relationship between the beginning of a contraction and the onset of FHR change.[6]

Periodic changes

Studies of FHR patterns during labor indicate that specific FHR changes are associated with contractions and appear to be a direct result of the mechanical effects of the uterine contraction on the fetus. Fig. 21-3 presents a diagram illustrating the effects of uterine contractions on the fetus. The mechanical energy of a contraction may produce fetal stress in at least three ways: (1) application of direct pressure to the fetal body, usually at the vertex; (2) occlusion of the umbilical cord; or (3) hindrance of venous outflow from and arterial inflow to the intervillous space.[6]

The FHR deceleration patterns appear to be the most clinically significant. It is important to identify the individual pat-

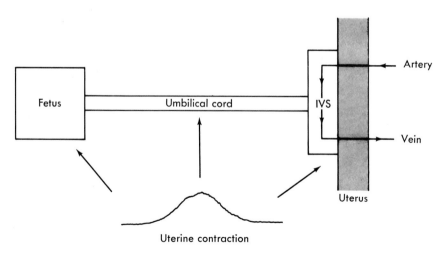

Fig. 21-3. Diagram of the effect of uterine contractions on the fetus. (From Hon, E. H.: An introduction to fetal heart rate monitoring, New Haven, Conn., 1969, Harty Press, Inc.)

terns. Fig. 21-4 illustrates the shape of FHR deceleration patterns. Three such specific patterns have been observed and are now used as standard nomenclature: (1) early deceleration, or head compression; (2) late deceleration, or uteroplacental insufficiency; and (3) variable deceleration, or umbilical cord compression (Fig. 21-5, *A*). The crucial fact is that these deceleration patterns may occur with any basal heart rate and may therefore be found within the normal accepted range of 120 to 160 beats a minute.

Early deceleration. The pattern of early deceleration of the FHR associated with head compression is presented in Fig. 21-5, *A*. This pattern is presently considered to be relatively innocuous and not related to fetal acid-base disturbances. It is probably due to a momentary increase in intracranial pressure. This increase stimulates the vagal center in the brain, resulting in the depression of FHR. This pattern, usually occurs when the patient is 5 cm. dilated or when the membranes rupture. Although this pattern is presently

considered to be reasonably benign, it is important to distinguish this pattern from the late deceleration pattern.

Late deceleration. The pattern of late deceleration of the FHR associated with uteroplacental insufficiency is given in Fig. 21-5, *B*. This pattern, found more frequently in high-risk pregnancies, uterine hyperactivity, and maternal hypotension, is ominous and associated with a decrease in maternal-fetal exchange. Uteroplacental insufficiency (UPI) is related to fetal hypoxia, usually indicates a depressed baby, and may occur any time during labor. Contractions can reduce or stop maternal blood flow through the intervillous space (IVS) by exerting direct pressure on the vessels and also by constricting the individual vessels. The IVS may be thought of as a safety reservoir containing oxygenated blood, from which the fetus can continue to receive oxygen even after an interruption of blood flow. Contractions alone usually will not produce hypoxia in the fetus.

Variable deceleration (Fig. 21-5, *C*). This is the most common FHR pattern associated

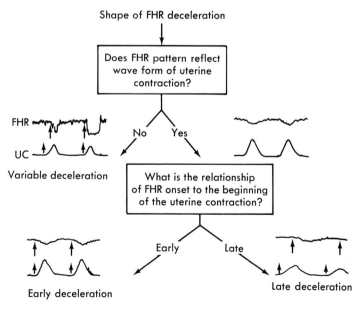

Fig. 21-4. Diagram for identification of specific FHR deceleration patterns. (From Hon, E. H.: An introduction to fetal heart rate monitoring, New Haven, Conn., 1969, Harty Press, Inc.)

with clinical fetal distress. It is probably caused by umbilical cord compression (CC). This pattern is usually not associated with fetal acid-base imbalance unless the FHR changes are frequent, profound, and prolonged. It may be found in conjunction with either early or late deceleration patterns or both. The position of the umbilical cord at delivery is an inconclusive indication of the possible compression that it may have undergone, since the position of the cord changes with the movement of the fetus. This deceleration pattern is usually alleviated by a change in maternal position. When this pattern is correctly identified many cesarean sections for fetal distress may be eliminated.

Baseline changes

The baseline FHR pattern is established when the patient is not in labor or in the interval between periodic FHR changes, which often is the same as the interval between contractions. Irregularity in the base line is considered a good sign, since it indicates that the fetus has a functioning, well-developed nervous mechanism controlling its heart rate. A smooth, or fixed, base line,

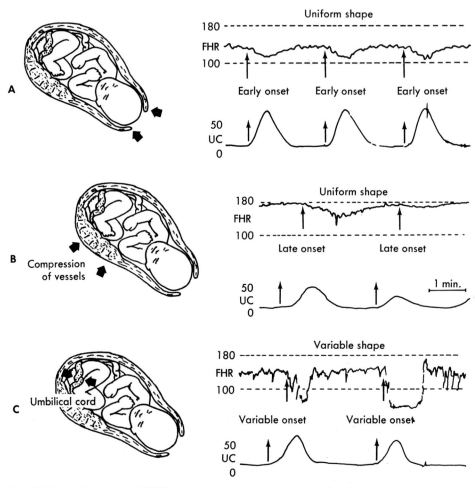

Fig. 21-5. A, Diagram of FHR pattern: early deceleration; head compression. **B,** Late deceleration; uterine placental insufficiency. **C,** Variable deceleration; umbilical-cord compression. (From Hon, E. H.: An introduction to fetal heart rate monitoring, New Haven, Conn., 1969, Harty Press, Inc.)

showing no irregularities, indicates that the nervous control mechanism of the FHR is not fully developed or has been blunted by drugs or fetal deterioration.[6]

An irregularity of 4% to 9% of the baseline value is acceptable. The FHR is controlled by the sympathetic nervous system, which tends to elevate the rate, and the parasympathetic (vagal) system, which tends to lower it. Each individual has his own characteristic rate, which can be determined during pregnancy.

Tachycardia. The fetal heart rate must remain above 160 b.p.m. for at least two complete contraction cycles for the baseline value to be considered as tachycardia. Moderate tachycardia exists when FHR is 161 to 180 b.p.m., whereas marked tachycardia exists in the range of 181 b.p.m. and up. Tachycardia is frequently found with conditions of immaturity, maternal fever, and minimal fetal hypoxia. The presence of tachycardia with no baseline irregularity and late deceleration (UPI) is ominous and a warning of acute fetal distress. Thus, the significance of this pattern depends on the presence of a deceleration pattern and baseline variation.

Bradycardia. Bradycardia results from the vagal effect on the fetal heart and may represent the effects of hypoxia on the fetal myocardium. In the absence of late decelerations (UPI) usually no fetal compromise exists, and a vigorous newborn is delivered. Bradycardia may be associated with congenital heart lesions.

TREATMENT OF FETAL DISTRESS

Understanding of the pathophysiological mechanisms is essential to successful treatment of fetal distress. Fig. 21-6 diagrams the treatment modalities used in response to the FHR patterns, late deceleration (UPI) and variable deceleration (CC). The main treatment modalities include (1) changing maternal position, (2) decreasing uterine activity, (3) correcting maternal hypotension, and (4) administering oxygen by mask to the mother.

Changing maternal position

This measure represents an attempt to remove pressure from the umbilical cord. In addition, the lateral position may decrease uterine activity. A change from supine to lateral position should be consid-

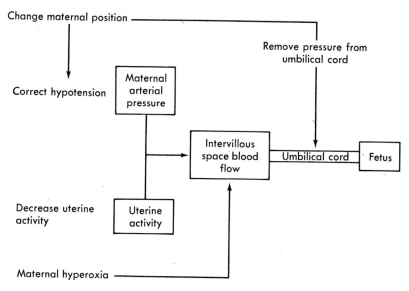

Fig. 21-6. Diagram of treatment modalities used to correct fetal distress (late deceleration and variable deceleration). (From Hon, E. H.: An introduction to fetal heart rate monitoring, New Haven, Conn., 1969, Harty Press, Inc.)

ered as an initial method to correct fetal distress; if the right lateral position does not correct distress, the left lateral position should be tried. This treatment modality should be initiated by the nurse, when the deceleration pattern has been observed. The nurse should note and record on the monitor's graph each position change. This will assist in the interpretation of data and will also help the physician to plan appropriate management. An additional nursing responsibility is to change the patient's position from the supine to the lateral, after each vaginal examination. On occasion, it may be necessary to place the patient in Trendelenburg's position to correct the fetal distress pattern after both lateral positions have been tried and when the graph of FHR reveals no correction of the deceleration pattern.

Decreasing uterine activity

Decreasing uterine activity will increase perfusion of the IVS. If oxytocics are being used, the amount and rate of the medication should be reevaluated. If the contractions are spontaneous, the reduction of contractility is difficult. In some research centers, a uterine depressant such as isoxsuprine hydrochloride may be administered.

Correcting maternal hypotension

Both systemic and local arterial hypotension will produce fetal hypoxia. Systemic hypotension may be corrected by the administration of I.V. fluids or blood, control of conduction anesthesia, and the avoidance of large doses of meperdine hydrochloride (Demerol). Local hypotension may be corrected by placing the mother on her side or by elevating her legs.

Administering oxygen

The administration of oxygen may increase the maternal-fetal oxygen transfer. A late deceleration pattern may often be alleviated by the use of oxygen, when maternal hypotension or excessive uterine activity is not present. The administration of oxygen to the mother can raise the fetal P_{O_2} level.[11] If the nurse institutes this corrective measure, oxygen should be administered by a tight-fitting mask at 6 to 7 liters a minute.

• • •

The use of the foregoing corrective measures to alleviate fetal distress will be beneficial in most patients. However, some situations of fetal distress will not respond to these treatments. Hon[6] states that persistent ominous FHR patterns for thirty minutes after the institution of the outlined therapeutic measures indicate that labor should be terminated operatively.

PATIENT'S RESPONSE TO FETAL MONITORING

Electronic fetal monitoring has been conducted for over a year at The Toledo Hospital, a community institution with 3,500 annual deliveries. There are both private and staff deliveries, and the hospital participates in a residency program. Corometrics equipment is used in both external and internal monitoring. Last October a monitoring project, sponsored by a grant from the Selma Collin Fund, was begun, allowing the procedure to be more fully developed and refined as a clinical tool. I was responsible for the implementation of monitoring in the delivery unit and for the collection of data. To date, 115 patients, both private and staff, have been monitored by either external or internal techniques and have been interviewed afterward. The sample is comprised of patients who have diagnosed high-risk conditions or who demonstrate clinical fetal distress during labor.

Procedure

The consent of the attending physician is required for internal monitoring; however, if the nurses decide to use external monitoring as an adjunct to their nursing observations, the physician's consent is not obligatory. The internal monitor is usually applied by the research nurse-midwife, an Obstetric-Gynecological resident, or by the private obstetrician.

The patient to be monitored by either technique was approached initially by the resident, the obstetrician, the nurse, or myself. This initial patient contact included the following points: the purpose of monitoring, an explanation and a description of the equipment and of the information it provides (a close check on how the baby

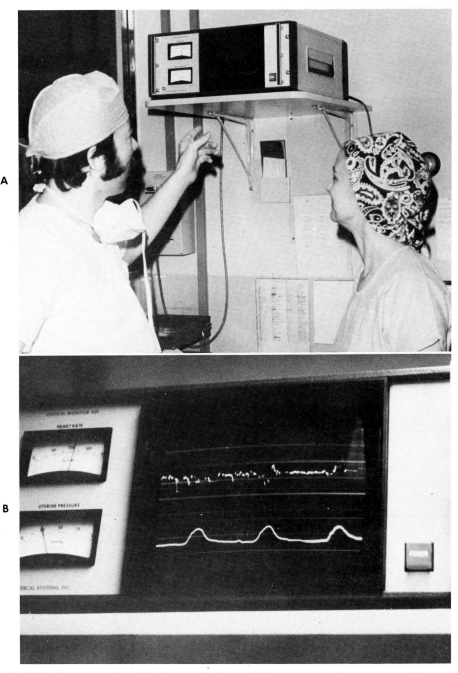

Fig. 21-7. A, Central monitoring unit located in nurses' station. **B,** Detail, central monitoring unit. Fetal heart rate and uterine contractions on oscilloscope located in nurses' station. (Photographs courtesy Thomas Blakowski.)

is tolerating labor), and a description of the procedure and of how the fetal heart-beat will sound. Every attempt was made to minimize the patient's concern that the baby was sick or in trouble. The patient was never coerced to accept the procedure. Rather the procedure was presented as an additional aspect of specialized care that was available to them at no extra cost. Whenever possible, the husband or family were involved in this discussion. In our experience with 115 patients, only two refused the procedure: one patient had a language barrier that caused misunderstanding, and the other was excessively anxious about labor.

In the study, the patient was moved to one of four labor rooms equipped for central monitoring, allowing the monitor data to be observed both on the printouts in the patient's room and also at a central oscilloscope located at the nurses' station (Fig. 21-7). The patient's equipment was brought into her room, and instrumentation was begun. The internal apparatus was applied with the patient supine and with her hips elevated on an inverted bedpan. The same precautions were observed as for a vaginal examination. The nurse was present to support the patient and to assist with the instrumentation. The external equipment was applied by the nurse with the patient in the supine position, which might be changed to the lateral posture later with only minor readjustments of the belts. Once the monitor was attached and was functioning well, the display on the print-out was explained to the patient and to her husband. They were taught to watch for contractions, for FHR, and for the distance between contractions. If the sound of the FHR was bothersome, they were shown how to turn off the speaker. Data for the chart were collected on an especially designated form, which was then completed with delivery findings and later analyzed by me. The next day I interviewed the patient to determine her response and to answer any questions that she might have.

Postmonitoring interviews

The initial responses of patients to the monitoring equipment during the first thirty minutes of application was used to categorize two groups. The positive group manifested feelings and made comments indicating that they were interested in new ideas and equipment, that they did not have this benefit with their last baby, or that they were pleased to have someone observing them with special care. Most of the patients in this group were also excited about hearing the baby's heartbeat, which seemed to be a strong motivation for their participation in fetal monitoring.

The second group had a negative initial response that was revealed at the time of interview. They said that they were frightened of the unknown or that they were concerned about harm to themselves or their babies. The request for permission to use the monitor led some patients to jump to the conclusion that they or their babies were already in jeopardy. Very few patients said that they were disinterested. Those who did were either very young and apathetic about the whole process or had been medicated and therefore were not responsive to their environment. Some of these patients were also well into the active phase of labor and not fully aware of their surroundings.

The later patient responses, after the first thirty minutes of monitoring equipment use, were more varied and therefore did not provide such concise groupings. Many saw the monitor as helpful because it told them when a contraction was coming so that they could be prepared or because it kept their husbands occupied. For some it seemed to hasten labor. The patients did not feel that monitoring made labor longer. For many the sound of the baby's heartbeat provided reassurance. One patient said that, although during her pregnancy she knew that the baby was well because she felt movement, during early labor she became certain only when she heard the heartbeat. Patients compared the fetal heartbeat sound to a washing machine, a horse race, or a fish tank pump. Some patients were more anxious at being monitored. These patients commented that they knew that "the end was near" or that the mere presence of the machine made them "jumpy." Occasionally, problems with electrical interference produced extraneous noises that at times were quite annoying. A few patients, as they entered the active phase of labor, were disturbed by the belts of the external monitor. In most cases, the patient's husband or family were more interested in the monitor and its data display.

Few of the patients had heard about fetal monitoring before they arrived in labor. Some saw the central unit when they went on the expectant parents' tour of the hospital. Occasionally the private physician mentioned monitoring to a few of his high-risk patients. Several of the patients had heard about monitoring either from the newspaper or from a local television interview describing my activities. Most of these patients had few if any questions about monitoring at the time of the interview. Usually they said that they had told or would tell their friends about the experience and also would recommend it to them if they had the opportunity to participate.

The postmonitoring patient interviews have provided some valuable data. Previously physicians and nurses expressed concern about the patients' tolerating the procedure. It can now be stated that the patients' and their husbands' responses were usually positive and appreciative. This information has increased the acceptance of the monitoring project by the private obstetricians, as well as by the delivery room staff. There is also a clearer understanding of how patients perceive the purpose of the monitor, and these data have been used to revise the information about the monitor given to future patients. We now realize how important that first contact is in creating patient acceptance of fetal monitoring. When their preparation was scanty or hurried, patients tolerated the procedure poorly. That the nurse's positive response, growing out of knowledge and approval, is critical to the success of the monitoring project and to the patient's attitude became obvious.

NURSING ROLE IN FETAL MONITORING: FACILITATOR vs. RESISTER

The patient's acceptance of fetal monitoring is often dependent on the nurse's support and personal reaction to the equipment. The nurse, because of an intimate contact with the mother in labor, is in an excellent position to initiate and facilitate fetal monitoring and thus to contribute to improved perinatal care. Often medical innovations are met by resistance from the nursing staff. This reaction may be based on lack of knowledge or outright resistance to change or technology. Because monitoring involves new equipment and may be used in medical research, nurses may think that it is not their responsibility to get involved. However, the nurse's role in fetal monitoring has three major areas of focus: the patient, the machine, and the labor and delivery staff.

The expectant mother

Before discussing nursing functions with the expectant mother in relationship to fetal monitoring, the nurse must have a thorough knowledge of the purpose of fetal monitoring, the reasons for monitoring, and the scope and limitations of the equipment. The nurse's primary responsibility is to prepare the patient for fetal monitoring, including a complete explanation of the procedure, the instrumentation, and the reason for monitoring. The nurse should emphasize the value of close observation in labor without alarming the mother over the baby's condition. To fulfill this responsibility, the nurse must know the patient and then decide on the best approach. Some patients will demand a fuller explanation, whereas others may be alarmed if too much detail is offered. The husband or the family member who is present with the mother in labor should be included in the interview with her. Both the patient and the nurse must remember that the monitor neither replaces the nurse nor increases the demand on nursing time, once the mother understands the procedure and the equipment is functioning properly. The laboring mother's need for comfort and supportive measures must be evaluated as usual and met appropriately.

Often the monitor makes it easier to help a mother with her contractions because the nurse is able to tell her when the contraction is beginning, when it is peaking, and when it is almost completed. The mother herself has access to this information by watching the graph. This provides the mother with information that helps her maintain control by breathing and relaxing appropriately. The nurse can instruct the husband to be an effective coach. Many of the parents interviewed after monitoring thought that the main objective of fetal monitoring was to provide information about contractions.

The nurse's contact with the patient being monitored does not terminate in the labor and delivery unit. I found that a visit to these patients the next day could be beneficial and significant. The visit is an excellent time to answer questions about the monitor and to discuss labor and delivery. The mothers also respond favorably to a visit from their labor room nurse, interpreted by them as "deluxe care." Nurses themselves recognize this important aspect of comprehensive, patient-centered nursing care. The postmonitoring session also provides an opportunity to present the mother with a small section of the tracing for her baby book.

When expectant parents visit the labor and delivery suite, the nurse should introduce them to the fetal monitor. This prelabor contact can be significant in facilitating an acceptance of monitoring. Usually patients with prior knowledge of fetal monitoring responded more favorably to the procedure.

Often nurses will say that a patient is a poor candidate for fetal monitoring. In these cases, my experience has showed that the nurse usually has failed to render supportive care to a patient who is frightened and tolerating labor poorly. Some of the mother's apprehension may be diminished by hearing the baby's heartbeat and thereby concluding that he is well. Thus monitoring can help the nurse to give good care. Fetal monitoring provides more accurate information about fetal toleration of labor. A nurse working in the labor area should want to use every available method to ensure the infant's well-being.

The machine

The nurse may be solely responsible for initiating external monitoring. If internal monitoring is used, the nurse must assist with instrumentation, including setting up the sterile equipment, attaching the light

to the endoscope, applying fundal pressure, flushing out the strain gauge, and attaching the leg plate. The nurse should also help maintain sterile technique. The nursing staff may be helpful in suggesting new implementations; their assistance in innovation is invaluable. Trouble with the rigid catheter guide spurred one of our nurses to suggest the use of a flexible rubber catheter, enabling a skirting of the presenting part, thereby achieving a more successful placement of the uterine catheter for obtaining the necessary pressure readings. Also, recognizing that a resident was having difficulty with the placement of the endoscope, a nurse brought him a sterile vaginal speculum, enabling direct visualization for attaching the fetal electrode. The maintenance of the equipment and ordering of supplies is a responsibility that the nurse may delegate to another staff member. Because of experience in charting, the nurse often is more skilled and sensitive to the need for keeping accurate records of every medication, change in position, procedure, and examination to be marked on the monitor tracings. These records are of invaluable assistance in interpreting the tracing. Monitoring will be more successful when the procedure is written clearly. The nursing staff, by becoming involved in the writing, can make a valuable contribution that will help to ensure ease of operation. This written procedure will also help all members of the delivery staff to become familiar with the equipment, thereby decreasing some of the apprehension associated with new equipment and hopefully increasing the use of the fetal monitor.

The staff

Fetal monitoring facilitates a close working relationship between the nurse and the physicians involved in delivery: obstetricians, anesthesiologists, and pediatricians. For a monitoring project to be successful, a medical-nursing team is essential, for often the nurse recognizes the need for closer observation in labor and is in a position to recommend the use of the monitor. The nurse is also the liaison between the various medical groups, informing the obstetrician about the FHR and contraction pattern so that he may plan appropriate management. The nursery nurse and the pediatrician should be notified during labor of fetal distress, so that they may then make adequate preparations to care for the newborn. The anesthesiologist should be informed of the fetal status so that he may administer the safest and most effective anesthetic to the mother; possible resuscitation of the newborn should also be anticipated.

CONCLUSION

The fetal monitor is an indispensable component of modern labor observation, contributing accurate information about the labor process and the progress of the mother and fetus. These data are essential to those physicians who must plan the management of labor and delivery, and to the nurse who uses the data to facilitate the management process. Fetal monitoring should be recognized as a challenge; the nurse should become knowledgeable about this new clinical tool in labor care. Using data about the fetus and uterine contractions as a basis for care, the nurse can make a significant contribution to ensuring fetal well-being during labor, delivering a healthy newborn, and reducing the fetal mortality rate.

References

1. ACOG Newsletter **15**:6, Aug., 1971.
2. Aubry, R. H., and Nesbitt, R. E., Jr.: High risk obstetrics. I. Perinatal outcome in relation to broadened approach to obstetric care for patients at special risk, Am. J. Obstet. Gynecol. **105**:241, 1969.
3. Babson, S. G., and Benson, R. C.: Management of high-risk pregnancy and intensive care of the neonate, ed. 2, St. Louis, 1971, The C. V. Mosby Co.
4. Day, E., Maddern, L., and Wood, C.: Auscultation of foetal heart rate; an assessment of its error and significance, Br. Med. J. **4**:422, Nov. 16, 1968.
5. Gruenwald, P.: Perinatal death of full-sized and full-term infants, Am. J. Obstet. Gynecol. **107**:1022, 1970.
6. Hon, E. H.: Introduction to fetal heart rate patterns, New Haven, Conn., 1969, Harty Press, Inc.
7. Hon, E. H.: Direct monitoring of the fetal heart, Hosp. Prac. **5**:91, Sept., 1970.
8. Nesbitt, R. E., Jr. and Aubry, R. H.: High-risk obstetrics. II. Value of semiobjective grading system in identifying the vulnerable group, Am. J. Obstet. Gynecol. **103**:972, 1969.
9. Proceedings of the National Conference for the Prevention of Mental Retardation through Improved Maternity Care, May 27-29, 1968, Washington, D. C., U. S. Dept. of Health, Education, and Welfare, Children's Bureau, Social and Rehabilitation Service.
10. Schifrin, B. S., and Dame, L.: Fetal heart rate patterns; prediction of apgar score, J.A.M.A. **219**:1322, March 6, 1972.
11. Wood, E. C.: Studies of the human fetus during normal and abnormal labor, Int. J. Gynecol. Obstet. **8**:867, Nov., 1970.

Bibliography

Bishop, E. H.: Ultrasonic fetal monitoring, Clin. Obstet. Gynecol. **11**:1154, 1968.

Caldeyro-Barcia, R., Méndez-Bauer, C., Poserio, J. J., Escarcena, L. A., Pose, S. V., Bieniarz, J., Arnt, I., Gullin, L., and Althabe, O.: Control of human fetal heart rate during labor. In Cassels, D. E., editor: The heart and circulation in the newborn (symposium), New York, 1966, Grune & Stratton, Inc., pp. 7-37.

Case, L. L.: Ultrasound monitoring of mother and fetus, Am. J. Nurs. **72**:725, 1972.

Hon, E. H., and Paul, R. H.: A primer of fetal heart rate patterns, New Haven, Conn., 1970, Harty Press, Inc.

Paul, R. H.: Fetal intensive care; intrapartum monitoring; case examples with self-instruction, Los Angeles, 1971, University of Southern California.

Roux, J. F., Wilson, R., Yeni-Komshian, H., Jassani, M., and Jordan, J.: Labor monitoring. A practical experience, Obstet Gynecol **36**:875, 1970.

Schneider, J.: The high risk pregnancy, Hosp. Prac. **6**:133, Oct., 1971.

Strickland, M. D.: Fetal assessment techniques; a challenge to the nurse practitioner. In Duffy, M., Anderson, E. H., Bergersen, B. S., Lohr, M., and Rose, M. H., editors: Current concepts in clinical nursing, Vol. III, St. Louis, 1971, The C. V. Mosby Co.

22

The maternity nurse clinician in practice

Mary M. Fowler

Although many articles are written about the nurse clinician by educators, administrators, and others, few are by the practitioner functioning in that role. This chapter is concerned with my activities as a nurse clinician in maternity and newborn nursing in a large military hospital.

Maternity nursing is more than the physical care of a woman and her infant. It is also involved with the stresses and conflicts that contribute to the crisis experienced by the mother and her family in the childbearing experience. Caplan has described pregnancy as follows:

> . . . a period of altered behavior; it is a period of disequilibrium compared with the normal state of the family; it is a period of emotional upset in the woman and often in her husband and other children. It is a period when there are problems, many of which cannot be adequately handled by the customary problem solving mechanisms*

Pregnancy is a period of maturational crisis. Maturational or developmental crises are ". . . periods of marked physical, psychological and social change that are characterized by common disturbances in thought and feeling."† Pregnancy is considered a normal developmental process. Furthermore, not all maturational crises of any one period are completed before the next period begins. The crisis of one developmental period may be superimposed on the next with the individual attempting to cope with the stresses of both.[3] A pregnant 15-year-old girl is engrossed in the common problems and desires of adolescence when she must also cope with stresses peculiar to pregnancy.

A variety of maturational problems are encountered in pregnancy. One of the most important of these problems is that "The woman is preparing for a completely new role. If this is her first baby she is moving from being a wife to becoming a mother."* She might worry that there will not be room for both her and the baby in her husband's affection or that she cannot be a successful mother and wife too. She might have feelings of ambivalence toward her pregnancy, her baby, or both. Other stresses of pregnancy are physical discomforts of the various stages of pregnancy, erratic mood swings, probable changes in sex drive, changes in body image, fear of labor, or fear of harm to or even death of self or baby.

Situational crises are also frequently encountered in pregnancy. Situational crises are said to exist ". . . whenever stressful events occur in a person's life situation that threaten his sense of biological, psychological or social integrity."†

A situational crisis might develop from any of the following circumstances:

1. A change of residence during pregnancy, especially if the move separates the mother from supporting relatives
2. A father who is not in the home during pregnancy or present at the time of delivery
3. A mother who is unmarried
4. A history of loss of a previous fetus or child

---

*From Caplan, G.: An approach to community mental health, New York, 1961, Grune & Stratton, Inc., p. 65. Used by permission.
†From Parad, H. J., ed.: Crisis intervention: selected readings, New York, 1965, Family Service Association of America, p. 73.

---

*From Caplan, p. 66.
†From Aguilera, D. C., Messick, J. M., and Farrell, M. S.: Crisis intervention: theory and methodology, St. Louis, 1970, The C. V. Mosby Co., p. 57.

5. A history of an abnormal or premature child
6. A recent death of a loved one
7. Several children in the family already, especially if the interval between pregnancies is very short
8. A medical problem that might have a deleterious effect on the outcome of the pregnancy

Although it is recognized that all these potential crisis situations are present in pregnancy and extend into the puerperium, health care personnel have not been too successful in finding ways to give the mother and her family the help they need. I believe the maternity care given in the medical center where I am situated is similar to care offered in most other large hospitals. The patients see a number of physicians in the course of their antepartal care. Large numbers of patients act as a restraint on both the physician and the patient. The physician does not take a personal history each visit, and the patient frequently states that the physician is so busy that she does not want to bother him with questions or ask for explanations. Patients frequently go home with unanswered questions. This causes needless worry and concern. The nurses and physicians who would like to function differently feel frustrated and fall into the established system of health care.

As an inpatient, the mother may encounter a separate staff (nurses and physicians) in the labor-delivery suite, recovery rooms, postpartum unit, and nursery. Communication between staff from each area is not always good. This lack of continuity adds additional stress on the patient.

As a nurse clinician, I am assigned as an additional member of the maternity service health team. I am directly responsible to the chief nurse in the Department of Nursing and am given the freedom to work as I see fit with patients in any area of maternity-newborn care.

Because of my availability on all units, I am viewed as one person the patients can contact at any time in their childbearing experience—one person who can *listen* to their problems and concerns, answer their questions, *listen*, give guidance, *listen*, explain procedures, *listen*, interpret physician's instructions, and, above all, LISTEN when they desperately need a confidential sympathetic ear.

The importance of listening can be demonstrated by this report of an interview with Mrs. C.

> Mrs. C stopped me in the clinic and asked to speak with me. She was very upset and unhappy. The physician she saw the week before had told her that her labor would be induced if she had not gone into spontaneous labor by that day. The doctor she had just seen decided that it would be inadvisable to induce labor at that time. Mrs. C was disappointed and angry. She could not understand why the doctors could not agree. She was allowed to talk and express her feelings freely. Her main source of anxiety seemed to be that she was afraid she would not get to the hospital on time. Her previous labors had been very rapid. She lives a distance from the hospital, and traffic can be heavy. I reviewed her chart and talked with the physician; with this information, I explained why the doctor did not want to induce labor then. She appeared satisfied but came back to the fear of not getting to the hospital on time. We discussed the early discernible signs of labor and explored the possible methods of getting help if time was pressing. Actually she had discussed this with the personnel of the dispensary near her and knew how to get help. Finally, she blurted out, "Would my baby just die if I delivered at home or in the car?" I explained that most babies would cry and breathe spontaneously after delivery. I told her how to clear the baby's mouth and nose of mucus, emphasized the necessity of keeping the baby warm, and told her to leave the cord intact and call an ambulance. She appeared very relieved. She said, "Is that all you have to do? I thought the doctor had to do something to the baby before it would breathe."

A thirty-minute conference with Mrs. C in which her feelings and anxieties were expressed and explored finally got to the basis of her extreme fear. Explanations and positive things she could do to help herself and her baby allayed her feelings of panic and gave her the needed confidence to await normal labor at home.

Sometimes nurses do not listen well enough or long enough to discern what the "real" problem is.[4] If I had tried to appease Mrs. C by assuring her that we had good physicians who were trying to help her, she would not have continued our discussion. I would not have known of her erroneous idea that her baby might die if delivered without medical help, and she would have gone home with the same fears and anxieties as she had when she came in.

(Mrs. C was delivered of a normal baby boy in the hospital.)

Continuity of care is another aspect of maternity nursing that is frequently lacking; it is important to all patients, but for some it is crucial. This is well demonstrated in the care of Mrs. W.

Mrs. W is an example of a person undergoing a profound maturational and situational crisis. Her ego strength and self-concept were so poorly developed that she was left with little ability to cope with the crisis of childbearing. She was reminiscent of the "apronstring" child as described by Looff in his book *Appalachia's Children*.[4] Mrs. W came from a poor home in a deprived rural area. She was a middle child of twelve children. She had little formal schooling and little social experience outside the family. She was extremely shy and fearful. Her husband was her only source of emotional support. She was ill equipped to cope with hospitalization and the indignities encountered as an obstetrical patient. The number of persons she had to meet was traumatic to her. Any stranger was a threat.

Mrs. W was admitted to the labor suite in early labor; she was frightened to the point of panic and would not allow anyone to touch her. The physicians thought that I might be able to help her. At first she rejected me, but as I stayed with her, accepted her behavior, and gave her support, she became more cooperative. I took her blood pressure and monitored the fetal heart. She would reach for my hand when a contraction started. Her record revealed that she had had no prenatal care. She told me that her husband brought her for her prenatal appointments and thought she was receiving care but she would spend an hour in the snack bar and did not go to the clinic because she was afraid and embarrassed. She was painfully shy and appeared overwhelmed by fear; she appeared bright and was very pretty. She would not look at me except when the contractions came. Then her eyes were panic stricken like those of a trapped animal. Her labor was painful but ineffectual. When the membranes ruptured, the amniotic fluid was stained with meconium. An x-ray pelvimetry revealed a contracted midpelvis; it was decided that a cesarean section was the best method of delivery. The decision and the procedure were explained to Mrs. W and her husband. She was still very frightened but cooperated as she was prepared for surgery. Her husband stayed by her side and walked to surgery with her.

A baby boy was delivered with Mrs. W under general anesthesia. She did not see her baby in surgery. Mrs. W was returned to the obstetrical ward from the recovery room the morning after surgery. She appeared subdued, quiet, and fearful but was trying her best to do exactly as she was told. She would ambulate, cough, and use the blow bottles as instructed. When I talked with her, she indicated that she would like to see her baby. When I returned from the nursery, she was sitting upright in bed and reached out her arms for her baby. I placed the baby on her lap and loosened the blanket. She stroked the baby's hair with one finger, brushed his cheek, and put her finger in his tiny fist. She commented: "This is my little Jimmy." She had told me that she would name him Jimmy if she had a boy. I left her alone with the baby for a few minutes. When I returned to take the baby back to the nursery, she kissed him lightly on the head.

I was very pleased with this healthy beginning of the mothering role. After I had gone, one of the staff nurses went to Mrs. W's room. In the conversation that followed, Mrs. W remarked, "Was that really my baby?" The staff nurse immediately reported the patient's question to the nursery. In view of her behavior when admitted to the labor room, both physicians and nurses interpreted the comment at face value. They thought Mrs. W really did not realize that the baby was hers and that she could not be trusted to care for him. I had seen Mrs. W with her baby. I knew her initial contact was normal and healthy. She was beginning the identification and claiming process. I believed she was really saying, "I can't believe that anyone as worthless as I am can have such a perfect child."

The physicians were reluctant but agreed that Mrs. W could go to the nursery and care for her baby under supervision. She was so pathetically shy and insecure that she could not chance making a mistake with the baby with all the nurses watching her. She would go to the nursery faithfully but could not progress beyond holding Jimmy. She would not feed or diaper him. The nursery nurses tried to reassure her, but they were anxious and really did not believe she could care for her baby. Mrs. W's husband was very attentive and concerned. He was confident that she could care for baby Jimmy. He explained that Mrs. W had never been away from home or met many people but she had helped care for her little brothers and sisters and her sister's children. When Mrs. W had recovered from surgery sufficiently to care for the baby through a rooming-in arrangement, I encouraged the physicians to let her have the baby to develop her mothering role in the privacy of her room. They were rather reluctant but agreed that the baby could be with Mrs. W while I was on the floor. A nursing care plan was developed to give her all the encouragement we could. We would answer any question, help with any care when asked, but otherwise we could not hover too close. We could compliment Mrs. W on any progress she made in caring for herself or baby Jimmy. Any help or suggestions were to be given in a helpful, positive way without implying that she had not done a good job. Mrs. W really did well with the baby when we were not supervising too closely. We would compliment her on how well the baby was eating, how clean and nice she kept him, and even on her appearance. We noticed if she washed her hair or put on a pretty gown. She responded well to this recognition of her personal worth.

One day when I visited Mrs. W, she was holding and gently rocking her son. I commented that

Jimmy seemed to enjoy the rocking. She replied, "We both do." This was a beginning. A few days later I told her she was doing a beautiful job of caring for her baby. She answered, "I think so, too, and he is gaining weight." Mrs. W had a complication of surgery that required her to be hospitalized for two weeks. Perhaps this was a blessing in disguise; she needed time to gain confidence in herself and convince the physicians that she was mature enough to care for her child.

Mrs. W had many problems, but we were primarily concerned with helping her through the hospitalization with as little psychological trauma as possible and with helping her develop confidence and proficiency in her mothering role. We were pleased with her progress. A referral was sent to the Navy Relief Nurse (public health nurse) for follow-through care when she was discharged from the hospital. At 4 months of age, Jimmy is a friendly, sociable baby. His mother is caring for him successfully.

All patients have a need for information, interpretation, explanation, or all three throughout their pregnancies. Many anxiety-producing situations can be alleviated if patients can get help with problems when they arise. Most of the patients receiving care at this hospital are away from supportive family and friends, and many of their husbands are assigned away from home for varying lengths of time. A crisis occurs more frequently when the usual emotional support is not available. One of my most important functions is to be a resource person to the patient in her childbearing experience; as a nurse clinician, I am one individual she can turn to for support or information about general concerns.

I meet with all patients at their orientation to antepartal care, explain my role, give them my phone number, and tell them when and where I can be contacted. I spend a part of each antepartal clinic day in the general waiting room answering questions or discussing areas of general concern. The patients have a great deal in common and participate well together. Many of their concerns can be handled in a group discussion. Typical concerns include the following:

1. How does labor start? When should I come to the hospital?

2. Can my husband be with me in the labor room? What kind of anesthetic or pain medication will I get?

3. Questions prefixed by "Is it normal?" "Is it normal to be tired all the time? To have pains in my side? To feel depressed sometimes?"

4. Questions on do's and don't's. Primigravidas especially are anxious about doing something that might harm their babies. "Can I swim? Bowl? Have sex?"

5. Hospital routine is another area for questions. "How long will I be in the hospital? I heard the babies are kept in the mothers rooms. How many visitors can I have?"

These types of questions can usually be dealt with in a group. Sometimes, though, I can detect deeper anxieties among the patients. If I do, I suggest a further private discussion. Sometimes the patient will ask to talk privately.

For example, we had been having an active discussion period when the group became quiet. To start the conversation again, I asked how many of them *really* planned this pregnancy. Four or five raised their hands. Others shrugged and halfway or definitely said, "No!' One lady said she was surprised. I looked at her expectantly. She added, "We have been married thirteen years, and this is the first pregnancy. Wouldn't you have been surprised?" There were varied comments around the room. When it was quiet again, she said, "May I make an appointment to talk to you. I'm so scared." We set up an appointment convenient for her. If this patient were concerned with the pregnancy itself, labor, and delivery, I would suggest classes in the Lamaze method and would continue to see her. If her anxieties were based on fear of motherhood or the changing family, I would help her as I can, but I could refer her to other help if indicated.

Frequently, patients will wait for me or stop me in the hall and indicate a need to talk. I have a room in the clinic available for conferences. It is not uncommon that the patient has just left the physician, and her questions are, "What did he mean by thus and so? Is there anything wrong?" Sometimes a patient will ask me to explain something to her husband.

I know the braver, more articulate patients are the ones who ask the questions or seek help. The timid ones, who need help the most, are likely to hold back. When

I can spot them, I make an effort to talk to them individually.

Many of the patients' questions and concerns are related to labor and birth. Birth is anticipated with both elation and dread. An informed patient usually has a more satisfying labor-birth experience than an uninformed patient. She is usually less fearful and can work with her labor more successfully. Patients and their husbands are encouraged to attend prenatal classes and classes in preparation for childbirth. They are given a tour of the entire maternity floor. In the labor and delivery suite they see the equipment and meet some of the personnel; policies and techniques are explained. They see the nurseries and the postpartum wards and are given time to ask questions. Husbands are encouraged to accompany their wives in any of these activities and may be with them in labor and delivery.

Patients need both physical and emotional support during labor and delivery, and individual care is a necessity. The aim of care includes not only the delivery of a healthy baby to a healthy mother but also a satisfying experience for the mother (and father if he is present).

After the excitement and drama of labor and delivery the puerperium is frequently thought of as anticlimactic, a period of recuperation. Rubin gives a much better description:

A complex state of the childbearing experience, during which the physical and psychological work of gestation and delivery becomes final. And during this stage, a new role, with a complete set of new tasks is begun—before the previous work is quite finished. What is past and what is future combine to form the composite present of the puerperium.*

Throughout history, cultures have had some provision for meeting the needs of new mothers. This may be done by taboos or tradition, but it offers support as the mother recuperates and begins to mother her child. Since the advent of early ambulation and rooming-in, we are inclined to give the mother responsibilities before she is ready to handle them. In the first few days of postpartum the new mother has

*From Rubin, R.: Puerperal change, Nurs. Outlook 9:753, 1961.

definite dependency needs. She needs to be cared for; she needs rest. Sleep deprivation is frequently a problem, especially when rooming-in is utilized. She experiences mood swings, cries easily, and is very concerned with her ability to be a good mother. She has a need to talk, especially about her labor and delivery. This appears to help her find meaning in the experience. The way her needs are met and the ego support that she is given will be reflected in the way she is able to mother her child. These are universal maternal needs. Any maturational or situational crisis may be superimposed. The mother may be a teen-ager herself. The baby might be premature or have an abnormality. These patients need additional help.

Frequently the nurse and physician focus on physical needs. When the mother and baby are cared for by the obstetrical and the pediatric staffs, some areas, such as breast-feeding, are neglected, or the patient may get conflicting information.

A large percentage of my time is spent with the postpartum patient and her baby. I make ward rounds and see every patient every morning. As I make the routine physical examinations, I can evaluate the patients' needs. By sharing my findings with both nursery and postpartum nurses, better care can be planned for each mother and baby. Following are other advantages in my making rounds:

1. The mothers know me from the clinic.

2. I am not as rushed on rounds as the physicians are.

3. I can answer questions or give suggestions on care of either the mother or baby.

4. Patients relate to me more freely because I am a woman and because I am not as authoritarian a figure as the physician is.

Although I discuss the referral of complications with the physician, I am free to make general decisions. An example follows:

Mrs. M was scheduled to be discharged. She appeared nervous and anxious about caring for her baby. When I talked with her, I found that her marine husband was on sea voyage; she had not lived here long enough to make close friends. She had expected her mother to be with her, but at the last minute she could not come. She was taking her baby home with no supportive person to help her. I suggested that she remain in the hospital another day and contacted the Navy Relief Nurse, who promised to see her at home the day after discharge. With this small amount of support and one more day in the hospital, Mrs. M appeared much more secure and was ready to go home.

Situational crises vary and must be dealt with individually. Mrs. B simply needed to talk.

After the birth of her fourth child Mrs. B had a tubal ligation. Two years after the tubal ligation she became pregnant. I asked what her feelings were when she found that she was pregnant for the fifth time. This was the opening she needed. She talked of her dismay and total rejection of the pregnancy, her thoughts of having an abortion, and her moral rejection of this solution to her problem. She had guilt feelings for even considering an abortion. She spoke of financial difficulties, her friends' attitudes toward her large family, and her own feelings concerning overpopulation. She talked freely, and an occasional comment or question reflected back to her was all she needed from me. However, she had a definite need to "talk out" her feelings. She was holding her baby close as she talked. Finally, she said, "I'm glad we have him now. We will find a way, won't we, son." As I left the room, she said, "Thanks for listening." It was therapeutic for her to be allowed to talk to a nonjudgmental listener.

The prime concern of a maternity nurse clinician is to make available the best possible care throughout the childbearing experience. If it is acknowledged that pregnancy is an unstable period when unsolved problems can become crisis situations for the mother and her family, then it behooves us as nurses to find ways to help with those problems when they arise. It is frequently not the complexity of the situation but the immediacy of available help that makes the difference. A simple answer to a question, a correction of an erroneous idea, a word of understanding, or an encouraging nod of approval can be therapeutic for a mother in the experience of childbearing and child rearing. I have concentrated my efforts on being available to patients as an effective listener, providing continuity of care to families, accepting the referrals of complex cases from the staff and planning nursing approaches with them, and carrying out group and individual counseling during all phases of the maternity services.

The progress I have made would have been impossible without the support of the administrative staff who gave me the time and freedom to develop this role. Cooperation by the medical and nursing staffs was another prerequisite. Their acceptance of the nurse clinician role was demonstrated by their willingness to refer patients and to cooperate with me in planning individual care.

References

1. Aguilera, D. C., Messick, J. M., and Farrell, M. S.: Crisis intervention: theory and methodology, St. Louis, 1970, The C. V. Mosby Co.
2. Caplan, G.: An approach to community mental health, New York, 1961, Grune & Stratton, Inc.
3. Lesser, M. S., and Keane, V. R.: Nurse-patient relationships in a hospital maternity service, St. Louis, 1956, The C. V. Mosby Co.
4. Looff, D. H.: Appalachia's children, Lexington, Ky., 1971, The University Press of Kentucky.
5. Parad, H. J., editor: Crisis intervention: selected readings, New York, 1965, Family Service Association of America.
6. Rubin, R.: Puerperal change, Nurs. Outlook **9:**753, 1961.

Bibliography

Clark, A. L.: Maturational crisis and the unwed adolescent mother, Nurs. Sci. **2:**121, April, 1964.
Henning, E., Martoglio, G., Quita, M., Reinbrecht, J., and Strickland, M.: A dynamic nursing appraisal of the puerperium. In Lytle, N. A., editor: Maternal health nursing, Dubuque, Iowa, 1967, William C. Brown Co., Publisher.
Kennel, J. H., and Klaus, M. H.: Care of mother of high risk infant. In Stern, L., editor: Clinical obstetrics and gynecology, New York, 1971, Harper & Row, Publishers.
MacPhail, J.: Reasonable expectations for the nurse clinician, J. Nurs. Admin. **1:**16, Sept.-Oct., 1971.
Menninger, K.: The vital balance, New York, 1963, Viking Press.
O'Grady, R. S.: Feeding behavior in infants, Am. J. Nurs. **71:**736, 1971.
Peplan, H.: Interpersonal relations in nursing, New York, 1952, G. P. Putnam's Sons.
Rudolph, S. H.: Notes from a maternity ward. In Lytle, N. A., editor: Maternal health nursing, Dubuque, Iowa, 1967, William C. Brown Co., Publisher.
Williams, B.: Sleep needs during the maternity cycle, Nurs. Outlook **15:**53, 1967.

23

Environmental influences on the fetus

Marie D. Strickland

Environmental influences that have a detrimental effect on the fetus are known.

What can the health care practitioner do about the problem?

HISTORICAL PERSPECTIVE

It is probably safe to assume that man has tried to offer explanations for congenital malformations ever since the first one occurred. Historical records have showed that, in very early times, the explanation was usually limited to one of interpretation, that is, the occurrence of a congenital malformation was usually viewed as either a good or a bad omen.

This was particularly demonstrated with the discovery and translation of the Summa Izbu, a stone tablet from ancient Babylonian times, around 600 B.C., which was consulted for the meaning of malformations. This tablet listed malformations, from head to foot, for both the right and left sides of the body and gave a specific meaning for each as demonstrated in the following excerpts:

If a woman gives birth and the right foot of the child is like the foot of a turtle, the enemy will plunder the possessions of your land.

If a woman gives birth and the child has no hands, the enemy will conquer the city where the birth took place.

If a woman gives birth and the right arm of the child is short, that land will become rich.[20]

Attempts to predict undesirable fetal effects have also been recorded. As early as 1155 B.C., during the Chou dynasty, Chinese women were warned that consuming "goat meat would produce a sickly child, while turtle meat would yield a short-necked infant."[27] In ancient Rome, pregnant women were told to abstain from eating wolves' flesh, with premature birth as a consequence, and that if they were to eat mouse meat, they would produce a child with black eyes.[26]

Not too many years ago the birth of a defective or mentally retarded infant was thought to be the result of an act of God or a "tainted" inheritance. Superstitious beliefs about pregnancy have prevailed since primitive and ancient times and still coexist in our present-day society, along with the technological advances that have brought us to the beginning of space exploration.

Maternity nurses have long been familiar with superstitions such as the following: if a pregnant woman were "to sit on one or both feet habitually, the baby will have club feet."[33] Pregnant women will frequently attribute their heartburn symptoms to an abundance of hair on the fetal head. This belief is further supported when coincidentally the infant is born with a thick crop of hair. However, no explanation is given when the infant is born with only a few wisps. Multiple gestations have stimulated superstitions such as that offered by a primitive tribe on British New Guinea, who believed that a woman might give birth to twins if she ate bananas from a tree containing two bunches.[25]

FETAL ENVIRONMENT DEFINED

Applied to the fetus, the term *environment* biologically includes the uterus, amniotic fluid, and those substances that pass through the placenta and enter the fetal bloodstream.[5] The importance and impact of its environment on the growth and development of the fetus should be easily recognized, but is not always.

The purpose of this chapter is to go beyond beliefs in omens, "tainted" inheritances, and superstitions and to present data that are now available to us about some known environmental influences and their deleterious effects on the fetus and neonate. It is my premise that, with the knowledge available today, the nurse practitioner can develop a more effective role in helping to reduce poor fetal outcomes from known environmental hazards.

SCOPE OF THE PROBLEM

It is paradoxical that, although 99% of all babies born in the United States today are delivered in hospitals, 250,000 infants are born each year with abnormalities due to faulty prenatal development. Of these, 126,000 have defects so obvious that they are recognized as mentally retarded at birth.[6] Besides these, authorities estimate that 500,000 stillbirths and spontaneous abortions are due to faulty prenatal development. An estimated 15 million Americans of all ages have one or more defects that affect their daily lives.[17] And these are not all of genetic origin; three fourths of the 6 million retardates in this country have no recognizable cause for their deficiency.

The cost is immeasurable. How can one place a dollar-and-cent value on the emotional trauma experienced by the parents who have a defective infant born to them? How do we help them cope with feelings of disbelief, anger, and guilt implied in their questions, "Why us? What did we do wrong?" How does one weigh the cost of the decision to institutionalize the infant or to keep it at home? How is it possible to measure the cost of disruption of normal family life because the infant requires special care and attention? How can one evaluate the anguish present when parents must explain the defect to siblings, friends, neighbors, and other family members? How does one estimate the financial burden of institutionalization or rehabilitation or both, perhaps over a long period of time?

Because of scientific advances, life is frequently prolonged in these children, so that now they may survive their parents, which necessitates long-range planning for the child's future protection. And certainly, tremendous sorrow may arise in parents when they cannot see their children enjoying life experiences like others. Their children may be thwarted from achieving educational and career goals, loving and caring relationships with mates, or the rearing of families of their own.

Many nurse practitioners have seen families literally destroyed under the weight of this type of crisis. In the last thirty years, some young couples in their childbearing years have demanded that childbirth be a family-centered experience. Basically this means that the husband be allowed to be present and to participate in the birth experience.

This is a positive step in strengthening the emotional bonds between a couple and their newborn. However, one must acknowledge that the labor process is but a brief period in the whole gamut of a full-term gestation.

The future road lies in preconceptional guidance—preparing young women and men for the childbearing years. Waiting until a woman suspects or is sure that she is pregnant can be too late. Our new (and yet not so new) focus ought to be that a pregnancy should be planned for from its conception to its termination, to try to ensure a more favorable fetal outcome.

PLACENTAL BARRIER CONCEPT

In the past, too much confidence has probably been placed in the placental barrier concept, expecting the placenta to protect the fetus from any environmental attack. The human placenta is complex in structure, simultaneously performing a number of diverse functions such as respiration, transport of nutrition to and excretion from the fetus, and endocrine exchange. Additional functions are probably protein and hormone synthesis and immunological and protective roles, as well as a number of aspects of intermediary metabolism.[8]

The structures across which transport occurs are known collectively as the feto-maternal placental barrier, or membrane. In the fully completed human placenta, this barrier is composed entirely of tissues of fetal origin. At different stages of pregnancy there are significant differences in the structure and thickness of the barrier.[8] It has been clearly established that the human placenta cannot be regarded as a simple semipermeable membrane allowing only passive transfer. Transport mechanisms in which there is coupling to placental metabolism are also involved and could be labeled active transfer. The rate of transfer of different substances such as gases, electrolytes, macromolecules, and even particulate matter will be varied. It even seems likely that the passage of many substances may involve cytoplasmic activity within the barrier itself.[8]

There seems to be little doubt that many deleterious substances in the maternal bloodstream cross over the placenta to the embryo and the fetus; however, the factors that determine the rate at which transport of these substances takes place at various times during pregnancy have not been clearly identified. It has been shown that the only types of molecules that are almost exclusively rejected by the placenta are those that are very large or that bear high electrical charges. Thus it is believed that the placenta should no longer be regarded as a barrier to foreign materials. Although the placenta does impede the transport of some substances, it facilitates the passage of others.[3] Although various aspects of placental function have been studied, more research on placental transfer and its relation to teratogenesis needs to be done. Most of the information available at present is related to late pregnancy and not to the embryonic stage, when teratogenic risk is the greatest.

Consequently, if the term *placental barrier* gives the impression to the health care practitioner or his patient that a protection of the fetus from chemical influences is provided, it is a misunderstood concept. Obviously, then, until more data are acquired it would be wise to promote caution during pregnancy, as will be explored later in the chapter. The fetus lives wherever the mother lives. Barnes[5] states that "the fetus does not live in some protected world behind a curtain of either iron or trophoblast."

CONCEPT OF TERATOLOGY

In the 1930s Hale, an American veterinarian, found that when a diet deficient in vitamin A was administered to pregnant sows, the piglets were born without eyeballs.[34] This was the beginning of mammalian teratogenic experimentation.

In the early 1950s the theory was first introduced that a fertilized ovum, normal to begin with, becomes defective only if a "catastrophe" overtakes it in the womb after conception. This catastrophe might result from a disease carried by the mother or from some other external force. This shock to the fetus has often been referred to as an *insult.* Currently, the terms *stress factors, stress agents,* and *teratogenic agents* are used. To date, scientists have been able to reproduce in their laboratories all the common defects with which human offspring are sometimes born. From this has developed the science of teratology.

Teratology is defined as the study of abnormal development that is directly concerned with the genesis of malformations. A teratogenic agent is defined as one capable of producing or developing monsters or malformations.

When a pregnant mammal is exposed to the effects of a teratogenic agent, the type of malformation and its incidence are governed by two major factors[34]: the timing and the intensity of dosage of the agent.

Of the two factors, the timing is probably the more important. It has been found that teratogenic agents administered before implantation of the blastocyst do not produce malformations. They may destroy, but not deform, the embryo. Since the rapidly dividing ovum is very fragile, the teratogenic agent can destroy the blastocyst during the period of maximum embryotoxicity. However, slight injuries have also been shown to be overcome without harmful consequences to the growing embryo because, during the segmentation stage, many cells retain their totipotency and damaged cells can be replaced by newly formed ones.[11]

Teratogenic agents will produce structural malformations in humans in the period after implantation, which occurs one week after fertilization and during the entire period of organogenesis. For an organ, the period critical for teratogenic ef-

Table 1. Fetal congenital malformation timetable

Gestational period	Significant fetal developmental activity	Known teratogenic agents	Fetal effects
1st week	Cell cleavage		Cyclopia Siamese twins
		X rays	Abortion
16th-22nd day	Limbs make their appearance as small buds on 21st day	LSD (?)	Defective limbs Chromosomal aberration
		Thalidomide	Phocomelia Blighting of limbs Missing arms or legs
20th-40th day	Heart and viscera outside body		Heart defects Heart displacement Malformation of viscera
4th week	Organogenesis		Tracheoesophageal fistulas
	Body cells undergoing rapid differentiation	X rays	Spina bifida Mental retardation
	Rudiments of eyes, ears, and nose make their appearance		
5th week	Eye lenses	Rubella	Cataracts Blindness
		X rays	Clubfeet Cleft palate Microcephaly
	Face		Cleft palate
	Anterior neuropore closes in brain	Aminopterin	Anencephaly
	Urinary tract		Beginning of urinary tract anomalies
6th week	Eye lenses, skeleton, heart, vascular system	Rubella	Cataracts Deformation of lower jaws, hands, or feet Heart disease
7th week	Main outline of body nearing completion		Cleft palate Failure of fingers and toes to grow Defective lungs or heart
8th week			Heart defects Stunting fingers and toes
9th week	Almost completely formed in human miniature	Rubella	Deafness

fects is at the time of its greatest mitotic activity. The period of maximum teratogenicity lasts, in the human, until the ninth week of gestation. Some teratogenic agents, like rubella, show an action preferential to specific organs.

After morphogenesis of an organ is complete, structural malformations cannot be produced by teratogenic agents; however, the fetus still may not be out of danger. For example, the differentiation of some organs, such as external genitalia, can still be harmed, and the central nervous system is still vulnerable in the last trimester of pregnancy, during which histogenesis of the brain takes place.

Table 1 lists some of the defects to which the fetus is vulnerable in the first nine weeks of its development. Many specific precautions can be taken during pregnancy to lessen the risk of congenital lesions and infant morbidity and mortality, but, unfortunately, many of these must be taken before a woman would ordinarily consult her obstetrician or know for sure that she was pregnant.

The latter fact imposes a responsibility on the health care practitioner (1) to keep abreast of new developments and information about teratogenic agents; (2) to help educate the general public about potential environmental hazards to pregnant women; (3) to become more active in preconceptional counseling, one aspect of which is educating young women before they come into their childbearing years about good health practices and the second, informing couples who are contemplating childbearing about the environmental or genetic factors and the social practices such as drug abuse that can be potential hazards to their unborn offspring; and (4) to be keen and alert in observations of the newborn. All defects are not obvious at birth. If you know the normal, presumably you will recognize the abnormal. It has been widely accepted that infants having one defect will usually have another one to accompany it.

INFLUENCE OF DRUGS

The study of the teratogenicity of drugs is in its infancy, being given impetus only by the tragedy of the thalidomide babies, which occurred in the early 1960s. Usually information about the adverse reactions of drugs on the human fetus has been learned in retrospect.

The teratogenesis of drugs is complex and depends on a number of factors: (1) the developmental stage of the embryo; (2) its genetic constitution; (3) the physiological and pathological state of the mother and whether she has such conditions as diabetes, obesity, hypertension, and toxemia, as well as inadequate liver function; (4) high susceptibility of the fetus to drugs, partly related to its lack of development of detoxifying enzymes; and (5) immaturity of the kidney in the fetus.[11]

Adverse reactions of drugs are more dramatic in the embryo than in the mother because the teratogenic effects are irreversible. The mother can recuperate more easily than the fetus from untoward effects, which for her might be manifested only by nausea, vomiting, diarrhea, or a rash.

For a variety of reasons, animal experimentation alone will not uncover all the threats to the human fetus, even though all the defects known to man have been duplicated in the laboratory. Since World War II we have become a "pill popping" society. The majority of people do not recognize that they are taking drugs. Many drugs such as aspirins, antihistamines, nasal decongestants, cough medicines, laxatives, and antiemetics are sold over the counter without prescriptions.

The findings from animal experimentation on the detrimental effects of drugs cannot be extrapolated completely to the human fetus. Frequently, large doses of medication that would not be palatable or feasible for human consumption have been used in the experimentation. Pregnant women naturally cannot volunteer to help determine how much of a dose of a specific drug is needed or which period of embryonic development is necessary for specific teratogenesis to occur.

In spite of these problems, however, the list of drugs having deleterious effects on the fetus and neonate continues to grow (Table 2). The thalidomide tragedy was a warning of the danger of prescribing untested drugs for pregnant women.

There are still many unanswered questions about maternal drug abuse and fetal effects. Whether chromosomal breaks occur in LSD users is a matter of dispute.[16] It may take two generations to learn whether there are mutational effects from this drug. As new psychedelic drugs continue to appear on the scene, fifty years hence who will remember which "mind-expanding" drugs were taken in the 1970s? Research is needed for long-term behavioral effects on the fetus as the result of maternal consumption of such drugs as LSD, heroin, methadone, and mescaline. Steroids are already known to affect the fetal central nervous system.[14] There is no way to predict what long-term adverse effects a drug may have on a fetus, as demonstrated by the discovery of cancer of the

Table 2. Effects of maternal medications on the fetus and neonate[5,7,23,30]

Maternal medications	Fetal or neonatal effects
Ammonium chloride	Acidosis
Androgens, progesterone, estrogen	Advanced bone age, masculinization of female fetus
Antihistamines	Anomalies
Chlorambucil	Anencephaly, abortion, multiple anomalies
Chloramphenicol	Neonatal death, Gray syndrome (failure to thrive)
Chloroquine	Death, deafness, or retinal hemorrhage
Coumarin	Fetal death or hemorrhage
Hallucinogens (LSD, mescaline)	Chromosomal breaks, aberrations, congenital defects
Methotrexate	Multiple anomalies, abortions
Narcotic drugs (heroin, morphine, meperidine hydrochloride)	Neonatal depression, CNS irritability, respiratory difficulties, brain damage, tremors, hemorrhage
Phenobarbital (in excess)	Neonatal bleeding
Propylthiouracil	Congenital goiter, mental retardation
Quinine, quinidine	Nerve deafness, thrombocytopenia
Reserpine	Anorexia, stuffy nose, lethargy, cyanosis, death
Sulfonamides (Kynex, Gantrisin)	Kernicterus
Salicylates (excessive)	Neonatal bleeding
Streptomycin	Nerve deafness
Thalidomide	Fetal death, phocomelia, deafness, cardiovascular, GI, and GU anomalies
Thiazide diuretics	Fetal thrombocytopenia (can be fatal)
Tetracycline	Discoloration of teeth, inhibition of bone growth in premature infants
Corticosteroids	Cleft palate, cleft lip*
Cyclamates	Cancer of bladder, chromosomal aberrations*
Erythromycin (estolate salt)	Liver damage*
Insulin shock	Fetal loss*
Meprobamate (Miltown)	Retarded development*

*Aberrations found only in animal studies at present and suspected in human beings on the basis of animal evidence.

vagina in the adolescent offspring of women who took diethylstilbestrol to preserve their pregnancies.[15] In the daily environment there is continuing exposure to all kinds of pharmacological and chemical compounds. The United States manufactures ½ ounce of pesticide per citizen per day. Some of it must be eaten or breathed in by pregnant women.[5]

A harmless drug may become teratogenic because of a toxic impurity or solvent to which it is added. Occupational hazards exist also, as evidenced by operating-room nurses' and nurse anesthesiologists' and anesthetists' having a high incidence of fetal loss due to residual volatile anesthetic agents in the operating-room environment.[12]

Prophylaxis

Based on information available today, what can the nurse practitioner do? It would be simple if we could follow Barnes's[4] suggestion that "the only complete protection would be to practice therapeutic nihilism for all females between the ages of 14 and 40." In other words, all women in their childbearing years should avoid taking any drugs at all. The difficulty here, as mentioned before, is that we seem to have become a drug-oriented society. Then how can this basic philosophy be implemented? Following are several measures that can be taken:

1. Educate women in their childbearing years to take only medications pre-

scribed for them, with the knowledge of their physicians, and, when pregnant, only with the knowledge of their obstetricians.

2. A drug history should be an integral part of a medical history for every pregnant woman. Many individuals are hesitant to reveal that they are drug abusers. Frequently this information is learned in retrospect, following delivery. Many individuals are unaware that they are taking drugs. A checklist of potentially hazardous drugs or classes of drugs could be developed to be included with the obstetrical history.

3. When a medication is known to have a teratogenic effect, it might be discontinued for the critical period of fetal development, or another nonteratogenic form of the drug might be substituted. After all, a drug may be essential and lifesaving for the mother.

4. Young people, prior to the time of childbearing, need to be educated about the potential hazards to their offspring if they become drug users or abusers.

5. Informational pamphlets, posters, and filmstrips could be developed, using graphic materials to illustrate detrimental drug effects on the unborn. The topic needs a well-organized publicity campaign.

INFLUENCE OF RADIATION

Radiation influences may be divided into genetic and somatic effects. The genetic effects involve the hereditary apparatus of the germinal tissue in the maternal or fetal gonad or both. They are prezygotic, occurring prior to pregnancy, thus implying a potentially adverse result on future progeny.

Somatic effects occur in the nonreproductive cells of the mother or fetus, irrespective of whether the impact is on the nucleus or cytoplasm. They are postzygotic, since they occur during the prenatal course of pregnancy, there is suggestion of a causal relationship with such gross changes as congenital malformations and leukemia.[5]

The principle of teratogenesis applies readily when a pregnant woman is exposed to radiation (Table 3). If she is exposed to a dose of 200 roentgen rays in the first nine weeks of gestation, the fetus will have structural malformations.[35]

Prophylaxis

The general public, as well as professional health workers, needs information about safe periods, when women in their childbearing years can be exposed to radiation without adverse effects. For most individuals, this exposure takes place in the form of x-ray procedures.

Women should avoid radiation exposure in the postovulatory phase of the menstrual cycle. The last menstrual period should be recorded on the x-ray slip. Roentgenograms in nonpregnant women should be taken during the menses or immediately thereafter. All too frequently, women are unaware that they might be pregnant, so that it is the health worker's responsibility to schedule them for x-ray exposure during a relatively safe period.

Since adverse effects can occur in the fetus even after organogenesis, radiation

Table 3. Radiation effects on the fetus[31,35]

Period of fetal development	Effects
Preimplantation period of embryo	All-or-none effect (blastocyst destroyed or normal embryo develops)
Period of major organ formation (up to 9th week)	Gross visceral malformations Skeletal changes (e.g., blindness, cataracts, spina bifida, reduction in size of brain, mental retardation, skull malformation)
Fetal period	No external malformations or death Profound brain lesions compatible with survival (e.g., microcephaly) Alters environment to cause cancer later in life (e.g., leukemia) Altered metabolism may damage genetic material of unborn offspring

should be avoided during pregnancy. Frequently pregnant women become anxious when a chest roentgenogram is ordered for them. The dangers can be negated when the abdomen is shielded by lead and rubber. Because of technological advances, exposure time can be reduced with fast films. The field size can be restricted to the exact area to be examined by the use of cones or light-beam diaphragms. It is also recommended that fluoroscopy be avoided during pregnancy, even though it is only 25 roentgen rays.[5]

However, radiation is a valuable modern tool of medicine. It may be necessary to utilize roentgenography as a lifesaving diagnostic aid and to present it as such to a pregnant woman and her family.

INFLUENCE OF MATERNAL INFECTIONS

The list of maternal infections that affect the fetus seems to grow annually (Table 4). Rubella, or German measles, is probably the best known for its teratogenic effects. In 1941, Gregg, an Australian, reported congenital malformations in children born to women who had had rubella in the first trimester of pregnancy.

In 1964, the United States had an epidemic of rubella to which 20,000 deaths in utero, as well as 20,000 birth defects, were attributed. The latter figure then rose to 30,000 because of delayed identification of defects.

Rubella seems to have a chemical affinity for certain cells. The defects appear to be due to a direct virus-cell relationship. It has been suggested that growth disturbance was due to the growth of the virus, which inhibted cell multiplication. The most common rubella-caused defects of early fetal development are eye defects, such as cataracts and glaucoma, cardiac lesions, deafmutism, and mental retardation. The defects that occur in later fetal development are microcephaly and central nervous system damage; some infants become carriers of the disease. Additional effects were seen in the incidence of prematurity and the failure to thrive syndrome.[22]

Prophylaxis

Whereas the ultimate goal would be immunization of the female population now that we have the rubella vaccine available, its successful achievement lies in the future. Emphasis is being given to the immunization of young school-age children because they are the potential source of infection for women in their childbearing years.

In 1966, a live rubella virus vaccine was developed, which has its limitation in not being able to be given to women in their childbearing years who might unknowingly be pregnant. In addition, there is the problem of educating the public about the dangers of rubella in pregnant women. Too many women still do not realize the serious consequences for their infants from a minimal rash experienced by the mother during her pregnancy.

Table 4. Maternal infections affecting the fetus or the neonate[5,9,24,28]

Maternal infection	Fetal or neonatal effects
Chicken pox, shingles	Chicken pox, shingles, increased abortions, stillbirths
Coxsackie B viruses	Myocarditis
Cytomegalovirus	Microcephaly, deafness, retinochoroiditis, mental retardation
Hepatitis	Neonatal hepatitis
Herpes simplex	Generalized herpes, death, encephalitis
Mumps	Fetal death, endocardial fibroelastosis, malformation
Nonspecific severe viral infections	Prematurity
Poliomyelitis	Spinal or bulbar poliomyelitis
Rubeola (measles)	Increased abortions and stillbirths
Rubella (German measles)	Blindness, deafness, failure to thrive syndrome, cardiac defects
Smallpox (variola)	Smallpox, increased abortions, stillbirths
Toxoplasmosis	Retinochoroiditis

All pregnant women should be urged to avoid contact with children who have an acute febrile illness, particularly when there is a known outbreak of rubella. Laboratory tests in the form of hemagglutination inhibition tests are available to determine immunization status or active disease. Whereas therapeutic abortion may be a choice if the presence of the disease is established during pregnancy, some couples may not see this as the solution for them.

The primary area of responsibility for the nurse practitioner seems to be education of the public about the dangers of rubella to the fetus and the promotion of the vaccination of children against rubella. Women of childbearing age can be given the vaccine when the possibility of pregnancy in the following two months is essentially nil. The latter condition requires the use of an effective birth control method or, in case of any doubt, abstinence from sexual relations prior to vaccination and for the two months following, which could present some difficulty in the husband-wife sexual relationship. However, if presented with the dangers to an unborn child, a couple might decide to abstain. Young women might be advised to have a rubella titer and subsequent vaccination if they are not immune, before marriage or taking on a sexual relationship that might result in an unplanned pregnancy.

Prophylaxis of any infection in the pregnant woman should be the same as for the whole population if a vaccination is available. Routine immunizations with live virus vaccines, however, should be avoided during pregnancy, except when necessary for rabies and cholera. A possible pregnancy should be explored before giving smallpox, mumps, measles, rubella, poliomyelitis, and yellow fever vaccines. This would seem to give additional support to the concept of planning for a pregnancy.

TOXOPLASMOSIS

A maternal infectious disease with detrimental fetal effects that has come into the medical and public eye recently, although it was identified thirty years ago, is toxoplasmosis caused by the *Toxoplasma gondii*.[1] The common theory is that the mother must have an acute infection while pregnant to cause congenital toxoplasmosis in the fetus.

Clinical manifestations of the disease in the fetus range from very slight to very severe effects. The end results are frequently indistinguishable from those brought about by other viruses, such as cytomegalovirus, rubella, and herpesvirus, or by erythroblastosis fetalis. These abnormalities include neurological damage that ranges from microcephaly to hydrocephalus, as well as chorioretinitis, pneumonitis, anemia, and hepatosplenomegaly with jaundice. Long-term effects have been seen as mental retardation, convulsions, and severe visual impairment.[1,3]

Diagnosis in the pregnant woman can be determined by a blood titer. Positive results indicate a need for titer evaluation and close examination of her infant to detect problems early. Infants who have had a positive diagnosis have been treated with sulfonamides and pyrimethamic and folinic acid successfully.[19]

Prophylaxis

Toxoplasmosis is acquired from the cyst forms found in infected meat.[19] One cyst can contain several hundred to a few thousand *Toxoplasma* organisms. One of these cysts is the minimal dose for infection. Prevention lies in not eating rare meat (pork, mutton, beef, or horsemeat). Meat should be cooked thoroughly.

Another source of the disease is cat feces. One oocyst found in cat feces contains eight sporozoites, a minimal infective dose and a significant source of the disease.[19] Pregnant women should be instructed not to have contact with cat feces and to avoid cleaning cat litter boxes because shaking dirty litter into the air can be menace also. When this information was made public, cat owners became incensed because they believed that their pets' existence was being threatened. The cats can be tested by a veterinarian for toxoplasmosis. They are more likely to have the disease if they hunt in fields or have access to rodents.

Undoubtedly, more research is needed in this area, but evidence supports the incidence of in utero acquired defects. The public, and particularly pregnant women, should be alerted to the dangers to the fetus from toxoplasmosis.

PSYCHOSEXUAL INFLUENCES

The question is often raised as to whether emotional disturbances in the pregnant woman have an effect on the fetus. There is evidence that maternal emotional disturbances can affect both fetal structural and psychological development.[21]

Chemicals within the mother's body pass on via her circulation and the placenta to the bloodstream of the fetus. This may not always be harmful but can stimulate its activity, causing a slight decrease in birth weight. The children of seriously disturbed mothers have been known to show psychological and psychosomatic irritability after birth.

There is evidence that the fetal nervous system can be permanently sensitized by its reaction to chemicals released during the mother's emotional upsets. Women have been known to be sterile or to have miscarriages during periods of extreme emotional stress. Nervous hyperactivity in the mother leading to excesses in certain hormones may affect the formation of the palate, resulting in a cleft palate.

The question has often been asked whether sexual intercourse can have a teratogenic effect on the fetus. No scientific evidence permits an unequivocal answer of yes or no. The discussion that follows is presented only to point out that this area needs more investigation.

Animals, even primates, abstain from copulation when the female is pregnant, but Western man does not. In early Judaic times, abstention from intercourse was practiced during pregnancy. Women were considered "unclean," but this may have been a protective measure to ensure population growth, when the observation was made that animals abstained.

Javert[18] found in his work with sterile patients and habitual aborters that miscarriages can follow orgasm. The habitual aborter has frequent orgasms. In Javert's study 25% of abortions occurred in newly wedded primigravidas, implying frequent sexual activity. Unmarried mothers seldom miscarry it is believed because the availability of frequent and regular sex is absent

without the presence of a husband or regular sexual partner.

Kinsey, in his work, postulated that the whole body suffered from a lack of oxygen during the sex act. The Masters and Johnson research has shown that oxygen intake cannot keep up with the body's requirements during sexual orgasm.[21] Monitoring devices demonstrated that uterine contractions occur during sexual foreplay that involves stimulation of the nipples. Uterine orgasmic tracings resemble contraction tracings that occur during the first stage of labor.

Are there implications here for the protection of the fetus? Newly pregnant women are rarely given advice to abstain from coitus unless they have a history of spontaneous abortions. Most professionals would argue that no scientific evidence supports this advice. The intent of this discussion is to point out that much research is needed in this area. Again, a pregnant woman could not be expected to volunteer her services for research in this area if she believed that sexual intercourse during pregnancy might be detrimental to her unborn infant.

INFLUENCES OF MATERNAL ORIGIN

Heavy cigarette smoking has been correlated with lowered fetal weight and prematurity. The babies tend to be shorter, besides lacking fatty tissue. Nicotine passes through the placenta into the body of the fetus, and carbon monoxide in the mother's blood reduces the amount of oxygen supply to the infant.[6]

One must also remember that there are dietary and other differences between smokers and nonsmokers and differences in personality, as well as degree of nervous tension.

Although it would most likely be difficult to get a heavy smoker to stop smoking, she might be motivated during pregnancy by the desire to protect her newborn to temporarily reduce her cigarette consumption. A young woman contemplating marriage and childbearing could be advised to give up smoking as part of preconceptional counseling.

Teen-age mothers and those over 40 years

of age have been found to have more incidence of complications such as toxemia with its common ensuing complication of premature delivery, with its frequent consequence of birth injury related to mental retardation and minimal brain damage.[6] There seems to be a snowballing effect.

Maternal aging has long been recognized as dangerous to the fetus. Placental insufficiency rises steadily with age and can be a cause of hypoxia. Parity increases with age, presenting its own dangers of malpresentations, breech deliveries, prolapsed cords, and Rh blood problems. Hydrocephalus, cleft lip and palate, and Down's syndrome have been closely associated with the aging factor.[4] The ovaries of a 6-month-old female fetus contain all the ova they will ever contain, but none will be released until puberty. The ova of a 40-year-old woman are really 40 years and 3 months old and have been exposed to a variety of stresses during that life period. In contrast, males do not produce sperm capable of fertilizing ova until puberty, and, in addition, the male continually produces a fresh supply of sperm.[32]

The reproductive period in women between the ages of 20 and 30 years seems to provide the optimum outcome for infants.[13] The ideal age for having a first baby is from 18 to 25 years, and being over 35 places the woman in a high-risk category.[2] The older primigravida often has a more prolonged labor because of greater cervical rigidity. There is also a tendency toward uterine ischemia, with the risk of hypoxia to the fetus. However, some physicians will not discourage a woman over 35 years of age from having a baby but would give her high-risk care.[2]

Maternal changes caused by syphilis, diabetes, and cardiovascular and other systemic diseases have long been known to have detrimental fetal effects. Toxemia, which develops only in the pregnant state, can lead to eclampsia and high fetal cost or loss.

In the future, more attention will probably be given to problems of ecology and how they may affect the pregnant woman and her fetus. In a newspaper series called "The Great Cripplers,"[9] Wei, an environmental-health physiologist at Berkeley, revealed the threat from high doses of mercury, manganese, and lead for pregnant women. The danger lies in damage to the nervous system in the fetus. Pregnant women were warned not to eat any sport fish. The warning was then extended to all women of childbearing age. One cannot overlook the role that nutritional factors may play in the cause of birth defects. Nutritional laboratory studies in animals and close observation of undernourished groups are providing important clues that may enable us to prevent some of the birth defects that are plaguing us.

Prophylaxis

Prophylaxis lies in the early recognition of maternal disease conditions and the implementation of an effective therapeutic regimen. There is a definite need for a more widespread acceptance and use of preconception medical examinations, evaluations, and recommendations. Women should be encouraged not only to seek prenatal care early, but also to remain under medical care. Although it might be desirable to urge young women to have their babies between the ages of 20 and 30 years, this may be an unrealistic goal for all women to achieve. It may well be that, with rapidly expanding knowledge about better medical management of pregnancies, young women could be encouraged to have their children between the ages of 18 and 35 years.

GENETIC INFLUENCES

One cannot leave the topic of fetal hazards without mentioning genetic influences on fetal development. The list of genetically determined fetal abnormalities, like trisomies 13 to 15, 18, 5 (cri-du-chat syndrome), 21 (Down's syndrome), and the inborn errors of metabolism like phenylketonuria and galactosemia continue to grow. The development of this aspect of the subject would require another chapter.

However, whenever possible, one must work toward the prevention or cure of a defect. At present, it is not possible to prevent the union of all harmful recessive genes because all sex cells carry a few (five or six) harmful recessive genes.

Although there is some genetic detective work and counseling available today, it may take a hundred years to see this type of disorders eliminated. There has not been common agreement as to what is a desirable or undesirable trait. What is harmful in the overt homozygous form may be protective or advantageous in the heterozygous form. Physicians, as well as families, need guidelines in this area.

Prophylaxis

The genetic counselor can play a variety of roles. He can provide significant information before marriage to couples who, by virtue of their familial history, have reason to be concerned about their future progeny.

The genetic counselor does not mandate whether or not they should have children. The counselor provides information as to the probable frequency with which a couple may have an affected child. The couple must then decide whether to take the chance by procreating.

Couples do have options. Using any of the reliable contraceptive methods available seems to be more acceptable than counseling regarding the choice of a marriage partner. For some couples, surgical sterilization, accepting the idea of irreversibility, seems the answer. Ideal candidates are those who are the proved carriers of a disease with a known rate of risk and those who hopefully have one or two normal children. The sterilization procedure should be done to the marriage partner who carries the defect. If the partner who carries the fault marries again, the chances for a defective infant again are present.[29]

In some situations, artificial insemination may be the answer. A donor must be selected who will not promulgate the defect. This choice can cause many problems, unless the couple can reach a mutual decision without reservations. There must be a strong stable marital relationship, and the husband must be willing to recognize the infant as his legal offspring and to accept the infant as his own in the parent-child relationship. On occasion, the decision will backfire, fanning feelings of inadequacy in the male, causing him to act out by rejecting the infant or his wife or both. The situation can be easily turned into a tragic rather than a happy, fulfilling one.

The last alternative is that of therapeutic abortion, particularly since abortion laws have become more liberal, permitting abortion for reasons other than to save the life of the pregnant woman. The decision can be based on scientific evidence now because of the amniocentesis technique. This procedure has been developed to aid in the prenatal diagnosis of genetic disorders. This technique can be used for conditions due to chromosomal anomalies and conditions due to mutant genes whose biochemical effects are demonstrated in amniotic cells or fluid. A third but less precise form of screening is used in the case of a mother who is a known heterozygote for a sex-linked disorder.[10]

However, the decision on abortion is not without its ethical and moral issues, as well as being an emotionally charged situation for the parents. They will need support from the nurse when they have made their decision.

The field of genetic counseling is only in its infancy. Much needs to be done yet in the whole area of genetic studies. Someday we will know the recipe for producing people—which traits should be promulgated and which discarded. We will also probably have the techniques developed to accomplish the discarding. These developments of themselves will generate other complex moral, psychological, religious, and social issues.

ROLE OF THE HEALTH CARE PRACTITIONER

Physicians and nurses must be committed to a basic philosophy that there is value in preconceptional planning. They must also believe that some birth defects are humanly caused and thus, with proper intervention, could be prevented, ultimately decreasing perinatal morbidity and mortality due to birth defects.

Unfortunately, many physicians and nurses do not have an orientation to the new field of fetology. Perhaps, then, the primary thrust belongs in basic medical and nursing educational programs to provide an introduction to this new field of medicine. New supporters of the concept cannot be recruited if they have not acquired basic tenets on which to base action in a program of prevention.

Once the professional worker is functioning in this area of practice, he has a responsibility to remain knowledgeable, by keeping abreast of current research and to attend conferences, workshops, and seminars devoted to the subject. The practitioner also has a responsibility to recruit and educate other professionals to the field of fetology.

The obstetrician must believe that his role is more than delivering a live baby. The demand now is that the infant should not only be alive, but also be able to develop a normal life after birth, a life that has value and meaning for the individual, as well as independence. Unfortunately, many physicians believe their responsibility exists only for the period beginning when a woman presents herself for prenatal care and ending with the delivery of the infant.

The public needs to be educated to expect more from health care. Some of this informational exposure is being made in the lay magazines. And some of our educated public is beginning not only to demand more, but also to wish to exercise more control over the outcome of their childbearing. Nurses can be contributors to the lay literature. Nurses have writing skills, as well as theoretical background; they have patient experiences that can enrich their resource material.

Nurses, because of the various positions they hold, can make significant contributions in planning for parenthood. They have access to adolescents through school nursing, sex education, and "marriage and family" courses in high school settings. Here preliminary information can be given about such topics as health care, drug abuse, venereal disease, smoking, and poor nutrition and their known and possible effects on offspring.

Nurses have access to couples in their childbearing years through community health programs, public health agencies, pediatric and well-baby clinics, antepartum and postpartum clinics, and courses on preparation for childbirth and parenthood. The nurse should not be an alarmist, but her actions should be geared whenever possible to preventive measures, such as implementing the following guidelines:

1. Women should be encouraged to have their children between the ages of 18 and 35 years.

2. The general population should be instructed to use no drugs unless prescribed by a physician. A woman contemplating childbearing should be instructed to take no drugs unless absolutely necessary and then only if her physician orders it. When pregnant, she should take drugs only with approval of her obstetrician.

3. Foster the concept of planning a pregnancy. Medical and gynecological evaluations should be done routinely. A genetic evaluation is indicated when the couples' familial or obstetrical history warrants it.

4. Women, either contemplating pregnancy or newly pregnant, should avoid exposure to infectious diseases. Whenever possible, women should be vaccinated against an infectious disease when there is no possibility of their becoming pregnant immediately thereafter.

5. Education in an adequate nutritional diet seems essential and should begin early in life, with particular emphasis on the adolescent years and again on the childbearing period.

6. Diagnostic x-ray films of or radiation therapy to the abdomen should be avoided in the woman during her childbearing years except when necessary as a lifesaving measure or when the woman is in her safe preovulatory period.

7. Couples may need help in selecting an obstetrician who is familiar with new research and techniques that are being developed to provide significant information about the status of the fetus.

8. Couples should also select physicians associated with reputable hospitals that can provide adequate services needed for good obstetrical and neonatal care.

9. Once the pregnant woman is under a physician's care, she should be urged to continue and to follow his advice.

CONCLUSION

The science of fetology is in its infancy. More scientific evidence is necessary to determine which environmental influences have a detrimental effect on the fetus, as well as the type of defect that will occur. This also implies that health care practitioners must keep abreast of new developments in the field and be resourceful as to how new findings can be used, so as to be of value not only for the individual but also for society. One must be cautious so as not to overreact, as new clues to defects are revealed. The key word at the moment is *prophylaxis,* supporting actions that will prevent the occurrence of congenital malformations or mental retardation. In the future, utilization of a wide variety of new techniques will be seen, such as embryo transplantation for better nuturing, miniscule fetal surgery to repair defects, altering of the genetic code to remove defects, medical treatment of the fetus in utero to counteract certain diseases, and more reliable sex-predetermining techniques to avoid sex-linked defects. The ramifications from these and other techniques like them are multitudinous and will cause serious moral, religious, and social issues for future generations.

References

1. Abramson, H., editor: Symposium on the functional physiopathology of the fetus and neonate, St. Louis, 1971, The C. V. Mosby Co., pp. 127-128.
2. Andrews, B. F., et al.: Identifying high risk pregnancy in time, J. Practical Family Med.: Patient Care **6:**26, 1972.
3. Assali, N. S., editor: Pathophysiology of gestation, vol. II, New York, 1972, Academic Press, pp. 284, 292.
4. Barnes, A. C.: Prevention of congenital anomalies from point of view of the obstetrician, paper presented, 2nd International Conference on Congenital Malformation, New York City, 1963.
5. Barnes, A. C., editor: Intra-uterine development, Phildelphia, 1968, Lea & Febiger, Publishers, pp. 362, 364, 367, 381, 383.
6. Beck, J.: Guarding the unborn, Todays Health **46:**39, 1968.
7. Benson, R.: Handbook of obstetrics and gynecology, Los Altos, Calif., 1971, Lange Medical Publications.
8. Boyd, J. D., and Hamilton, W. J.: The human placenta, Cambridge, 1970, W. Heffer & Sons, Ltd., pp. 286, 288, 290.
9. Carey, F.: The great cripplers, New York Post, 37, Oct. 15, 1971.
10. Carter, C. O.: Practical aspects of early diagnosis, Early Diagnosis of Human Genetic Defects, Health, Education and Welfare Publication (NIH) 72-75, p. 17, 1970.
11. Ciba Foundation: Fetal autonomy, London, 1969, J. & A. Churchill, Ltd., pp. 245, 250-251.
12. Cohen, E. N., et al.: Anesthesia, pregnancy and miscarriage, Anesthesiology **35:**343, 1971.
13. Eastman, N. J., and Hellman, L. M.: Williams' obstetrics, ed. 13, New York, 1966, Appleton-Century-Crofts, p. 6.
14. Fuchs, F., M.D.: Future of fetal pharmacology, unpublished paper, closing lecture at International Symposium on Fetal Pharmacology, Stockholm, Sweden, Dec., 1971.
15. Herbst, A., Herbst, A. L., Ulfelder, H., and Poskanzer, D. C.: Adenocarcinoma of the vagina, N. Engl. J. Med. **284:**878, 1971.
16. Hsu, L. Y., Strauss, L., and Herschhorn, K.: Chromosome abnormality in offspring of LSD users, J.A.M.A. **211:**987, 1970.
17. Hurley, L. S.: The consequences of fetal impoverishment, Nutr. Today **3:**3, Dec., 1968.
18. Javert, C.: Spontaneous and habitual abortion, New York, 1955, McGraw-Hill Book Co., Inc., p. 219.
19. Kimball, A. C., Kean, B. H., and Fuchs, F.: Congenital toxoplasmosis; a prospective study of 4,048 obstetric patients, Am. J. Obstet. Gynecol. **3:**211, Sept. 15, 1971.
20. Leichty, E.: The omen series—Summa Izbu, Nutr. Today **3:**10, Dec., 1968.
21. Limner, R.: Sex and the unborn child, New York, 1969, Julian Press, Inc., pp. 15, 22.
22. Lin-Fu, J. S.: Rubella, U. S. Department of Health, Education, and Welfare, Public Health Service Publication No. 2041, p. 3.
23. Little, W. A.: Drugs in pregnancy, Am. J. Nurs. **66:**1303, 1966.
24. Monit, C.: Viral infections of the human fetus, London, 1969, Macmillan & Co., Ltd.
25. Montagu, A.: Embryological beliefs of primitive peoples, Ciba Symposium, vol. X, Jan.-Feb., 1948, pp. 994-1008.
26. Mussey, R. D.: Nutrition and human reproduction; historical review, Am. J. Obst. & Gynec. **57:**1037, 1949.
27. Nixon, W. C. W.: Diet in pregnancy, J. Obst. & Gynaec. Brit. Emp. **49:**614, 1942.
28. Overall, J. C., Jr.: Virus infections of the fetus and newborn infant, J. Pediatr. **77:**315, 1970.
29. Reed, S. C.: Counseling in medical genetics, ed. 2, Philadelphia, 1963, W. B. Saunders Co., p. 278.
30. Riley, H. P.: Fetal and neonatal toxicity of drugs, Pediatr. Currents **17:**1, 1968.
31. Rugh, R.: Effects of x-rays on the human fetus, J. Pediatr. **53:**531, 1958.
32. Smith, G.: Amniotic fluid karotypes show fetal abnormalities, Hosp. Top. **50:**45, May, 1972.
33. Wesh, D. M.: Old wives tales about OB, R.N. **30:**64, July, 1967.
34. Woollam, D. H.: The effect of environmental factors on the foetus, J. Coll. Gen. Pract. **8** (supp. 2):35, Nov., 1964.
35. Yamazaki, J. N.: A review of the literature on the radiation dosage required to cause manifest central nervous system disturbances from in utero and postnatal exposure, Pediatrics **37** (supp. 37):877, 1966.

Bibliography

Adamsons, K., editor: Diagnosis and treatment of fetal disorders, New York, 1968, Springer-Verlag New York, Inc.

Rorvik, D. M.: Brave new baby, New York, 1971, Doubleday & Co., Inc.

24

Concerns, conflicts, and confidence of postpartum mothers

Edith G. Walker

All disciplines involved in health care seek knowledge concerning people and their behavior. Each profession can perceive from its own vantage point the experiences, know-how, and help of its members, and can appraise the situations in which it hopes to be helpful.[13] Health care workers search for data about people's challenges and concerns and seek to identify the elusive factors of self-confidence that enable them to cope with their problems and transcend their circumstances. Health care personnel identify human potentials and encourage personal development as they foster good physical and mental health.

Parenthood has been identified as a crisis by many writers. The stormy transition to parenthood has been studied by LeMasters,[9] Dyer,[5] Hobbs,[7] and Jacoby.[8] Rubin[12] described the postpartum period as one of the most distressful in a woman's life. Others have also discussed the problems of new mothers. Adams[1] studied the early concerns of primiparous mothers and identified many of the problems they had regarding infant care activities, as well as their need for professional help. Henning[6] reiterated the need of the postpartum mother for professional help.

A study by Carpenter and his co-workers[4] indicated that mothers need reassurance about their ability to care for their baby. In a study in Toronto, Carpenter[3] found multiple problems of primiparous mothers and the need for assistance in the first three months after the birth of a baby. Marshall[10] pointed out problems of mothers in the early puerperal period and suggested that most of these were amenable to nursing intervention. In her study of the depression of postpartum mothers, Anderson[2] identified clues that were possible indicators of depression of the mother, such as cumulative fatigue, helplessness when the baby cried, and feelings of inadequacy in giving care to the baby. She noted how important it was to mothers for fathers to share in the care of the babies. The value of having help from their own mothers varied among the subjects in this study. Rossi,[11] a sociologist, characterized our American family system as consisting of isolated households with little help from kin. She also indicated that middle-class mothers are frequently confronted with full-scale mothering before they are ready for it. Her article raises many questions. What kinds and amounts of help do mothers in low-income groups have? Are there other factors in the background of mothers that prepare them for the mothering role? Are there others who will assume the mother-surrogate role?

Because of their relationship with and proximity to families, nurses have unique opportunities to identify stress factors as they observe mothers in their growth into new roles and relationships. Nurses recognize that mothers respond to the crisis of parenthood in many individualized ways, and they can try to identify both the previous experiences that mothers have had that prepared them for the mothering role and the concerns and conflicts arising from the new role. Additional knowledge is needed, in particular, about the capabilities of mothers, how they cope with their problems, and who supports them. What gives a mother the confidence to move forward in the tasks and experiences that confront her? The helping process is a complex one, and to develop individual potentials, fortify strengths, and provide the kind of care that is needed, the nurse must begin where the person is.

Concern for the health of mothers and babies was the impetus for a study I did of postpartum mothers. The data from the literature indicate a multiplicity of factors that affect the transition of the mother during the puerperal period and further emphasize the complexity of the problem. The study I undertook focused not only on the concerns but also, and more particularly, on the coping methods and the support mothers received during the postpartum period after discharge from the hospital.

A STUDY OF POSTPARTUM MOTHERS

The sample of 100 mothers included fifty-one married black patients and twenty-five unwed black patients, who attended either the postpartum or family planning clinics in a midwestern university medical center, and twenty-four married white patients returning for a postpartum visit to the offices of obstetricians in a private obstetrical-gynecological group practice in a New England city. Mothers were either primiparas or multiparas who had been delivered vaginally of normal, full-term babies.

An interview schedule was used to obtain data. All interviews took place between the third and eighth week postpartum. Each interview lasted one-half hour. The following questions were asked of the mothers:

1. Would you tell me about your baby in the first week after you brought him/her home? Were things any different in the next few weeks?
2. Would you tell me about yourself in the first week after you came home from the hospital? Were things any different in the next few weeks?
3. (Asked about each incident mentioned in response to 1 and 2.)
   a. How did you manage?
   b. Did anyone help you?
   c. How did they help you?
   d. What would have made it easier for you?
   e. Did you anticipate any of these problems?
4. How are things going now?

Most of the necessary background information was obtained from the patient's records prior to the interview. The mothers were distributed by parity as follows:

	PRIMIPARA	MULTIPARA
Black—married, clinic patient	13	38
Black—unwed, clinic patient	18	7
White—married, private patient	16	8

The married clinic patients were 15 to 40 years of age, with an average of 22 years. The ages of the unwed clinic patients ranged from 14 to 32 years, with an average of 19 years, whereas those of the private clinic patients were 17 to 30 years, with 26 years as the average. The average number of years of education for the married clinic patients was 12, compared to 9 for unwed clinic patients and 12 for married private patients.

After about the tenth interview I realized that mothers who had many siblings expressed feelings of adequacy in handling the baby. Of the black married mothers, the range of siblings was 0 to 10 (average, 5.6), with 18 mothers having 6 or more siblings and 10 mothers having 10 or more siblings. In the unwed black mothers group the range of siblings was 0 to 15, with an average of 5.5 Of the white mothers, the range of siblings was 0 to 6, with an average of 2.2.

Concerns about the baby

In asking the mothers to "Tell me about your baby," it was assumed that they would mention *first* what concerned them most. Every mother whose baby had a complication mentioned this first. Complications mentioned included colds, diarrhea, milk allergy, bleeding cord, and diaper rash. Sixty-four of the mothers mentioned that the baby slept well or slept poorly and cried a lot. Forty-two percent of the babies cried the first week, particularly during the night hours, indicating that this is a common and disturbing problem. Mothers felt helpless when confronted with the crying of their infants. Twenty-seven mothers mentioned being concerned about how the baby took his feeding. These responses indicate the importance of complications and the sleeping and eating behavior of the babies to the mothers. Following are examples of such comments:

The screams of the baby were unnerving.

He slept during the day and cried at night.

She had her night and day confused.

She stays awake at nights.

He is greedy.

She is wonderful—slept all night.

One mother mentioned that during the first few nights she put on the lights, turned on the radio, changed the baby's diaper and position, and rocked him until he slept.

Concerns about self

Mothers identified additional areas of concern when asked to "Tell me about yourself." Concerns of the mothers in relation to self were physical complications and conflicts confronting them. Two of the greatest concerns of the mothers about themselves were painful perineum and fatigue. Most of the physical complaints other than fatigue were improved or were gone after the first week. Only eleven of the 100 mothers were breast-feeding, and none of them related any of these problems. Another interesting point was that the number of psychological complaints such as depression, tension, and fears reported was higher for white private patients than for black clinic patients.

COPING WITH SIBLING RIVALRY

The number of mothers who mentioned sibling rivalry, 36 of 61 who had other children, indicated the enormity of this problem. One mother who had six other children ranging from 6 to 18 years of age spoke of her problems with the children.

Everyone wanted my attention. I had never been away from them, and they wouldn't eat while I was in the hospital. Every one had problems. The oldest girl (18) resents growing up. She and the 6-year-old boy were the worst.

Many mothers would say that the other children were not jealous of the new baby but would then go on to describe behavior that gave evidence of resentment of the baby. Some of the responses of the mothers to the resentment of the other children would indicate that this is an area that should be introduced in the anticipatory guidance of mothers-to-be. Symptoms should be described and intervention planned. One mother said:

I still have problems with my 6 year old. He is afraid to go to bed and to take a bath. He won't look at T.V. I don't know what to do.

Another mother told the following:

My 2-year-old little girl was jealous. She didn't like the baby being in her crib. I took her out a month before. She keeps saying "my crib." I took her off bottles; now she steals the baby's. Things got worse. She pinched the baby and stuck her fingers in his eyes. I had to send her to my mother's to stay.

Little comment is needed on this situation; this mother needed guidance very much.

Sibling rivalry was more pronounced in families who had toddlers and when mothers had had no children for at least five years.

Supportive help

Among the black married mothers, all had help with the new baby; forty-five of the fifty-one had two or more sources of help in the home. Of the black unwed mothers, three had no help, ten mentioned a single source, and twelve had two or more sources. Of the white mothers, three had no help, nine had a single source, and eleven had two sources. Most of the mothers seemed to appreciate the help, but a few did not want it. The three unwed mothers who lacked help spoke of fatigue. The white mothers with no help made comments:

I needed help, but nobody could do it right anyhow.

I took care of the family, house, and two horses the first week. The second week I was tired, depressed, and had no appetite.

I like doing my own work. I washed the floor, took care of the family, and was very active. The second week I went to the hospital for heavy bleeding.

Many mothers who had help were openly appreciative of the support given to them by others. Support is said to be the third hand and involves understanding, care, and help.[15] The concentration of support within the family is a readily identifiable strength. The warmth, the fortitude, the love, and other healthy elements of family functioning as described by Stitt[14] were indicated in these responses by mothers.

I felt I'd be proud of my baby, and I am.

A mother of six with newborn twin boys said:

My husband grabs one kid and feeds him, and I feed the other. The 5 year old pampers the 1 year old. My husband learned from me how to cook. In bad weather he's home from his construction job, and he scrubs the kitchen floor. My girl friends stay on Sundays when my husband and I go out.

The children all help.

A delightful 21-year-old mother with three children showed wisdom beyond her years.

My mother-in-law and aunt helped the first week, and my husband helped after work. I told my husband "no baby blues this time, I love my family and you even more." I can't go out like I used to, so I just sat down and talked to myself. I'm young, and I have plenty of time to go out. I breast-feed my baby. I always have food on the table even if my dishes pile up.

I was sick the first week. My husband rubbed me down. He cooked and kept house. On the fourth week I cooked and did the laundry, but he still kept the house clean.

My family and in-laws all help. My husband helped with the kids. The fourth week I was on my own, but on weekends he fixes breakfast and feeds the kids so I can sleep late.

Following are comments of unwed mothers:

When I first saw her, I didn't want her. The second night I couldn't believe she was mine. The fourth night I couldn't wait till she came. Now I don't leave her unless it's real important, and then I miss her. I didn't have any help at home, so it was hard. I got tired of looking at the four walls; now I can take her out.

The baby's father and his mother and my mother and sisters all help.

One of the joys of the study for me was to be able at the conclusion of an interview not only to intervene with suggestions for some of the problems but also to share my perception of strengths within the mother and family.

Most of the mothers sought help in illness but were more lax in seeking health supervision. The clinic mothers had a history of broken appointments. Clinic mothers who had their postpartum checkup in the family planning clinic were more likely to keep the appointment than those attending the postpartum clinic. Only one mother mentioned that the nurse helped her. The mothers apparently did not see the nurse as a teaching person but only commented, "If I had known. . ."

Summary

Many problems of the postpartum mothers were identified through the inter-

views that have significance for nurses. These include the following:

The crying and feeding problems of babies
Need for assistance with breast-feeding
Lack of knowledge of mothers concerning child growth and development and infant care practices
Sibling rivalry
Physical problems of mothers, especially fatigue and painful perineums
Emotional problems
Need for support from others

The interviews revealed many positive factors and strengths within the mother and family that nurses should focus on in the assessment process. The way that mothers responded with unique behavior calls attention to the need for assessment of the *individual* mother to determine her abilities, strengths, and confidence in dealing with her concerns and conflicts.

CLINICAL APPLICATION OF THE DATA

This particular study of the postpartum mothers was presented recently to the nursing staff in a large women's hospital in New England, with ninety beds for maternity patients, 106 bassinets, an outpatient department with two satellite clinics, a regional newborn intensive care unit, and a large gynecological service. The presentation was made at the same time that a proposal for the development of a program for family-centered maternity care had been submitted by a committee of the nursing staff. As a result, I and a university undergraduate student were added to the membership of that committee. We shared the common goal of providing nursing care and services that would better meet the needs of new parents during the hospital stay and after they returned home. Thus a vital opportunity for service and education to work together on a common project for the improvement of patient care developed.

A program of family-centered maternity care has been developed in three phases. At the present time Phase II is in the process of development.

PHASE   I Pilot program
PHASE   II Formulation of guidelines staff conferences and education
PHASE III Implementation of the program

The pilot program was started in a

NURSING ASSESSMENT AND CARE PLAN FOR THE MATERNITY PATIENT

Mother

Number of siblings	Concerns	Nutrition	
Experience with	Perineum	Diet	
children	Breasts	Restrict fluids	
Problems	Afterpains	Force fluids	
Surgical	Fatigue	Juices	
Medical	Backache	No ice	
Social	Headache	I & O	
Emotional	Insomnia	Voiding	
Language	Daily care	Output	
Mother-infant	Bath	Bedpan	
interaction	Initial bath	B.R.P.	
	Bed bath	Bowels	
	Shower	Enema	
	Care of perineum	Suppository	
	Perineal care		
	Self-care		
	Medication		
	Sitz bath		
	Thermolite		

Baby

Good
Not good
Anomalies
Transferred
Expired
Mother informed
To be placed
Circumcision (boy)
  Yes
  No
Feeding
  Breast
  Formula
  Schedule
  On demand
  Needs help

Other:

MATERNITY PATIENT TEACHING NEEDS

Personal care

Pericare
Breast care
Bathing; hair washing
Depression
Fatigue
Medication and effects

Newborn

Initial examination
Baby bath
Feeding; burping
  Breast; bottle
Dressing
Ways of holding-handling
Care of cord
PKU test

Care of circumcision
Sleep patterns
Crying
Individual responses
  of babies
Sibling rivalry

Discharge plans

Does patient have necessary equipment for baby?
Are living arrangements adequate?
Does mother have help at home?
Does mother need help with family planning?
Help needed with _____

Referrals

VNA pediatrician
Social service
Well-child conference
Clinic appointment
Family planning
Homemaker's service

		Boy		
Age:	Marital status:	Girl	Rh = Rh — RhoGAM	
Adm. No.:	Name:	Adm. date:	Del. date:	M.D.:

twenty-bed wing of a maternity floor and continued for a period of three months. A team of interested staff nurses under the leadership of a professional nurse was involved in the care of the mothers and also assisted them with newborn care. Areas of assessment and teaching relating to the concerns of the mother about herself and her baby and his care were organized into a checklist, which was based in part on the needs identified in the study described.

The mothers on the unit could attend the regular group classes and conferences held in the teaching room, or sharing room, as it is often called. An evaluation questionnaire to determine patient satisfaction was given to mothers. Responses indicated that patients were pleased with the increased personal interaction with the nurse.

The following teaching care plan for the newborn was developed for use by the floor and nursery nurses.

From the experience of the pilot project, definite ideas emerged that served as guidelines for further planning.

1. There is a need for a professional nurse who will assume the leadership role with responsibility for nurses and nurses' aides who also are caring for maternity patients.

2. There is a need for staff education in preparing personnel to assume a greater role in the assessment of the patients and identification of problems and teaching needs.

3. The *Nursing Assessment and Care Plan for the Maternity Patient* (p. 234) and the *Maternity Patient Teaching Needs Plan* (p. 234) were made a part of the nursing Kardex. The *Teaching Care Plan for the Newborn* below was inserted into the newborn cribs for use by the floor and nursery nurses.

4. The sharing of knowledge between parents and nurse is the most effective method of learning. There is additional value in group sharing through parent conferences, coffee klatches, and group demonstration classes. During this sharing, the nurse should try to help parents identify their own strengths.

5. Use of audiovisual tools as well as a health library with books and pamphlets that are readily accessible to mothers is valuable. Teaching sessions over closed-circuit television should be a part of the entire program.

6. A parents' manual with suggestions for the postpartum period and child care is useful as a reference to the mother when she goes home.

7. Information concerning homemaker service should be available in the parents' manual.

8. Development of better referrals is necessary, so that patients, both private and clinic, could be seen by the visiting nurse in the community.

9. Evaluation of the effectiveness of the program should be ongoing.

The Visiting Nurses Association in this

TEACHING CARE PLAN FOR THE NEWBORN

                        Date   **Initial nurse**

Initial examination of baby by mother
Ways of holding-handling
Feeding—breast or bottle; burping
Dressing infant
Sleep patterns
Care of cord
Care of circumcision
Baby bath
Crying of newborn
Individual responses of baby

Please indicate if teaching is not needed or desired by mother.

city is an agency whose functions are to provide nursing care for the sick in the home as well as health promotion services. There is a staff of eighteen nurses. A report of the study of postpartum mothers and the changes in their care through the development of a family-centered maternity care program was given as inservice education to the visiting nurses. The idea of using a nurse's checklist that would include the assessment of both the mother and baby and a teaching plan concerning mothers' personal care and conflicts, as well as their knowledge and concerns about the baby, engendered a lively discussion. The staff suggested the inclusion on referral forms of more specific data about the mother and baby, which would alert the public health nurse to the needs of the mothers and provide for a follow-up of the teaching that had begun in the hospital.

CONCLUSIONS

Several points emerged from both the study itself and the utilization of the data in a clinical setting. It was evident that unstructured interviews could supply much useful information for improving patient care. Much of the information concerning needs and problems of postpartum mothers confirmed what others have shown. What was new, however, was the identification of the strengths of the mothers themselves and the resources they used to meet their problems. This information in turn provided clues for teaching and care programs within the hospital setting and the community. By anticipating problems and identifying potential strengths, the nurse could help in the prevention of stress for families in the postpartum period.

References

1. Adams, M.: Early concerns of primigravida mothers regarding infant care activities, Nurs. Res. 12:72, Spring, 1963.
2. Anderson, E. H.: A study of postpartum depression: Implications for nursing, ANA Clin. Sessions 10:10, Spring, 1964.
3. Carpenter, H.: The need for assistance of mothers with first babies, doctoral dissertation, Teachers College, Columbia University, 1965.
4. Carpenter, H., and Staff of the East York-Leaside Health Unit: An analysis of home visits to newborn infants, Toronto, 1960, East York-Leaside Health Unit.
5. Dyer, E. D.: Parenthood as crisis: A re-study, Marriage and Family Living 25:196, 1963.
6. Henning, E., Martogleo, G., Quita, M., Reinbrecht, J., and Strickland, M.: A dynamic nursing appraisal of the puerperium. In Lytle, N., editor: Maternal health nursing, Dubuque, Iowa, 1967, William C. Brown Co., Publishers.
7. Hobbs, D. F.: Transition to parenthood: A replication and an extension, Journal of Marriage and the Family 30:413, 1968.
8. Jacoby, A. P.: Transition to parenthood: A reassessment, Journal of Marriage and the Family 31:720, 1969.
9. LeMasters, E. E.: Parenthood as crisis, Marriage and Family Living 19:352, 1957.
10. Marshall, V. A.: Problems of the early puerperium, master's thesis, Yale University, 1970.
11. Rossi, A. S.: Transition to parenthood, Journal of Marriage and the Family 30:26, 1968.
12. Rubin, R.: Maternal care in our society, Nurs. Outlook 11:519, 1963.
13. Shaw, F. G.: Reconciliation, a theory of man transcending. In Jourand, S., and Overlade, D. C., editors: Disclosing man to himself, New York, 1968, Van Nostrand Co.
14. Stitt, P. G.: Helping medical students to find the strength in people, Children 13:104, May-June, 1966.
15. Stockwell, M. L., and Nishikawa, H. A.: The third hand. A theory of support, JPN and Mental Health Services 8:7, May-June, 1970.

25

Planned change in a hospital maternity service

Nancy A. Lytle

ORGANIZATIONAL CHANGE

Planned change in the relationships between a hospital maternity and gynecology patient service and a maternity and gynecological nursing faculty of a school of nursing has been implemented as a result of "An Experiment In Nursing." The experiment was undertaken at Case Western Reserve University with the cooperation of the administration and the Department of Nursing at University Hospitals of Cleveland during the years 1966 to 1971. Planned change is "a deliberate and collaborative process involving a change agent and a client system which are brought together to solve a problem or, more generally, to plan and attain an improved state of functioning in the client system by utilizing and applying valid knowledge."* This chapter describes the enabling mechanisms that led to the implementation of a number of planned changes in providing maternity and newborn nursing care at Mac-Donald House, the maternity and gynecology service of University Hospitals of Cleveland.

The experiment was prompted by the commitment of the Frances Payne Bolton School of Nursing faculty "to provide a productive and stimulating clinical learning environment for undergraduate and graduate students of nursing, fulfill its obligation to society, make a contribution toward alleviating the alleged manpower shortage in nursing, and help to reduce the gap between available knowledge and its application."* Commitment to the concept of academic leadership for nursing was the stimulus underlying the experiment.

A diagram showing the organizational relationships between the School of Nursing and the University Hospitals is presented in Fig. 25-1.

An agreement was reached whereby the School of Nursing was invested with the authority and responsibility for controlling the quality of nursing care, nursing education, and nursing research in the five clinical services of University Hospitals. This control was to be exercised by the appointment of clinicians who would practice, teach, and have responsibility for the nursing care and the appointment of nurses competent to engage in inquiry. By action of the boards of trustees of the university and University Hospitals, responsibility for nominating personnel for selected positions of leadership in the nursing department of the hospital was also placed in the School of Nursing.

New types of faculty and hospital staff appointments were introduced to reflect new responsibilities assumed by faculty members and by leadership personnel in the hospital. Joint hospital and university appointments were established for persons who held positions in both institutions simultaneously. Clinical directors of nursing, each of whom served as director of one of the five specialty services of the hospital and chairman of the faculty group of a particular nursing specialty in the school,

---

*From Bennis, W. G.: Changing organizations, New York, 1966, McGraw-Hill Book Co., p. 91. Used with permission.

*From Schlotfeldt, R. M., and MacPhail, J.: An experiment in nursing, implementing planned change, Am. J. Nurs. **69:**1018, May, 1969.

held joint appointments, as did some nurse clinicians.

Appointments as clinical faculty members were given to competent hospital practitioners who discharged the responsibilities of their position in ways that significantly influenced nursing practice, the education of undergraduate and graduate students, and the research programs of the school. Appointments as associates in nursing in the hospital were given all faculty members whose teaching, practice, and research activities required use of the clinical resources of the University Hospitals.

Differentiation of roles through the development of role expectations for hospital personnel in accordance with their qualifications and competencies and the proper use of an individual's expertise were viewed as two ways of helping produce maximum

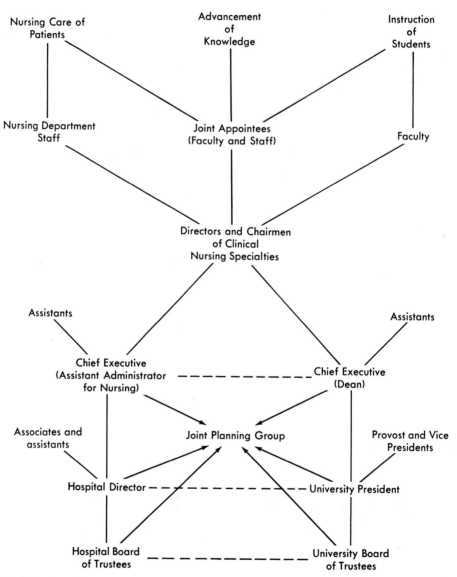

Fig. 25-1. Organizational relationship between the School of Nursing and the University Medical Center, Cleveland, Ohio. (From Schlotfeldt, R. M., and MacPhail, J.: Am. J. Nurs. 69:1018, 1969.)

effective achievement of practitioners. New position categories and titles were developed so that new role expectations could emerge, as illustrated by changing the head nurse position and title to that of Senior Clinical Nurse, with the expectation that the nurse would be encouraged and assisted to focus her time and attention on establishing and implementing standards for patient care. It also become the expectation that the Senior Clinical Nurse would assume the major role in formulating goals for patient care in collaboration with her nursing associates. To make it possible for this nurse to meet new role expectations, a unit manager system was developed. Division coordinator positions were established on each patient division. Persons holding these positions assumed responsibility for the clerical and managerial functions that have been traditionally performed by a head nurse and her associates. It was found that persons other than nurses could perform equally well the tasks of procuring, maintaining, and storing supplies and equipment; transcribing physician orders; and exercising the control of traffic and other numerous tasks viewed as supportive to members of the nursing staff.

Educational needs of incumbents and newly employed personnel were met by revising the existing centralized orientation and staff development programs, especially in the area of leadership development for registered nurses.

THE MATERNITY AND GYNECOLOGICAL NURSING PRACTICE COUNCIL

Freedom to determine the means by which close collaboration could be facilitated between the faculty of the School of Nursing and the staff in leadership positions in University Hospitals was provided the directors of nursing and their associates. In the fall of 1968, a few months after activation of the experiment in the maternity and gynecological specialty, the Director of Maternity and Gynecological Nursing called a meeting to discuss the experiment's concept of academic leadership in nursing and how this concept might become operational in this specialty service

located in MacDonald House at University Hospitals. Persons invited to the meeting were all members of the faculty who held associate appointments in University Hospitals or persons in leadership positions in the hospital who held clinical faculty appointments in the School of Nursing. The latter group consisted of the Assistant Director of Nursing, nurse clinicians in joint appointments, and clinical supervisors. The decision to form an organization that would formalize the implementation of the academic leadership concept and foster collaborative relationships between practitioners in the specialty was made at this initial meeting of the group.

A Maternity and Gynecological Nursing Practice Council was formed in January, 1969. The stated purpose and functions of the group are presented here:

Purpose:
  Define maternity-gynecological nursing practice. Make recommendations to the Director of Maternity-Gynecological Nursing based upon the study of:

Functions:
  1. Standards of maternity-gynecological professional and technical nursing practice
  2. The nature of maternity-gynecological nursing practice
  3. The scope of maternity-gynecological nursing practice
  4. Situational reality (e.g., existing phenomena, work group characteristics, roles, work patterns, authority structures) in maternity-gynecological nursing practice
  5. Teaching-learning needs and opportunities in and for maternity-gynecological nursing practice
  6. Maternity-gynecological nursing practice in relation to trends in health care
  7. Health issues and the contributions of maternity-gynecological nursing practice to the community at large

Membership in the Council was extended to persons who attended the initial meeting. All these persons elected to join the Council, although membership was not considered mandatory. Each group member, including the director of nursing, was to have equal voice and vote. A chairman, secretary, and treasurer were to be elected yearly for a one-year term. Visitors such as graduate students in nursing, the Project Director of the Experiment in Nursing, the Dean of the School of Nursing, and the Assistant Administrator for Nursing were welcome to attend the Council meetings at any time. Regular evening meetings were scheduled once a month. Meetings of ad hoc committees of the Council were to be held in accordance with the task to be accomplished. It was expected that professional nurses employed in the hospital service and students would be invited to serve on ad hoc committees of the Council. Purposes and functions of the Council were to be reviewed yearly. To date, no revisions have been made, and they stand as just outlined. Thus professional nurses employed by two private institutions, only a few of whom were employed by both institutions, formed and have maintained a group for academic leadership in a hospital specialty service.

Recommendations of the Nursing Practice Council are submitted to the Director of Maternity and Gynecological Nursing. Action to accept and delegate responsibility for implementation rests with the director in her role as administrator of the service and chairman of the maternity and gynecological faculty group. Frequently, a staff or faculty member volunteers to assume responsibility for implementing a recommendation.

Professional personnel and also undergraduate and graduate students studying maternity/gynecological nursing may refer their concerns regarding nursing practice to the Council for consideration. The first two projects undertaken by the Council involved problems identified by the two groups. There were no nursing policies and guidelines for the care of women in labor or for the breast-feeding mother and infant. Inconsistencies frequently occurred in the care provided patients. Professional nurses were unclear about the role they were to assume, both with labor patients and with breast-feeding mothers. Prompt action by the Council to clarify the role of the nurse and the nature of nursing practice was indicated.

A subcommittee of the Council was appointed. The committee's first task was to prepare definitions for policies, guidelines, and procedures. While committee members worked to complete this task, the nurse clinician with joint responsibility for nursing practice and the instruction of students in the labor and delivery unit reviewed the literature and developed a rationale for the nursing care of patients with spontaneous and induced labor. The director of nursing agreed to assume the same type of assignment in the area of breast-feeding. The subcommittee then prepared the policies and guidelines for practice in the two areas and submitted them to the Council for action.

Prior to and during the preparation of the policies and guidelines for nursing practice, the nurse specialists and members of the subcommittee conferred frequently with their medical colleagues. Particular effort was made to seek medical input when the knowledge base was being assembled. Many conferences were held with the obstetrician charged with administrative responsibility for care on the labor and delivery and postpartum divisions and with the pediatrician administratively responsible for newborn care in the nurseries. The purpose of these conferences was to discuss the roles and responsibilities that nurses and physicians should assume with respect to practice in the areas under consideration. Although the nursing staff and faculty exerted much effort to include physicians at every point in the deliberations, communication, although maintained, was often strained. Our physicians, who traditionally had made decisions regarding the "what and how of nursing practice," were now conferring with a group of competent nurse practitioners who held the belief that they had the right and obligation to delineate the nature of nursing practice and the proper role of the nurse. Eventually, these highly committed physicians and nurses did resolve their differences. Agreement was reached on the essential elements of patient care. The physicians gradually began to realize that competent nurses are willing and capable of sharing responsibility for patient safety and programs of health care.

Nursing care of patients having spontaneous or induced labors

Nursing policies for the care of women having induced labors and guidelines for the assessment of women having spontaneous and induced labors were completed during August, 1969. These recommendations were promptly accepted by the Director of Maternity and Gynecological Nursing. Medical concurrence with the policies was immediate. The obstetrician with whom we had conferred at length during the formulation of the policies assumed an active and supportive role in helping obtain acceptance of the policies by private and resident physicians. A carefully coordinated staff development program was activated for nursing personnel on each shift in the labor and delivery unit. We hoped by this means to assure that the nurse's role was understood and practiced in accordance with the policies and guidelines. Faculty members assumed responsibility for conveying the information to students. The nurse clinician and the assistant director of nursing functioned to help reduce the nursing and medical resistance to change in the nurse's role. But it was several months before we could state with a degree of certainly that all nursing personnel were implementing the policies and that physicians understood and accepted the role assumed by nursing personnel.

The nursing practice policies for the care of women with oxytocic induced labors during stages one and two stipulated that nursing action was confined to the administration of oxytocic drugs such as buccal, intranasal, and intramuscular oxytocin when the patient's physician was present. Nursing responsibility for the care of patients receiving intravenous oxytocin was described as maintaining the flow at the rate ordered (after initiation) by the physician when nursing assessments indicated normal progress. Signs and symptoms of possible complications in the condition of the mother or fetus such as prolonged uterine contractions and late or variable deceleration of the fetal heart rate were noted as requiring prompt action by the nurse to slow down or discontinue the rate of the intravenous flow and to obtain the assistance of the physician in immediate attendance.

The guidelines for assessing patients in labor described precisely the baseline observations nursing personnel were expected to make, including the frequency of these observations. Patient data pertaining to vital signs, periods of uterine relaxation and contraction, physical characteristics such as condition of patient's skin, uterine elevation or dipping, and sensations experienced by the patient were identified as essential in planning nursing action.

One small segment of the *Nursing Practice Guidelines for Assessment of Patients in Labor* is reproduced in Table 5 to illustrate how the material was organized and our initial effort to isolate certain patient behaviors to be noted by the nurse.

The policies and guidelines formulated by the Nursing Practice Council have been implemented on our labor and delivery division for almost two and one-half years. The role of nursing personnel in the care

Table 5. Nursing practice guidelines for assessment of patients in labor

| Nursing assessments of _____ | Observations | Assessment period | | Abnormal variations to be reported | Possible complications associated with abnormal variations |
		Patients with spontaneous onset of labor	Patient with oxytocic induced labor		
Behavior characteristics of patient	Facial expressions Physical activity during and between contractions Direction of attention (extroversion or introversion) Vocal tones Degree of anxiety	On admission, every half hour during first stage of labor, and every 5 minutes during second stage	Same	Increasing restlessness Increasing anxiety Inability to control behavior during labor	Uterine dysfunction Tetany Impending uterine rupture Malpresentation C.P. disproportion Abruptio placentae Toxemia Exhaustion

of women in labor is clearly delineated and consistently followed. Access to printed materials that outline minimal standards for assessment of the labor patient and the fetus by nursing personnel and students has facilitated improvements in the quality of care patients receive. Practitioners, present and future, are stimulated to make nursing judgments. They apply broadly based knowledge in depth in decision making about individual patients. Increasingly, personnel and students exhibit self-directed behavior in the labor and delivery room that is indicative of professional nursing practice. Teaching effectiveness for students and personnel has increased with the introduction of materials that speak to the nature of nursing observations with a particular patient population.

Nursing care of the breast-feeding mother and infant

The second accomplishment of the Nursing Practice Council was the preparation of materials for use in instituting a program of care for breast-feeding mothers and infants. The Council recommended acceptance of policies and guidelines for use by nursing personnel and an instruction brochure for distribution to breast-feeding mothers. The recommendation was accepted by the Director of Nursing. Prompt concurrence for institution of the breast-feeding program was obtained from the Nursing Council and the Medical Council, the two bodies charged with responsibility for the nature and the quality of professional practice in University Hospitals.

The nursing policies that were developed are included herein because it is believed that nursing's contribution to the establishment of successful breast-feeding will be realized only when nurses request and are granted the responsibility and authority outlined in our statement.

University Hospitals of Cleveland
MATERNITY AND GYNECOLOGICAL NURSING
POLICIES
THE CARE OF THE BREAST-FEEDING MOTHER
AND HER INFANT

1. The registered nurse shall assess the infant's physiological readiness for breast-feeding and the mother's readiness for

breast-feeding. The registered nurse shall take appropriate action. This includes
a. Deciding when the infant is ready for his first feeding.
b. Deciding when the mother is ready to learn to breast-feed her baby.
c. Instituting an on-demand feeding schedule after securing order from physician.
d. Helping the mother to learn to breast-feed her baby.
2. The registered nurse is responsible for helping breast-feeding mothers to establish an adequate supply of breast milk. This action includes
a. Providing mothers with necessary information.
b. Assisting mothers when their babies are ready to nurse.
c. Supervision of the mother in the regular stimulation and emptying of the breast.
d. Instruction in and supervision of manual expression of breast milk.
e. Instruction in and supervision of the use of a manual breast pump as necessary.
3. The registered nurse shall initiate action with breast-feeding mothers for the purpose of preventing painful breast engorgement and sore nipples. This action may include
a. Providing mothers with appropriate information.
b. Supervision of the mother in maintenance of low milk pressure in breasts.
c. Taking the baby to feed when he is hungry and the mother's breasts are filling or her breasts should be stimulated.
d. Modifying breast-feeding techniques to minimize engorgement or sore nipples.
e. Clean, warm, moist applications prior to manual expression.
f. Reporting breast engorgement or sore nipples to the physician.

Prior to implementation of these breast-feeding policies, several mothers reported the following:

I found some of the nurses unsympathetic to a nursing mother. One nurse remarked right before my baby was brought to me for the first feeding, "Your baby probably won't like your milk." She might have meant to be helpful, but I wasn't in the mood for this type of joke or indirect guidance.

The only criticism I have about the care is that the nurses were inconsistent in the advice they gave to a breast-feeding mother.

The nurses were much too rigid about night feedings, especially for breast-feeding mothers— but then one nurse told me the baby couldn't come out for feeding unless the doctor wrote the order.

I wanted and needed more guidance than I got about breast-feeding, and I always had to ask questions before anybody gave me information. It was a couple days before I realized I could increase the feeding time per breast beyond the 5 minutes my doctor recommended.

The results brought about by planned change, the formulation of policies and guidelines, and some intensive staff education prompted new mothers to send us these comments.

The help the staff gave me when I was first learning to breast-feed my baby was very much welcomed and of good quality. I feel the care has improved since I worked here five years ago and since I had my last baby two years ago.

All the people helped me with breast-feeding, but I thought a few people were outstanding in their patience, knowing the help I needed before I was aware I needed it and generally making my stay pleasant.

One of my roommates had trouble breast-feeding. Everyone helped, no one ever discouraged her, and an effort was made to have the same nurses help her on each shift.

I really appreciated the nursery personnels' suggestions and help in *schedule flexibility.*

People were interested in me and my baby and our adjustment to one another. Not only did they give me the booklet on breast-feeding, but my questions were always answered so that I never felt confused. I found everyone just pleasant and helpful.

I had my last baby two years ago. At that time no one seemed interested in me or my baby. I received no explanations or instructions about what I could or could not do and what I should be doing for myself and the baby. This time I was greatly surprised at the general overall improvement in nursing care, especially the help I received in feeding my baby.

I felt more confident about feeding the baby and being ready to manage at home because I was helped over some troubled times. The entire staff, not just the nursery nurses, helped me adjust.

In the two years since I was last here, for what-ever reason, there is much improvement. This time there was consistency in what personnel, doctors, and nurses told me about breast-feeding. More nurses were confident and professional enough to "let down" on the rigidity of the rules, which let in room for individual care and loving care. This was very heartwarming.

After eighteen months' experience with written policies that permit independent nurse action in the care of the breast-feeding mother and infant, an attempt was made to assess their value. The conclusions reached were as follows:

1. A coordinated program of care designed to meet the needs of a breast-feeding mother and infant results when nursing and medical practitioners collaborate in the reallocation of responsibility for patient care and formal channels of communication are utilized to convey this action.

2. Registered nurses change their behavior and initiate independent action with increased frequency when provided with nursing care policies that sanction independent functioning.

3. Registered nurses are motivated to seek out additional opportunities for independent nursing action after successful experience with a breast-feeding program that promotes independent decision making based on collection of patient data and the use of care principles.

4. Nurse-patient interaction and patient competence and confidence are enhanced when new mothers have access to information and are involved in decision making associated with the breast-feeding process.

5. Greater flexibility in the feeding schedules of all infants and especially breast-fed infants occurs when nursing personnel begin assessing each mother and infant prior to delivering nursing care.

6. The quality of education provided for future professional nurse practitioners is improved when students practice in a setting where nursing care standards are explicit and independent nursing action is an expectation.

INNOVATIONS IN PATIENT SERVICES
Maternity continuity clinic

Improving the quality of care provided patients attending the hospital prenatal clinic and fully utilizing the potential of health professionals has been the goal of both nurses and physicians. It is recognized that pregnant women who are in good health and expected to have a normal pregnancy require a different type of health care than that usually provided in most physician-conducted clinics.

Our group believed that a qualified nurse clinician with graduate preparation in maternity nursing could be effective in organizing and conducting a health care program for pregnant unmarried adolescents and others.

Medical consultation could be obtained if the patient's condition was found to deviate from the normal. Furthermore, if warranted, the condition of each patient could be evaluated by a physician immediately prior to her estimated date of confinement. Resident physicians were available to assume responsibility for conducting the labor and delivery and to provide health supervision for the delivered mother and the newborn infant. Consultation services were also immediately available from the social worker and the dietitian.

On presenting the idea to members of the Maternity and Gynecological Nursing Practice Council, we were encouraged to proceed with finalization of a program to utilize professional nurses in the delivery of primary health care to healthy pregnant women. The placement of a nurse clinician in the clinic to be responsible for delineating the scope of nursing practice, setting standards for care, delivering care, and instructing and guiding other nurses in the delivery of primary health care was viewed as appropriate and necessary. The Council further recommended that continuity in patient care be assured by having the same nurse provide care for a patient throughout her pregnancy and by having this nurse make suggestions for nursing care during the intrapartal and postpartal periods, as well as making at least one follow-up visit during the patient's hospitalization. In making the recommendation that the scope of nursing practice include making independent judgments about the delivery of health care to healthy pregnant women, Council members realized that this was a departure from a prevailing idea that only nurses with midwifery preparation are qualified to assume responsibility for the delivery of care to healthy pregnant women.

As a result of the collaboration between physicians and nurses, a new approach was taken to the utilization of professional health personnel in the prenatal clinics. Nursing personnel now make independent judgments as they provide comprehensive health care to healthy pregnant women. Since the fall of 1970, when the Continuity Clinic began, 159 women have received health care from the nurse clinician or her one associate. We now are preparing all registered nurses employed in the obstetrics and gynecology clinics to carry a case load in the Maternity Continuity Clinic. As a result, we hope to increase the number of women who can be accommodated. In addition, we anticipate that nursing care provided all patients attending the clinics will improve.

Students studying maternity nursing are exposed to role models who serve as primary health practitioners and who make independent nursing judgments. They assume varying degrees of responsibility for the delivery of patient care in the Maternity Continuity Clinic, depending on the objectives of their program of instruction (undergraduate or graduate) and their motivation and competence. Evidence gathered by physicians and nurses in a predominately service clinic suggests that broad-based comprehensive patient care is being delivered, communication between nurse and patient is therapeutic, and patients are satisfied with the care received.

Activities for mothers

The creation of a hospital climate responsive to individual differences of new mothers remains more a dream than a reality on most maternity services. Members of our nursing staff concluded after careful study that involving mothers directly in decision making about how they spent their time while hospitalized was a workable approach to recognizing individual differences and meeting the conscious learning needs of new mothers.

An *Activities for Mothers* sheet was prepared and distributed to mothers on their admission to the postpartum and newborn division. Two types of information were presented: specified hours when infants in the nursery would be taken to their mothers for handling and feeding and the visiting hours for family and friends. Opportunities for flexibility in the infant feeding schedule, extended visiting by infants in their mothers' rooms, teaching activities for groups of mothers such as luncheon roundtable discussions and classes on infant care and family planning, father visiting, and guest meal service were all listed and described. Thus the activities available at certain hours or certain days of the week were stipulated.

One-to-one nurse-patient communication that involved providing mothers with guidance, instruction, explanations, and interpretations necessary for decision making and progress in the mothering role was considered a part of comprehensive postpartum nursing care.

Nursing personnel assessed the physical condition of each mother and infant, paying particular attention to maternal behavior that suggested "taking in" or "taking hold" motivation and readiness to learn or a need for rest and reflection. Using this patient data and any other that might provide cues as to a patient's perception of herself in the maternal role, a professional nurse discussed with each mother her plans for the organization of her day. Nursing intervention was instituted throughout the day whenever it seemed appropriate and helpful to a particular mother. It was the mothers, however, who made the final decision with respect to how they spent their time.

The *Activities for Mothers* sheet is a mechanism for removing the restrictions often imposed on mothers and the staff by "the schedule" of a maternity unit. Its use has had the effect of stimulating nursing personnel to respect the rights of new mothers and to consider their wishes when providing them with nursing care. Our standard for postpartum nursing care has changed, and the quality of care has improved.

This approach to the delivery of postpartum nursing care was a gradual process and involved the combined thinking and work of a group consisting of several senior clinical nurses, a nurse clinician, the part-time instructor of mothers' classes, a faculty member, the director, and the assistant director of nursing. This group met once a week for about six weeks while "brown bagging" their lunch to discuss the learning needs of new mothers and to evaluate the adequacy of efforts in this area of nursing practice. Teaching activities for staff and private patients throughout the pregnancy cycle were carefully reviewed. Information from the literature was introduced, provocative questions were raised, and personal observations and experience were shared. It was not long before group members were expressing innovative ideas for patient teaching activities appropriate for all new mothers or for a special group of mothers, such as unmarried adolescents.

Luncheon roundtable discussions for mothers led by a knowledgeable professional nurse possessing competence in group process was the idea of a senior clinical nurse. This nurse prior to the luncheon meetings had been inactive in patient teaching; this function was low on her priority list. Her suggestion to provide mothers an opportunity to express and discuss their concerns received the enthusiastic acceptance of the group. This nurse then volunteered to assume responsibility for getting the roundtable discussions started, including the problem of obtaining the acceptance and cooperation of physicians, the dietary department, the nursing staff members, etc.

Innovative ideas are generated and new and different approaches to the delivery of patient care are instituted when maternity nurses interact in a setting in which knowledge forms the basis for nursing practice, the quality of nursing practice is evaluated on a regular basis, and competent nurse practitioners stimulate and support, but do not control, practice.

Father visiting program

Encouraging husbands to share their wives' labor experiences has been a practice at our hospital for several years. Many couples also share the joy of their child's birth. On the other hand, fathers were assigned the role of spectator when they visited their wives and infants in the maternity division.

The concept of family-centered maternity care was operational on our maternity divisions only insofar as mothers benefited from extra hours spent with their babies after the morning and/or afternoon feeding period. Models demonstrating expectations of the mother or father role with newborn infants were absent in this traditionally oriented environment. Nursing personnel perceived themselves as responsible for carrying out physicians' orders and satisfying the basic physical needs of mothers and infants.

Believing that new parents had a right to early contact with their infants, as well as individualized instruction, and that nursing personnel had a responsibility to provide it, the Director of Nursing and her associates designed an experimental program of care that would involve the mother and father, but especially the father. To gather information as well as to prepare the personnel for change, it was proposed that a pilot study be conducted. The primary purposes were (1) to ascertain father and/or parent interest in direct father-infant-mother contact and (2) to determine the feasibility of establishing a father visiting program under the auspices of the existing staff.

Preliminary planning for the introduction of the study included communication with members of the medical and nursing personnel who would be involved. The Senior Clinical Nurse on the private patient division where it was believed the study could be done was fully acquainted with the purposes and plan of the study. With no hesitation, she offered to assist with any necessary arrangements. It was indicated during this initial discussion that decisions which might involve changes in patient care services delivered on her division would be preceded by the elicitation of recommendations from her.

Pediatricians were enthusiastic in their support and offered their services in working out the details and barriers to conducting the study; obstetricians were not. We interpreted their responses as being suggestive of apathy and wonderment that nursing wished to bother with something like father visiting and parent instruction when there were many problems requiring attention, such as poor staff morale on the maternity divisions, too few registered nurses, and limited success in recruitment of competent personnel. We listened to the obstetricians and attempted to explain our reasons for developing the proposal; we also indicated our desire to obtain their cooperation if we decided to conduct the study. No obstetrician expressed unwillingness to cooperate should the study be conducted.

Members of the Maternity and Gynecology Nursing Practice Council recommended that the pilot study be done. They further stated that collecting information about father motivation and reactions to a structured program of care could contribute to developing a rationale for nursing intervention with new fathers.

Persons charged with administrative responsibility for the obstetric and gynecology service—the Medical Director, the Director of Nursing who proposed the pilot study, and the Hospital Administrator—agreed that the study should be done. The Medical Director and the Hospital Administrator both assumed active roles in informing physicians regarding details of the study.

After full acceptance of the proposed pilot study was gained, a number of materials were prepared to introduce the experimental program and to collect the desired information. They consisted of the following:

1. *Message for New Mothers and Fathers*—distributed by the nursing staff after the mother had been delivered of a living, full-term newborn infant. It briefly explained the program, the reasons for conducting the study, and the procedures to be followed by the fathers and mothers. Since fathers could also request guest meal service for dinner with their wives prior to the 6 P.M. infant feeding period, information about this service was included.

2. *Message for Visiting Fathers*—material distributed to fathers who chose to visit during the 6 P.M. infant feeding period. The purpose was to outline procedures to be followed during the visiting period and to indicate the freedom afforded fathers to initiate the type of infant contact they desired. The availability of nursing assistance was mentioned, as were possible in-

fant contact activities. One procedure described was that of scrubbing and gowning; another was the plan for fathers to take their infants from the nursery and wheel them in their cribs to the mothers' rooms. For each instruction an explanation was given. Emphasis was placed on the need for fathers to be free of a respiratory infection. Included also was a statement regarding the questionnaire that would be distributed to them.

3. *Memorandum to Nursing Personnel*—issued by the Director of Nursing to describe the purposes and procedures of the study and the role and activities of the study personnel. It also presented the goals of nursing care as being: (1) to foster family unity, (2) to promote the establishment of a father-infant relationship, (3) to promote feelings of confidence in new parents, and (4) to provide opportunities for new parents that develop the ability to recognize and meet the care needs of a newborn infant.

4. A questionnaire to be answered by fathers who participated in the program. Their reactions to direct contact with their infants and to the assistance given by the nursing staff were solicited.

5. A nursing record of instruction and/or assistance given to each participating father, including a report of the father's behavior with his infant, to be completed by the nurse.

Prior to the initiation of the study, informal group meetings were held with nursing personnel to discuss the father visiting study, to answer their questions about the planned program of care and the prepared materials, and to examine their feelings regarding the program. Generally, the idea of fathers being present and participating during an infant feeding period was well received. Personnel who would be working during the hours when fathers visited had the opportunity to view a video tape recording made of father-mother-infant-nurse interaction. Both professional and nonprofessional personnel responded to the tape with enthusiasm. Many of them offered to assist in making the study a success. The importance of feedback from them during the study was emphasized at this time. However, we were conscious of

the fact that three registered nurses who had worked on the division for many years had adopted a "wait-and-see" attitude.

Responsibility for organizing and conducting the study was shared by the Director of Maternity and Gynecological Nursing and her assistant, since no special funds were available to finance it. The month of January, 1971, was chosen as the time period to conduct the study. One undergraduate student was available for employment as a nursing assistant, and two graduate students could be employed as registered nurses on a part-time basis during this month. Employment of the students supplemented the personnel available to care for the mothers and infants. In addition, each evening one student could be scheduled to assist with the father visiting study. For twenty-five consecutive days, during the 5:30 to 7 P.M. period, a study staff of two individuals, the Director of Nursing and one student—either graduate or undergraduate—or the Assistant Director of Nursing and a student, were available to instruct and to provide nursing assistance to fathers participating in the program.

Fathers of all infants hospitalized on one maternity division were offered the opportunity to participate in the father visiting program. Participation was voluntary; on some evenings 88% of the fathers visited during the 6 P.M. feeding period. Included were both first-time fathers and fathers with two or more children. Out of a possible 119 eligible fathers, 78, or 70%, elected to participate. Of the participating group, 87% returned the questionnaires that had been distributed to them.

Analysis of the questionnaire responses indicated that most new fathers decided to participate in the visiting program because they had a personal need: "to touch daughter and she me," "to know what our son looked like, felt like, and how he was getting along," and "to see, touch, and get acquainted with my son." They had a personal wish "to share wife's experience," and "to take advantage of the wonderful opportunity to spend time as a family." About one sixth indicated that they decided to participate "to make my wife feel and see how interested I am in the baby," "at the urging of my wife," and because "wife thought I'd enjoy it—I did." The remaining fathers attributed their participation to "learn from a nurse firsthand how to handle the baby," "to handle child in presence of experienced personnel, to gain technique and confidence before going home," "to pick up points from the nurses," and "to learn correct way of baby care from beginning."

Over one half the fathers who participated in father visiting described the most satisfying aspect of the program as having a chance to be "close to baby" and "to hold and see baby." The feeling of being part of a family was important to the next large group of fathers, who found it satisfying to "meet the baby with my wife and getting the feel of having a baby to care for again," "to hold the baby, the three of us together," and "just being that near to son and wife at that time." Several fathers expressed satisfaction about "taking baby to my wife and feeling trusted when doing it" and "having a nurse show me a few things about baby care."

The most unsatisfying aspect of the father visiting program was reported as "none" by more than half the fathers. Approximately one sixth indicated that other family commitments prevented them from participating in the program more often. The features that were unsatisfying to a few fathers were maintaining clean technique, handwashing, gowning, and returning their babies to the nursery so that other persons could visit their wives.

Fathers described themselves as feeling loving, tender, happy, and fearful as they touched and handled their babies for the first time. Staff members who noted the facial expressions of the fathers added feelings of joy and pride to the list of feelings fathers experienced.

Analysis of the nursing action records indicated that all fathers either requested or were observed as needing instruction in handling or feeding and burping the baby. Although the nurses moved in slowly in an effort to allow each father freedom to decide what he wished to do when with the baby, the fathers desired and utilized the instruction provided by the staff. Usually attempts were made to draw the mother into the conversation so that three adults participated in the teaching-learning act. Fathers, even those who visited nightly, expressed minimum interest in going beyond holding and feeding the baby. The first evening visiting time was usually spent looking at and holding the baby.

During the first seven days of the study a few members of the regular staff made overtures interpreted as indicating interest in and eagerness to become involved in the care program. Two staff members, one a nurses' technical assistant (aide) and one a licensed practical nurse, stated that they felt capable of and would like to participate in the program. Their services were utilized on a selected basis.

On the basis of the findings, it was concluded that fathers would find a father visiting program satisfying and would elect to participate in it if the program were offered on a permanent basis. It was apparent also that all nursing personnel, with the exception of three, were ready to accept the program and to develop their competence for this type of nursing care.

Six weeks after the termination of the pilot study, a second-year graduate student, completing preparation for practice as a nurse clinician, undertook the task of preparing the nursing staff for involvement in the father visiting program. The care program was offered on a regular basis two nights per week—Wednesday and Sunday—because these were the evenings when the majority of fathers visited during the pilot study. Shortages in personnel prevented further expansion of the program at that time. The graduate student's experience of planned change, the problems encountered, and the modifications made in the program are being prepared for publication.

Today, one year later, recruitment of competent registered nurses is no longer a problem, and all registered nurse positions on maternity divisions are filled. Morale is high; personnel are competent to teach and guide mothers and fathers as they experiment with and adjust to the responsibilities of parenthood. The nursery on the division where the study was conducted has been remodeled to include several small nurseries, and mother-infant care is individualized. Personnel have just completed a plan to offer father visiting several hours each day. Planned instruction and supervision by the nursing staff will be included as part of each new father's first and, perhaps, second visiting period, depending on individual need and request.

Our experience suggests that new mothers wish to be learners, not teachers of their husbands. No husband indicated that he preferred to learn from his wife. We have found that fathers can move in fast and begin to assume control in the care of the new baby, leaving the unsure mother out of the caretaking activity. Nurses frequently intervene at this time to facilitate communication between the new father and mother and to promote a feeling of confidence in *both* of them. Fathers with other children and often first-time fathers are observed to leave the hospital before regular visiting hours are over if the father-infant-mother contact that preceded the regular visiting hours was satisfying. Consequently, we do not expect the number of hours when fathers visit to be appreciably increased. An increase in the number of hours available for father visiting will offer parents greater freedom in organizing their own time schedules. We anticipate that fathers will begin attending more of the group teaching activities organized for mothers; a few already have. Fathers have been offered the opportunity to talk about their own concerns and problems associated with parenthood. We anticipate that the request for this activity will increase. What we will offer and how we will offer the service will be carefully planned and evaluated with personnel on each division.

Nursing personnel on the division where 50% of the patients are unmarried are now planning to institute a father visiting program for both the married and unmarried fathers.

Students, undergraduate and graduate, and new personnel from all maternity divisions observe, participate, and learn from the fathers who serve as change agents in our hospital.

SUMMARY

Maternity nurse practitioners committed to the concept of academic leadership for nursing introduced planned change in a hospital maternity service. This group of nursing specialists was one of five specialty groups at University Hospitals of Cleveland who assumed new roles and relationships as part of "An Experiment In Nursing" conducted by Case Western Reserve University in collaboration with University Hospitals. Innovations in nursing practice and education and an increase in investigative endeavors in nursing were the expected outcomes when the Director of Maternity and Gynecological Nursing and her associates in the school and in the hospital were given the opportunity to exercise leadership at a policy-making level on matters related to maternity nursing practice.

Knowledge was the basis for action, which involved nursing personnel according to their competence and potential in planning and decision making. The general plan was to influence the activities of nursing personnel toward goal setting and goal achievement. Commitment to the advancement of practice in the specialty involved the systematic gathering of data related to the change process, the inclusion of patient and family member response to nursing interventions, personnel and student response to the establishment of new and/ or different standards for patient care, the creation of new roles for nurse practitioners, and provision for educational experiences to promote competency in practice.

Four principles applied in the administration of the maternity and gynecology service facilitated planned changes in nursing care.

1. All communication, verbal and written, directed to nursing and medical personnel was focused on promoting understanding of action to be taken or requests for a specific type of performance by nursing personnel.

2. The ability or potential of nursing personnel to meet current role expectations or anticipated changes in role expectations was continuously assessed.

3. Efforts were made to establish congruence between suggested or requested action for patient benefit and the practice goals of members of the staff.

4. Ideas submitted by nursing personnel after the use of problem-solving techniques were utilized to influence the performance

requested or expected of nursing personnel.

Reactions of personnel to planned change on this maternity service is illustrated in the following statement made by a licensed practical nurse when she was honored for 25 years of continuous employment on a maternity division: "There have been some wonderful changes at University Hospitals, especially at MacDonald House. It is a wonderful, happy place to work, especially for young nurses who want to learn. I am grateful for the new things I am always learning."

The maternity nurse leaders served as role models, teachers, counselors, problem solvers, investigators, and colleagues. They displayed the traits of perseverance, courage, insight, and tact. Equally important was the commitment, enthusiasm, and optimism they displayed when confronted by apathy, dissatisfaction, regressive behavior, and acute shortages of personnel, including faculty and leadership persons.

Planned change reported in this chapter suggests that competent maternity nursing specialists cope successfully with the realities of the present while planning for the future. Maternity nurses employ nursing leadership when they (1) involve others in decision making, (2) assist personnel to make hidden and impending problems visible, (3) deal constructively with problems or consequences not predicted, (4) establish priorities after comprehensive assessment of related factors and significant variables, (5) create two-way communication channels, and (6) engage in continuous evaluation and systematic study.

References

1. Bennis, W. G.: Changing organizations, New York, 1966, McGraw-Hill Book Co.
2. Schlotfeldt, R. M., and MacPhail, J.: An experiment in nursing, rationale and characteristics, Am. J. Nurs. **69:**1018, 1969.
3. Schlotfeldt, R. M., and MacPhail, J.: An experiment in nursing, introducing planned change, Am. J. Nurs. **69:**1247, 1969.
4. Schlotfeldt, R. M., and MacPhail, J.: An experiment in nursing, implementing planned change, Am. J. Nurs. **69:**1475, 1969.

26

Is abortion murder? Two Catholics reply

Anne Lally Milhaven
John Giles Milhaven

DILEMMA OF A NURSING ADMINISTRATOR
Anne Lally Milhaven

The care of a patient having a therapeutic abortion presents a problem if a nurse objects to abortion on religious and moral grounds. As a profession, nursing rarely deals with moral issues that are in conflict with the nurse's professional role. Thus the nursing literature does not meet head on religious and moral objections that present obstacles to the nurse's giving supportive care to a patient having a therapeutic abortion.

As the nursing head of a large obstetrical-gynecological department at the time that the abortion law was liberalized in New York City, I faced the problem of staffing a new unit for therapeutic abortion patients. This chapter will focus on one of my most difficult problems, dealing with the nurse who sincerely believes that abortion is murder. My husband, a specialist in Christian ethics, will analyze the nature of this religious objection from the viewpoint of Roman Catholic teaching, since most nurses who hold this belief are Roman Catholics. Hopefully the nursing profession can draw on the discipline of religion to gain insight into this troublesome issue.

The nursing department of which I was the head served the maternity, pediatric, and gynecological needs of 200 patients. On liberalization of the New York State law relating to abortion, a twenty-eight-bed unit was established for abortion patients. Plans were made to accept sixty to seventy patients each week. Efforts to recruit personnel from both within and without the department were difficult. The reasons given for hesitation and reluctance ranged from general moral scruples to a conviction that the abortion program was intended as racist genocide to the kind of emotional conflict that one nurse described: "I cannot support patient A in one room struggling to save her pregnancy and then walk into the next room and support patient B 'getting rid' of hers." Sometimes one suspected reasons other than the moral objections given, as in the case of nurses who later had abortions themselves. One could conjecture that often the true motives underlying the moral grounds given were something less serious, such as fear of the judgment of peers.

What I found most difficult to deal with, however, was the sincere person who objected to abortion on moral grounds determined by religious faith. Not only did this prevent some nurses from having anything to do with the abortion patient, but it also affected nurses who did agree to work with these patients. Their feelings were sometimes manifested by punitive and reproachful treatment of the patient. Since I found this religious objection the greatest obstruction to supportive nursing care of abortion patients, I gave it considerable scrutiny and tried to understand it.

In the first place, I discovered that one can easily underestimate the obstacle a religious conscience can create to abortion. Nursing administrators suggest that a nurse should in personal life act according to conscience but in professional life respect the beliefs of the patient and recognize the right of the other person to act according to them. However, the obstacle a religious conscience presents is usually the belief that abortion is murder, that is, the direct killing of an innocent human being—no less murderous than beating a 2-year-old child to death. To a nurse holding such a belief, it is irrelevant to speak of respecting the beliefs and rights of the patient. No nurse can be expected to admit that a patient has a right to murder or, even if she does have, that the nurse should respect that right and support her in the murder.

To one not sharing the religious convictions of the nurse, the comparison of abortion with murder and beating a child to death seems ridiculous; yet the comparison is the heart of the objection of many nurses in part because it constitutes the core of the official abortion position of the Roman Catholic hierarchy. This identification of abortion with murder explains why many religious persons offer a further antiabortion argument that is unintelligible to those who do not share their beliefs. They argue that acceptance of abortion can lead to acceptance of other kinds of killing in society, not only of the unborn, but of others such as the sick, the aged, and the insane. The argument is logical if you accept the premise. If abortion is murder, then permitting abortion opens the door to other types of killing. If society is willing to permit one form of murder, what will prevent the acceptance of others if the demand is great enough? This is why religious objectors to abortion claim that legalizing abortion leads logically to situations such as that which ended in the gas chambers of Auschwitz.

As a result, therefore, of the premise that abortion is murder, most attempts to meet this objection within the nursing profession are irrelevant and useless. Psychology, counseling, seminars, and reminders of professional responsibility are of no use unless one can somehow deal directly with this religious conviction. But how *can* one deal with it? Nursing, for all its many-faceted competence, is not professionally equipped to settle religious questions.

VIEWPOINT OF A CHRISTIAN ETHICIST
John Giles Milhaven

I should like to suggest that the situation is not hopeless. Not everything connected with religion is private, personal, and incapable of being discussed objectively. Many religious people today appreciate and use the analyses coming from a relatively new but already established discipline used in many American universities. This approach involves examining religious questions in a critical, objective, and scholarly manner. As to departmental location within the university, it is found under different names, but most often that of Department of Religion or Department of Religious Studies. The same discipline, however, may be utilized by a scholar in another department (e.g., history or philosophy). In any case, this professional inquiry into religion is recognized as a secular one in a secular university, and yet the inquiry is often carried on from a view sympathetic to the religion considered, a situation that was unprecedented before World War II. A large number, probably the majority, of those who take the courses and read the professor's publications do so, not only from academic curiosity, but also out of a personal interest in religion. Many educated Christians and Jews are familiar with the names of at least some of the scholars in this field, for example, James Gustafson (Yale), Jacob Neusner (Brown), Joseph Fletcher (Virginia), Maurice Freedman (Temple), John Noonan (California), Paul Ramsey (Princeton), Joseph Fichter (Harvard, Princeton), and Robert Francoeur (Rutgers). Books like Fletcher's *Situation Ethics* and Neusner's *The Way of Torah* are used by discussion groups in churches or synagogues.

On the other hand, secular professions also avail themselves of the expertise of these analysts of religion. A prime example would be the members of the medical profession who have consulted the system of medical ethics developed by these thinkers. Physicians read Noonan's *Contraception,* Ramsey's *The Patient as Person,* and Fletcher's *Morals and Medicine.* Specialists in religious studies are members of the staff, the board of directors, and the fellows of the completely secular, medically oriented Institute of Society, Ethics, and the Life Sciences, located in Hastings-on-Hudson, New York. At the Medical Ethics Workshop at Dartmouth College in the summer of 1972 the faculty included William May, Chairman of the Department of Religion at Indiana University, as well as the previously mentioned Paul Ramsey. In planning the forthcoming medical school, the Division of the Biological and Medical Sciences at Brown University is consulting the Department of Religious Studies on a regular basis in regard to the ethical education of its future medical students. It is noteworthy that both *Time* and *Newsweek,* in their recent articles on medical breakthroughs in genetics, quoted university-based specialists of religion for perspectives on the ethics of genetic engineering and control, which are now becoming possible.

Obviously, the point that I intend to make is that nursing, too, could consult the discipline of religious studies and perhaps gain objective and helpful perspectives on the religioethical objection to abortion under discussion in this chapter. Not that the religious ethicists form a consensus on whether or not abortion is moral. In fact, they offer a wide spectrum of different positions, as *The Morality of Abortion,* a collection of essays put out by the Harvard University Press, illustrates. Therefore a nurse having religious objections to abortion could not be argued with on the grounds that all the professional religious ethicists would disagree with her. Some come to conclusions similar to hers.

However, another approach to the problem is suggested by the fact that many who have the particular religioethical objection that we have been discussing, that abortion is murder, do so because they are Catholics and therefore hold "the Catholic position." But is this *the* Catholic position? Could the discipline of religious studies clarify for nursing whether there is not some misunderstanding or oversimplification here? To answer the question, one might first look for some research into the Christian tradition similar to that carried out by Rabbi David Feldman into the Jewish tradition. The Rabbi traveled over Europe, spending many hours in old libraries. From the records that he found, he was able to document the fact that the rabbinical tradition was more liberal on abortion than many Jews had believed.

But similar historical research into the Catholic or Christian tradition will not help to loosen the knot of the present-day Roman Catholic objection. As is well known, such research has been done and has established that the Christian tradition did not universally endorse the present Catholic view. Church leaders universally condemned abortion, but some did so on the grounds not that it was murder but that it was a form of contraception, at least in the first few months of pregnancy. Often, too, the condemnations of abortion found in the tradition give no grounds. The modern proponents of the thesis that abortion is murder cannot and do not claim that this was the general view of the Christian, or Catholic, tradition.

The hard core of the present-day insistence that abortion is murder is primarily an appeal to human reasoning based on scientific data. The reasoning is intended to prove that the fetus is a human being from conception (or implantation) on and that therefore any direct killing of it is murder. Catholics are by no means the only group today who accept this reasoning, but they are probably the largest one that does, since the Catholic hierarchy has made it abundantly clear that this is the principal and decisive argument proving that abortion is murder. Since many and perhaps most Catholics do not even try to follow the steps of this highly technical and philosophical argument, they accept it simply because they have confidence in "the Catholic position." But in what sense is accepting this argument essential to *the* Catholic position?

In recent years, recognized Catholic moralists such as Farley, Springer, Donceel, Wassmer, and myself have been pointing out that the argument is not valid and does not clearly prove that all abortion is murder. The Reverend Charles E. Curran, associate professor of moral theology at the Catholic University of America, past president of the Catholic Theological Society of America, and past president of the American Society of Christian Ethics, notes that "on the particular moral question of abortion there is now and will be increasingly in the future a diversity of opinion even within Roman Catholicism" and that "it will be increasingly difficult in the future to speak of *the* Roman Catholic teaching" on a question like this. Perhaps the most impressive illustration of the ongoing shift in Catholic thinking is a recent study that won for a Catholic ethicist the prestigious

Thomas More medal for "the most distinguished contribution to Catholic literature in 1970." The book is *Abortion: Law, Choice, and Morality* by Daniel Callahan. As Callahan tells it, he began his research intending to write a book defending the traditional prohibition of abortion. After four years of investigation and reflection, his opinion had changed. His position is a nuanced, complex one, but he does not hesitate to say simply that "there are no automatic moral lines to be drawn against abortion," and that, although abortion laws are needed, "they should be free enough to place the final decision in the hands of the pregnant woman." As these statements imply and Callahan explicitly affirms elsewhere in the book, he does not find convincing any of the arguments that abortion in the early months of pregnancy is murder. In brief, among recognized Catholic moralists and ethicists it is not *the* Catholic position that abortion is murder. This fact, however, is directly evident only to those who read scholarly volumes and professional journals dealing with moral theology and Christian ethics; yet might it not be a helpful fact to know if a nurse is trying to deal with this particular religious objection of conscience?

I am sure that many are familiar with another evidence that *the* Catholic position on abortion is dissolving, that is, the growing number of Catholic professional persons who automatically refer women seeking an abortion to colleagues. One finds this phenomenon among Catholic physicians, lawyers, counselors, and other professionals. The fact that they refuse to use their professional skill to help the women directly shows that they are still conscience bound, but that they do refer the women to someone else shows that they no longer consider abortion to be murder. The previous reasoning applies here, too: if a woman came asking for lethal medicine to give her 2-year-old child, would they refer her to someone who could help her to do this?

I hope that the preceding analyses have cast some light on the complex state of the Roman Catholic objection to abortion without arousing controversy. In brief the uncontroverted facts about the Catholic objection to abortion are as follows: (1)

the official foundation of the objection is that abortion is murder; (2) the proof of this foundation is drawn, not from the Bible or the consensus of Christian tradition, but from human reasoning on the pertinent scientific data; and (3) a growing number of recognized Catholic moralists and professional people doubt the validity of the proof that abortion is murder.

The Roman Catholic hierarchy still officially prohibits abortion. Consequently, even though the reason officially given for the prohibition is questioned by informed and responsible Catholics, the female nurse of that persuasion, like other such women, still has to ask herself whether she is obliged to refrain from having an abortion. She may well answer affirmatively, deciding that she is obliged to obey church authorities blindly. Whether this is the right answer for her is a delicate, controversial, and personal question, which will not be discussed here.

However, as to the attitude of this same nurse to other women having abortions, I should like, speaking as a Catholic and a moralist, to suggest some leading questions. The Catholic nurse who now sees reasons to doubt that abortion is murder but who feels personally bound to obey the authoritative church position might ask herself whether she has the right to impose this religious obedience on a patient. As we noted earlier, it is one thing for her to refuse to cooperate in what she clearly sees to be murder. The nurse that we are talking about, however, no longer sees it thus, and it is another thing for her to refuse nursing care to a patient simply because the patient is doing what the nurse's church forbids. The nurse has a right to expect people to respect her felt obligation to obey her church, but should she not, in turn, respect the conscience of her patient who does not feel this religious obligation? Would not such respect free the nurse to fulfill her professional responsibility and give full supportive care to those who are following their consciences in seeking an abortion?

In brief, the fact that the basis of the Catholic objection to therapeutic abortion is that it is murder has a boomerang effect in moral reasoning. Its thrust at first seems insuperable. How can one expect a nurse to cooperate in what she believes to be murder? Further study, however, reveals good reasons for a Catholic to doubt this equating of abortion and murder. The issues thus may change for a Catholic from one of cooperation in murder to one simply of obedience to authority; it is certainly open to discussion whether in this case the Catholic nurse is obliged to impose this obedience on the patient.

Bibliography

Callahan, D. J.: Abortion: law, choice, and morality, New York, 1970, The Macmillan Co., Publishers.

Donceel, J. F.: Immediate animation and delayed hominization, Theological Studies 31:76, 1970.

Farley, L. O.: The meaning of life and divine transcendence. In Proceedings of the Twenty-Third Convention of the Catholic Theological Society of America, Washington, D. C., 1968.

Feldman, D. M.: Birth control in Jewish law; marital relations, contraception, and abortion as set forth in the classic texts of Jewish law, New York, 1968, New York University Press.

Fletcher, J. F.: Morals and medicine, Boston, 1960, Beacon Press, Inc.

Fletcher, J. F.: Situation ethics, Philadelphia, 1966, Westminster Press.

Milhaven, J. G.: Toward a new Catholic morality, New York, 1970, Doubleday & Co., Inc.

Neusner, J.: The way of Torah, Encino, Calif., 1970, Dickenson Publishing Co., Inc.

Noonan, J. T.: Contraception; a history of its treatment by the Catholic theologians and canonists, Cambridge, 1965, Harvard University Press.

Noonan, J. T., Jr., editor: The morality of abortion; legal and historical perspectives, Cambridge, 1970, Harvard University Press.

Ramsey, P.: The patient as person; explorations in medical ethics, New Haven, Conn., 1970, Yale University Press.

Ramsey, P., and Wilson, J. F., editors: The study of religion in colleges and universities, Princeton, N. J., 1970, Princeton University Press.

Springer, R. H.: Current theology: notes on moral theology: July, 1969-March, 1970, Theological Studies 31:476, 1970.

Wassmer, T.: Questions about questions, Commonweal 86:418, 1967.

Welch, C.: Religion in the undergraduate curriculum: an analysis and interpretation, Washington, D. C., 1972, Association of American Colleges.

Medical-surgical nursing

with an introduction by
Betty S. Bergersen
Margery Duffey

The material in this section is an assort-
ment of facts, attitudes, and opinions concerning the need for knowledge about (1)
illness and trauma and their effects; (2)
the ill individual and his physical and
psychological responses, as well as his life
style; (3) the cause-effect relationships of
the external social and physical environment on illness and trauma and ill behavior; and (4) prevention and positive modes
of intervention.

The chapters discuss the conventional, as
well as more recent concerns for providing
effective and particularized patient care.

Severe burns, cervical cord injury, and
chronic, obstructive lung disease and their
sequelae continue to be of major concern
to health professionals. Much remains to
be done to prevent unnecessary sequelae
and to decrease disability, while maximiz-
ing productivity and capitalizing on capabilities.

Although touch is recognized as an important means of communication, and a
few studies have been conducted on the
nurse's use of touch, the patient's perception of touch has been neglected. Day's
chapter is undoubtedly a forerunner of
more intensive investigation into this vital
area.

Change is constant, and from it new perspectives emerge. Malcolm's chapter stresses

the need for individuals, their families, and health professionals to foster change and growth to meet life's challenges or to bring about the changes that they would like to see occur. Perry's chapter stresses the need for patients with chronic obstructive pulmonary diseases to develop new life styles and ways of coping with stress to subdue or eliminate cyclic physiological and psychological stress phenomena. Bock's chapter on skiing and nursing heralds a new area of practice for nurses, particularly for the primary care agent.

27

Toward health through growth

Nancy Malcolm

What can a nurse conclude when all the familiar types of nursing intervention have been attempted and a family remains in its chronic and cyclic unhealthy condition? Should one conclude, as is common, that illness and unhappiness for some persons are inevitable and irreversible? As a nurse in such a situation, I could not. So I turned from the "sick" models I had been taught and decided to focus on growth and health.

I started seeing the family at the request of another nurse who had been the family's therapist for two years in the outpatient department. That nurse had been with the family through some crises that included hospitalizations for both the husband and wife. When she transferred the family to me, they were in a noncrisis period and were attempting to reorganize when I began seeing them.

The couple, Phyllis and Bob, had each been married once before, and between them they had nine children. Seven of the children were still at home, their ages ranging from 1 to 18 years. Bob was a chronic alcoholic, who had been treated under numerous programs. Phyllis had had four short-term psychiatric hospitalizations over the previous six years with various diagnoses, such as hysteria, manic-depression, and schizophrenia. Initially I was meeting with Phyllis in her home about once a week. She had expressed a need for information on growth, development, and discipline of the 1-year-old because it had been so long since she had cared for a small child. These discussions also led to consideration of the conflict that Bob and Phyllis were having because she thought that Bob was disciplining the children too harshly. Another area of discussion and problem-solving was their efforts to reestablish their friendships and social contacts, which had been severely affected by Bob's periods of alcoholism and Phyllis' psychiatric hospitalizations. The third area of discussion involved ways in which Phyllis could encourage Bob to continue going to Alcoholics Anonymous meetings.

Bob and Phyllis then bought a house across town near Bob's parents. Soon the family was experiencing many more pressures: Bob began to worry about finances because of house payments and irregular work; Bob's parents began criticizing his decisions and bad financial management; and Phyllis' mother was also criticizing the couple. I met with Bob and Phyllis a few times in the out-patient department, and we attempted to problem solve with regard to the financial situation. Bob described Phyllis as being like a child, unable to make decisions, discipline the children, or be careful in spending money. Phyllis described Bob as having drunk periods when he became aggressive, domineering, and threatening to the entire family. During these times, both Phyllis and the children were frightened, believed that they could not please him, and never knew what behavior to expect from him. She said that he never showed affection to or approval of her or the children.

Bob's drinking increased, and he was admitted to another detoxification unit through the assistance of his AA sponsor. While he was an inpatient, he and Phyllis went to a couples' group one evening a week. These sessions with other couples having similar problems seemed to help them verbalize what they expected of each other and what kinds of things put each of them under pressure. When Bob was released, the three of us met again regularly with the goals of helping Bob learn to express affection and approval and encouraging Phyllis to make some decisions and support Bob's limit-setting with the children.

The financial and parental pressures became worse, and once again Bob started drinking. Again their patterns of behavior became apparent. When she became extremely fearful or anxious, such as when Bob's drinking became worse, she would respond either by getting physically sick or by mentally withdrawing from the situation as shown by her no longer doing housework or managing the children. In this state she could not eat or sleep but would smoke incessantly and wander from room to room, wringing her hands and staring into space. When Bob was drunk, he would accuse Phyllis of being "crazy" and of running around with other men, neglecting the children. Since the accusation was partially true, she believed him, and this contributed to her depression and to her negative feelings about herself.

I discussed the family situation with my supervisor, the psychiatrist in the outpatient department. He said that he thought that both Bob and Phyllis were dependent people, who had a "sick cycle." When one was doing well, the other would be sick for a while. As the sick one began to progress, the other would sicken and have dependency needs. The psychiatrist was convinced that Bob and Phyllis both needed "mothers" on whom they could be dependent and that AA could serve that purpose for Bob and my support could do the same for Phyllis. This advice produced frustration and conflict in me. I did not think that I had sufficient knowledge of psychoanalytic dynamics to be able to encourage such a dependency relationship. Also, I was uncomfortable with it. I had the underlying belief that Phyllis was capable of managing by herself. I believed that I had failed with Bob and that I could not help him.

The lack of progress with previous interventions caused me to consider how else I might approach the situation. Also, if I was frustrated and defeated by the situation, I could imagine how the family must feel. About this time, I heard Jourard[2] speak at a Minnesota League for Nursing convention. His primary thesis was that people "sicken," or become sick mentally or physically, when they do not change or grow with the demands of changing circumstances. "When people outgrow a way of being in their world, and when the structure of their world is no longer conducive to vitality, zest and growth, they sicken. When they sicken, rather than re-invent themselves and their world, they go to a hospital."[*]

Jourard's statement certainly described the life situation of Phyllis and Bob. They needed to become aware of new possibilities for their lives and to build new hope. Ideas for ways to actualize potentials for hope and change came from the writings of Otto, who emphasized that the families themselves must identify their strengths and then choose particular ones to develop further.[4] Although I had previously tried indirectly to reinforce in Bob and Phyllis characteristics that I perceived as strengths, they were too caught up in their problems even to be aware of, much less derive comfort and hope from, my attempts. I had to find ways to help them identify their strengths. More important, in focusing on strengths and growth, I had to take the risk of not trying to intervene in their problems and weaknesses. But I had already worked with them for a year in problem solving in relation to their difficulties and had not seen any lasting changes. Bob was still drinking and Phyllis dependent, childlike, and often withdrawn from reality. The risk of ignoring the problems and symptoms did not seem to be any greater, and, by ignoring the problems, no contradiction in approach would be presented such as, "Yes, you have strengths, but they don't do you much good in terms of the reality of your situation with its many problems."

I began by explaining to Phyllis the approach that I wanted to try. The next thing we did together was to take an inventory of her strengths, according to her perceptions. The strengths that she believed herself to possess were a sense of humor; the ability to manage a household, especially considering the number of children; and good mothering capabilities, such as affection-giving, limit-setting, and disciplining, despite Bob's assessment. She also believed herself to be articulate and fairly attractive and likable. I strongly reinforced this evaluation, based on my own perception of Phyllis. At this time Bob was in and out of the

home in various stages of drunkenness, so that I was unable to work with him.

The next few weeks, in each of our conferences, we would discuss various incidents of the week and how Phyllis had dealt with them. In each case we would discuss why and how what she did was a strength or ability. As time passed, she became more and more confident and at one point said that, even if there were undesirable consequences to her decisions, she would just have to make new ones in relation to those consequences. This evidence of her learning was exciting to me.

Phyllis could remember that, in her early teens, her family made her feel inadequate and that she was not a good person. As an adult, this feeling continued, and she was influenced to believe that she could not live without a man to manage her life and make decisions for her. During the course of our sessions, she began to overcome these feelings and expressed surprise at her own actions and attitudes toward herself. These changes occurred in spite of a deteriorating situation with her husband. Finally, after Bob inflicted a particularly severe drunken beating on herself and the children, Phyllis decided to leave him. She managed the move, the setting up of a new household, the eventual divorce, and the child rearing, facing the problems with increased competence, both in her perception and mine.

About a year later, during a discussion with Phyllis, she spontaneously began to do some evaluating of her abilities and her life situation. Several times during the conversation, she remarked on how much she thought that she had grown and was continuing to grow and learn. She had used the term *growth,* and, since I had never actually used the term in my conversations with her, I believe that this is her perception of the process that has happened in her. Evidence that she began making her own growth plans was that she said that she had come to the conclusion that it would be good for both her and the children if she could find a job. She said that working would give her a chance to interact with adults and to contribute income for taking care of her family and that it would give the children a chance to begin learning to take responsibility for each other and for running the household. Later she said that she discovered that it was necessary for the whole family to learn to communicate and plan together and that this improved their family feeling and contributed to their unity.

Phyllis said that going to work was also a help because she learned that she could get along with people and that, for the most part, people liked her and that these facts gave her confidence. She added that recently her teen-age children were becoming critical of her and that she was able to deal with the criticism because her experiences had taught her that, although she had faults, she also had many good personality characteristics. Further evidence of Phyllis's growth and health is that she has not had any more psychiatric symptoms, with the exception of one very short exacerbation. At that time she responded quickly after I once more reinforced with her the growth principles by which she had changed her life. Another outcome that

---

*From Jourard, S. M.: On personal growth, Minn. League Nurs. Bull., p. 4, Sept., 1970.

was significant to me was that, contrary to the psychiatrist's opinion, Phyllis did not need to be a person dependent on a mother figure. Besides gaining a different view of herself as a person, she had learned a process by which she could manage her life in an independent fashion.

THEORETICAL PERSPECTIVE

During and since this experience with Phyllis, I have further developed some theoretical perspectives in applying concepts of growth to the need for knowledge about health. This need to develop knowledge and interventions that will encourage and nurture health in individuals has become essential. For too long we have focused our energies on gaining knowledge about illness. Knowledge about health is comparatively nonexistent.

Certain observations can be cited to account for this lack of development. The entire medical-social system has been developed around illness. The energy of the system has been expended in systematizing knowledge, technology, and actions to confront the demands of illness in people. The idea that health is the lack of illness in itself further contributed to the concentration on illness. Health workers' philosophies about man's capacity to change and philosophies concerning the course of illness have no doubt hindered scientific consideration of health.

Some recent pressures and trends indicate a readiness within and without the sick-care system to develop the concept of health. One of the first such trends was the emphasis on the need for primary prevention in illness, coupled with development of the idea that, if individuals are given knowledge about factors that contribute to health maintenance, they will change their behaviors accordingly. The concept of providing greater emphasis on primary prevention has even stimulated the nursing profession to state that nursing education might develop the two alternatives of *episodic* and *distributive* as separate educational tracts.

The holistic view of man has also received attention from the health professions, stimulating a shift of emphasis from signs and symptoms and medicines and treatments to an awareness of the whole man, not just his illness. Many health professionals have realized that much of the therapy that has been used for psychosocial problems has not made significant and lasting changes in individuals, but rather seems to have contributed to the cycling and recurrence of their problems. This realization has promoted the development of new approaches that are aimed at enabling persons to mange their lives in their current situations. Examples of this include behavior modification, reality therapy, and the widely popular sensitivity groups. These changing viewpoints and approaches have led to further exploration of the conceptual area of health.

THE RELATIONSHIP OF GROWTH TO HEALTH

One of the most promising ways to begin this exploration of health is to consider the concept of growth. If promoting health has been the process of eliminating and ameliorating illness and disease, or "patching up," then perhaps promoting growth is that which goes beyond patching up and removing illness. Jourard has defined growth as follows:

> Growth is the disintegration of one way of experiencing the world, followed by a re-organization of this experience, a re-organization that includes the new disclosure of the world. The disorganization, or even shattering, of one way to experience the world, is brought on by new disclosures from the changing being of the world, disclosures that were always being transmitted, but were usually ignored.*

Jourard further identifies three parts of the "cycle" described as follows: "A growth *cycle* calls for (a) an acknowledgement that the world has changed, (b) a shattering of the presently experienced 'world structure' and (c) a restructuring, retotalization of the world-structure that encompasses the disclosure of changed reality."†

---

*From Jourard, S. M.: Growing awareness and the awareness of growth. In Otto, H. A., and Mann, J., editors: Ways of growth, New York, copyright 1968 by Herbert Otto and John Mann, The Viking Press, Inc., pp. 2, 3. Reprinted by permission of Grossman Publishers.
†Note the similarity of Jourard's definition of growth to the elements of the crisis model as proposed by Hill, R.: Generic features of families under stress. In Parad, H. J., editor: Crisis intervention; selected readings, New York, 1965, Family Service Association of America, pp. 32 to 35.

Signals of the need for growth

Jourard[2] explains that needs for growth occur when one's formed ideas, or concepts, about ourselves, about other people, or about our environment, or the reality we experience, change from within or when pressures external to the person demand that his concept change. Frequent indicators that the person's concepts have changed or that reality has changed and is therefore demanding changed concepts are such common experiences as failure in a particular task, or project, experiencing boredom with one's life or activities, or experiencing frustration or conflict with others. The need for growth can even be signaled by surprise at someone else's behavior or by learning something new about how others perceive you. The developmental tasks of various chronological stages trigger demands for growth and may or may not be associated with some of the indicators previously discussed.

The case that follows points out explicitly how a health and specifically a growth perspective differs from others in working with people, and it illustrates to some extent the signals of a need for growth.

Terry is a 19-year-old single girl with an 11-month-old baby daughter, named Debbie. After the delivery of the baby, Terry had a "nervous breakdown" and was hospitalized in a private psychiatric hospital for three months. Apparently, one of the factors contributing to the breakdown was the fact that Terry wanted to relinquish the child, but Terry's mother wanted to keep the baby. While Terry was hospitalized, the baby was placed in a foster home. Terry's mother works and is alcoholic, and Terry's father is dead.

When Terry came home from the hospital, her boyfriend broke up with her. At this point Terry attempted suicide and was subsequently hospitalized at a metropolitan medical center and then seen on an outpatient psychiatric basis. She was assigned to a group and placed on medications such as trifluoperazine hydrochloride (Stelazine) and benztropine mesylate (Cogentin).

Once home, Terry's baby was returned to her, and Terry decided that she wanted to keep her baby. Terry's mother and the baby's foster mother greatly criticized Terry's care of the baby, and the foster mother expressed a desire to adopt the baby. Terry decided to stop taking her medications because she did not want to be dependent on them and because she believed that she had hallucinations when she took them. The psychiatrist in charge of her outpatient psychiatric group said that Terry could not come back to group meetings unless she took the medication. Terry misses the group meetings but does not wish to take the medication.

In this example, three perspectives might be defined and would provide guidance in selecting nursing interventions. However, the first two are each limited in some way, and the third, the growth perspective, clearly illustrates its potential to enable the patient to maximize her strengths and potential as a human being. The traditional approach based on the perspective that Terry is mentally ill was not working with Terry. With this approach, the goals of the nurse were to encourage Terry to take the medication and return to the group therapy sessions. The nurse would also evaluate Terry's care of the child (in view of the criticism) and would consider the possibility of encouraging Terry to give up the child.

Another approach based on the perspective that Terry was in crisis and going through the grief process is an adequate approach but neglects much potential in the situation. For example, Terry is grieving due to loss of esteem from her mother, the foster mother, and the psychiatrist and from loss of the relationships with her boyfriend and earlier with her father. Therefore the nurse would assist her in the stages of grief and loss to promote resolution of the grief. Not only is the concentration primarily on past, unhappy events, but little attention is given to her developments as a person and the positive aspects of the events that she is experiencing.

A third approach would be based on the perspective that Terry is a learning, growing individual with certain personality strengths that can be even further developed. From this view Terry is a very sensitive teen-ager who has attempted to have an intimate relationship but has had difficulty. The breakdown and suicide attempt could be seen as the overreactions of a sensitive person. She would need encouragement to attempt to form new close relationships based on an understanding of her need for such relationships and discussion of ways to accomplish this goal. The decision not to return to the group and not to take the medications could be seen as a teen-age effort to be independent and to grow toward health. On the basis of this approach, the nurse would reinforce these efforts toward independence and decision making, assist in the reality of learning child care, and reward her for doing a good job in the midst of a difficult situation.

Each of these perspectives could be carried out in further detail with more specifics. Obviously, there might be areas of overlap among these three perspectives and, in the process of encouraging growth, some aspects of the other two perspectives might need to be included. The growth perspective would promote a positive effort toward the developmental task of learning about intimate interpersonal relationships, realistic expression of emotional reactions to life events, arriving at a satisfactory balance between independence and dependence, and the formulation of new goals.

The process of facilitating growth

The definition of goals and the plan of action based on the growth perspective is a process accomplished jointly by the helper, or professional, and the person experiencing growth. This facilitating or nursing process contains the traditional elements of assessment, hypotheses, interventions, and evaluation. The emphasis on growth results in different assumptions about an individual's behavior and therefore different assessments, hypotheses, and interventions. Some of the assumptions are that persons will seek their own highest level and that they are aware of what is possible for themselves and would like to pursue those possibilities. One also assumes that they can identify some of the barriers to reaching their goals and have some ideas about what can be done to achieve them and are capable of making decisions regarding their lives. Another assumption is that when they are actively and effectively working on their goals, their illness, or maladjustment, will not get worse and may improve. To illustrate, some questions that the helper might use to accomplish the process are as follows:

1. If anything were possible for you, how would you like your life to be?
2. What would need to happen to achieve this goal?
3. Of these things, which could you do now?

4. What would be the first step?
5. What can I, the helper, do to help you accomplish the first step?

Nursing interventions

Although individuals vary in their goals and the methods that they choose to achieve them, a helper could use or suggest a variety of specific interventions to facilitate the accomplishing of the person's growth task. For example, as already mentioned, a significant intervention is to help an individual decide on and articulate a goal or goals and a program of action to achieve the goal. Perhaps the greatest growth for a person would occur if he established some new personal goals or goals outside the self, such as for his family or some community group. The intervention might be to devise with the person or family ways to practice or carry out a new behavior, attitude, or role that might require discussion of ways to allocate reciprocal roles or tasks. Perhaps outdated, unexpressed, or new attitudes or concepts could be explored or changed through discussion, making collages or drawings, placing posters in the home, role playing, or deliberately practicing some psychocybernetic principles.[3] The nurse or helper might need to arrange artificial or real experiences designed to increase awareness or enjoyment of themselves, other people, or the environment.

An intervention that brings surprise and helps individuals is to take inventory of the person's strengths with him or with his family and perhaps evaluate only positive experiences on a weekly basis. The family may also want to try this among themselves and tell each other the strengths that they perceive. They might also tell an individual what they think will be possible for the person in a few years if he continues to use his strengths. Otto[4] calls this process *strength bombardment*, which develops assurance, confidence, and self-esteem in the family members.

Otto has written and studied extensively in the area of strength development and growth, both for individuals and groups. Most recently he has written a guide for groups of families who want to grow together. He is suggesting that this is one alternative type of communal living experience. In the guide he describes some activities that groups of families can use to develop strengths and encourage growth. Many of the activities can be adapted to individuals or single families. The titles of some of the activities will indicate their nature and relationship to growth. The details of these activities may be found in his book *The Family Cluster: a Multi-base Alternative.* A few of the activities are Depth Unfoldment Experience (DUE Method), Sex Stereotype Removal, The Minerva Experience, The Creativity Festival, The New Environment Adventure, and The Joy of Being Party.[5]

Occasionally the role of the helper is to encourage an individual to pursue or permit his own growth. The person desiring growth must suspend or change ongoing activities, commitments, and projects and become aware of other activities and possibilities. Jourard[2] points out that the person needs to reinvent or renew himself by pursuing a new project, taking a vacation, traveling, developing a new friendship or relationship, fasting, or practicing yoga or Zen meditation.

Results of growth

The aim of both individual and group interventions is to encourage development of personal awareness, of personality strengths, and of an environment in which change is desirable and fostered. To some extent the individual should learn a process of growth—becoming aware of when growth is needed, formulating a plan of action, and evaluating the results. One or several observations may indicate that growth has taken place. Joy and a feeling of hope, optimism, and well-being are generated. New or renewed self-confidence, along with increased awareness of challenge, should result in an increased amount of risk-taking behavior. The person will probably experience more congruence between his own behavior and the values he holds or his aspirations. He may appear to be able to have genuine fun, or he may have an increased sense of humor. He will definitely experience a decrease in negative experiences of boredom, conflict, frustration, or disappointment.

Hindrances to growth behavior

If the growth approach to health has this many benefits, what prevents professionals from using it more extensively, and why do not more persons develop growth plans for themselves and their families? No doubt the answers are complex, but some may be articulated and, having been recognized, could be resolved more effectively. Social sanctions play a major role in inhibiting professionals from using this approach and in preventing individuals from pursuing growth goals. For example, stereotyped expectations of roles of health professionals, dictating an obligation to "cure the sick" inhibits them from concentration on health, growth, and positives to the degree necessary. Such concentration would probably be most effective if the health worker were permitted to exclude, or ignore, illness and its symptoms, but such behavior would possibly be considered unethical or irresponsible.

The person experiencing a need for growth also has individuals around him who have stereotyped expectations for his behavior. Certain prescribed behaviors must be performed by persons in the mother, farther, child, single adult, or elderly adult roles. New behaviors that are part of a growth plan are met with resistance by others perhaps because insecurity and uncertainty as to what will be required of them are aroused. Sometimes this resistance is related to socially imposed values or goals. For example, in a hospital patients are expected to conform, to be dependent, and to some extent to be childlike. In situations such as the hospital, patients have insufficient social power to resist these values and support the motivation to grow. In families and school, children and adolescents frequently have insufficient social power to behave in ways that would be growth producing.

Environmental conditions often prohibit growth by limiting the observation of strength either by the person himself or by the health professional. For example, the role expected of the hospital patient may not allow for expression of behavioral strengths; therefore they may not be observed and subsequently developed. The same oversight may prevent his receiving feedback regarding his strengths and developing changes as a person. Environmental or social conditions that include poverty probably have a deterrent effect, as well as limit the available possibilities. More study of the limiting effect of poverty needs to be done to understand fully its relationship to growth. Physical disability might also have a limiting effect on personal growth, although this would have to be carefully assessed.

Perhaps one of the greatest hindrances to growth is the fact that, if a person recognizes his strengths or areas in which he wants to grow, he must take responsibility to make changes. This responsibility is threatening because risk-taking and exploration of new possibilities is required. The process might involve forming new relationships or changing old interpersonal relationships. A certain amount of fear of the unknown or of exposing weaknesses may exist.[1]

Despite these hindrances and difficulties, health professionals should view the exploration of health and growth as an opportunity for their own expansion and development. The signals of a need for professional growth are evident in the frustration with lack of progress in the chronic and psychosocial illnesses in our society. I am convinced that we must begin to facilitate a true science of health. As Selye has written:

> The secret of health and happiness lies in successful adaptation to the ever-changing conditions of the globe; the penalties for failure in this great process of adaptation are disease and unhappiness.*

*From Selye, H.: The stress of life, New York, 1956, McGraw-Hill Book Co., p. vii. Used with permission of McGraw-Hill Book Co.

References

1. Crerar, P. A.: A descriptive study of psychiatric patients' strengths perceived by psychiatric nurses and psychiatric patients. In unpublished Master's Plan B paper, Minneapolis, 1968, the University of Minneapolis, pp. 42-44.
2. Jourard, S. M.: On personal growth, Minn. League Nurs. Bull. 13:4, Sept., 1970.
3. Maltz, M.: Psycho-cybernetics, Englewood Cliffs, N. J., 1960, Prentice-Hall.
4. Otto, H. A.: Developing family strengths and potentials. In Otto, H. A., and Mann, J., editors: Ways of growth, New York, 1968, The Viking Press, Inc., pp. 77-85.
5. Otto, H. A.: The family cluster; a multi-base alternative, Beverly Hills, Calif., 1971, Holistic Press, pp. 9-22.

28

The patient's perception of touch

F. Ann Day

Prior to the nineteenth century, the main function of the nurse was to provide routine care and comfort to the patient. However, since the time of Florence Nightingale the emphasis has shifted to one of ever-increasing competency and involvement in the technical skills of nursing, with a concomitant decrease in emphasis on the caring, comforting aspects of nursing.[20] A large number of today's nurses relate to their patients by providing them with efficient, technically competent care, communicating with them, for the most part, while carrying out required nursing procedures. There is evidence that nurses give lip service both to the desirability of getting back to the patient's bedside and to improving their verbal and nonverbal communication skills.[1] However, even when given the opportunity to fulfill these desires, they seem to construct barriers such as performing additional administrative work or nonnursing, nonprofessional tasks, thereby preventing meaningful interactions with patients.[3]

Goshen[9] states that the nursing profession must become technologically sophisticated, or it will go "out of business." He believes that automation will free the nurse to perform "more valuable, more humane functions." If this is so, the nurse must be prepared to give up the comfort of many technical, administrative functions and return to the caring, comforting aspects of nursing.

Olson[16] writes ". . . what happens in nursing depends not only on nurses caring, but on how they show that they care." Touch, as a form of nonverbal communication, has great potential for demonstrating the nurse's care for and interest in the patients. Pluckham[18] remarks that "Years ago nurses were more inclined to communicate with their patients through touch than they are today." Communication by means of touch may reach the patient when verbal communication does not. It is thus unfortunate that touch is not used more extensively.

Jourard, in *The Transparent Self,* says:

> But if I touch him, especially if I touch him or if he touches me, he takes on a dimension of reality more real than if I just see or hear him. And he is more real if I smell and taste him. But perhaps he is more real if I touch him.*

Thus, for the nurse and the patient, using touch provides another dimension of communication, one that has perhaps the greatest potential of providing the patient with the support and comfort he requires.

A study was undertaken to investigate the circumstances under which medical-surgical patients see touch as being a desirable nursing intervention and to discover whether the use of touch is acceptable only in times of stress, as a part of everyday contact with the nurse, or only after a good patient-nurse relationship has been established. In addition, it was deemed to be of interest to nurses to discover what difference, if any, exists between medical and surgical patients in their perception of the desirability of touch and whether the age of the patient or the sex of the nurse has any bearing on the acceptance of touch.

DEFINITION OF TERMS

Nonverbal communication. *Nonverbal communication* is defined as communication other than by speech or the written word. The type of nonverbal communication to be discussed in this chapter is the use of touch.

Touch. *Touch,* for the purposes of this

---

chapter, is defined as physical contact between the patient and the nurse that does not involve the carrying out of direct physical care, such as holding a patient's hand, patting the patient's shoulder, and placing a hand on the patient's head.

THE IMPORTANCE OF TOUCH

"Tactile sensitivity is one of the primary modes of communication and orientation."[8] Probably the earliest and most elemental experience of the unborn human is a tactile one.[4,5,8] The amniotic fluid, through which the sound of the mother's heartbeat is magnified, provides a warm, pulsating environment for the fetus. During labor, it is squeezed and pushed and generally subjected to great pressure—all of which are tactile experiences. "Thus the baby's perception of the world is built upon and initially shaped by tactile experiences."[8]

From the time they are born, babies need to be touched and held:

It is through body contact with the mother that the child makes his first contact with the world, through which he is enfolded in a new dimension of experience, the experience of the world of the other. It is this bodily contact with the other that provides the essential sources of comfort, security, warmth and increasing aptitude for new experiences.*

Ruesch[19] remarks that the infant learns to associate pleasure with being touched, carried, talked, and played with. Without this type of stimulation the child will become emotionally retarded, apathetic, depressed, and unresponsive. Frank[8] states that ". . . denial or deprivation of primary tactile experiences may be revealed as crucial in the development of personalities and character structure. . . ." Montagu[15] believes that inadequate cutaneous stimulation in infancy may lead to a propensity for upper respiratory tract disorders in later life. He reports a high incidence of asthma among persons who, as young children, were separated from their mothers and thus, presumably, received inadequate tactile stimulation.

Dominian,[5] in his discussion of touch, notes that virtually all children run to the safety of their mothers when they suffer pain or trauma. They receive comfort and reassurance from the touch of their mother's hands on the affected part and by the caressing she gives. Thus touch becomes a crucial experience in the relief of pain and discomfort that carries over into adulthood.

As the child grows older, cultural prohibitions begin to appear.[3] He soon learns that there are parts of his own and others' bodies that are not to be touched. Davis[4] calls this a "tactile code." Because of this code, touch, especially in North America, is used sparingly when only warmth and compassion are to be conveyed, due to the sexual connotation placed on it in the North American culture. Persons in this culture generally do not like to be touched or bumped. They even apologize when they inadvertently touch someone. Apparently touch is considered an intrusion or violation against the self.

As Farrah[6] reported in her study, there is little information regarding the use of touch as a form of communication in nursing. Nursing textbooks simply record its use as a form of nonverbal communication.[13,17,21] Lewis[12] suggests that "There is particular need for recognition of the communication properties of touch, and a need for nursing research in this area." Peplau states, "The development of consciousness of tools used in nursing includes awareness of means of communication; spoken language . . . and the body gesture." She then goes on to say, "The nurse's gestures in relations with patients show how she feels about a particular patient or some aspect of his care."* None of these writers, however, mention how this form of communication may best be used or taught.

Both Dominian[5] and Montagu[15] comment on the need for body contact during times of stress. The need for security, reassurance, and comfort are constant human emotional requirements. These needs are activated and increased at times when sur-

---

*From Montagu, A.: Touching: the human significance of the skin, New York, 1971, Columbia University Press, p. 80.

*From Peplau, H. E.: Interpersonal relations in nursing, New York, 1952, G. P. Putnam's Sons, pp. 289, 306.

vival is threatened. Undoubtedly, persons, when faced with illness and hospitalization, have needs for security, reassurance, and comfort; thus physical contact becomes highly important for the patient's well-being.

In spite of these needs for security, reassurance, and comfort, Farrah[7] remarks that, although touch is a routine part of nursing procedures involving the physical aspects of care, it is used less frequently in situations involving the emotional, supportive aspects of care. In the only study of the use of touch with medical-surgical patients in current literature,[7] the reported use of touch by nurses was much higher than was predicted. Touch ranked as the third most preferred behavior out of five possible nursing interventions; when accompanied by a verbal response, it was reported to be the most preferred nursing intervention. However, it was stated that there may be some discrepancy between the nurse's reported use of touch and actual behavior in the clinical setting.

NURSES' USE OF TOUCH

"Touch is the fundament of being-in-the-world, for it is the vehicle par excellence by which the person locates himself in space-time."[3] Patients being touched by the nurse and feeling free enough to reach out and touch in return may be reinforcing their own sense of reality and hopefully, at the same time, receive comfort and reassurance. Touch, when seen as a caring, supportive gesture, will reduce distance between persons: it will break down invisible barriers that the individual erects around his "self." However, individuals differ in their tolerance of this type of contact; thus the nurses must be cognizant of their use of touch. Due to their cultural backgrounds, previous experience, and social maturity, patients may see the touch gesture as hostile or comforting, threatening or reassuring. Mercer[14] remarks that touch has many meanings. It can be an acknowledgment of a person's presence, a display of love, an act of aggression, an arousal of sexual desire, or a desire for comfort and a feeling of physical closeness. Nurses must be aware of the possibility that patients and nurses may misinterpret each other's gestures.

Just as patients differ in their ease in touching and being touched,[11] so do nurses. Touch should be used only to the extent that both nurse and patient feel comfortable using it. It should be used appropriately for the situation, so that its use will not degenerate into the same type of meaningless gesture as some of the trite verbal phrases used by nurses in talking to patients.

Johnson[10] cites three basic concepts in the use of touch:

1. Nonverbal behavior, particularly touch, has a potential for being the most meaningful form of communication.

2. Communication is improved when nonverbal behavior is accompanied by appropriate verbal behavior.

3. Nonverbal behavior can be misinterpreted.

Although touch is a positive form of communication, it does have a negative aspect. Touch may be interpreted by some patients as a homosexual or sexual advance and by others as a threat to their integrity. Johnson[10] mentions the effect that a female nurse in the same age group or younger may have on the male patient. Touch should be used only to the extent that it does not pose a threat to the patient and that the nurse is comfortable in using it.

In using touch as a form of communication its use must be congruent with both verbal communication and other forms of nonverbal communication such as gestures, facial expression, and the use of space. The patient would be inclined to doubt the nurse's sincerity if, when ostensibly offering comfort and support with a touch gesture, the communication was coupled with an angry expression, an immediate physical withdrawal, or a harsh, curt voice.

Touch is an integral part of nursing care when used thoughtfully and with full awareness of the many implications of its use: it has great potential for the establishment of meaningful communication patterns between patient and nurse. When used with the appropriate facial expression or verbal communication or both, touch is also a powerful tool for conveying emotions. Sympathy, kindness, and compassion may all be conveyed by a light touch on the arm, by holding the patient's hand, or by placing an arm around the patient's shoulders.

Ideas may also be communicated by using touch. Concern for the acceptance of the patient may be conveyed by the use of touch. If the nurse withdraws from the patient because of not accepting or caring for him, the patient will be able to tell this most easily by the way the nurse touches him—probably more easily and quickly than through verbal interaction.

An exploratory survey of ten medical and ten surgical patients was undertaken to determine how patients perceive the use of touch as a mode of nursing intervention. A set of eight slides was prepared depicting various patient-nurse interactions, all but one involving touch. The slides showed patients ranging in age from 25 to 79 years, as well as nurses of both sexes, whose age range was 23 to 36 years. The slides were shown through a small slide viewer; all the patients in the survey saw them in the same order. They were asked to interpret the scene and state what they did or did not like about the interaction and why and under what circumstances they would like this type of care given to them.

This projective testing method was chosen because it was believed that the subjects would respond more freely and meaningfully to this technique than they would to a more direct method such as a questionnaire. It was thought that the subjects would find this method interesting, thus be more willing to express their feelings with less deliberation. The responses of the subjects were tape-recorded to avoid loss of data.

Slide one. Slide one depicts an elderly man being helped to walk by a male nurse whose hand is on the patient's right arm. The nurse appears attentive to the patient.

This action was seen as a supportive, helping one by all subjects. One subject, a 54-year-old woman, stated that perhaps the nurse was giving too much support but generally agreed with the others that when one was beginning to walk again after surgery, especially if one is older, this type of support is comforting. The nurse's hand on the patient's arm was seen as an appropriate means for giving support and as signifying that the nurse was interested in and protective of the patient. Although five

subjects (two medical and three surgical) stated that holding the patient's arm was not necessary, they did not see anything wrong in the physical contact itself. They stated that the patient might have more confidence in himself if the nurse just walked beside him, rather than giving physical support. They saw a possible danger that, by depending on the nurse, the patient might retard his own recovery.

Slide two. Slide two shows a young female nurse sitting beside an elderly man's bed, holding his hand and apparently talking to him. Patient and nurse are looking intently at one another.

All but three of the seventeen subjects (two surgical and one medical) saw the nurse as sincere in her desire to communicate with the patient.

This situation was also seen as supportive and helping, although with some qualifications. The subjects saw this as most desirable for the older, depressed, lonely patient. For the most part, the women saw this interaction as one that their families could provide. A 52-year-old man said "the nurses have something better to do than sit and hold my hand!" However, a 54-year-old man with a diagnosis of acute leukemia stated "it helps to be touched by the human hand, other than to be poked at." A 25-year-old man stated that this was a direct attempt to give "personal contact." He differentiated between personal and professional contact by stating that personal contact involved giving moral support to the patient, whereas professional contact consisted of routine physical care. He stated that personal contact was good for older people but that he also would find it comforting. Regarding the same slide, a 63-year-old man stated that he believed this to be a supportive measure for the patient but that, "There should be no misunderstanding about what it means." He claimed that this interaction was more appropriate for the older patient but that it would be acceptable for younger patients if they were very ill. A 27-year-old woman who had undergone a partial pancreatectomy stated that the nurse was "letting me know she was reaching out to help me." All subjects agreed that the interpretation and importance of touch depended on the patient-nurse relationship. Also general agreement was that the action of a nurse sitting at the bedside and holding the patient's hand would be appropriate and desirable if the patient were having a great deal of pain or were depressed and lonely. Of the three subjects who did not see this nursing intervention as desirable, two did not think that the nurse was being sincere. The third subject, a 27-year-old former nurse, thought that this touch gesture would make an elderly patient feel loved and wanted but stated that she herself did not like this type of hand contact.

Slide three. In slide three, a middle-aged woman is lying in bed with a nasogastric tube in place. A female nurse is standing beside the bed, and no body or eye contact is occurring between the nurse and patient. Although all subjects agreed that the patient looked either fearful, anxious, angry, apprehensive or desperate, all but one subject saw the nurse as helpful or comforting. The latter woman, a surgical patient, interpreted the nurse's action as fear provoking or threatening to the patient. All other subjects implied that the patient was at fault, stating "nothing the nurse could do would help; she is that type of patient," and "she probably won't accept any help." The subjects stated repeatedly that patients should not be frightened of a nurse, that the nurse is interested only in helping patients, that nurses are there to help, and that the nurse attempts to comfort patients. One wonders if the subjects were reluctant to make any negative comments about nurses or if they have been so conditioned to regard nurses as tender, loving, and kind that they were reluctant to see them in any other light.

Slide four. Slide four shows a young woman lying in bed with a female nurse sitting beside her, holding her hand. They are looking at each other.

All subjects agreed that the situation depicted in the fourth slide appeared to be supportive and comforting to the patient. With the exception of the same two subjects who did not like this type of physical contact for themselves, all agreed that they would be comforted, especially in times of stress or depression, if the nurse held their hands. One subject, a 32-year-old man, stated that the nurse was being "beneficial"

and that "When the nurse spends time talking to you, the pain is not so bad." Another subject stated that "The patient is reassured: the nurse has taken time to listen." Still another subject said that "When you are feeling really low, it is nice to talk to somebody." However, most subjects commented that this did not happen often—that the nurses were "too busy."

Slide five. In slide five, a male nurse is assisting a young woman to walk. His arm is placed around her back.

Twelve of the seventeen subjects saw the situation depicted in the fifth slide as a positive action on the part of the nurse. These twelve, nine of whom were surgical patients, agreed that the nurse was being "supportive" and "helpful" to the patient. One subject stated that this action gave the patient "confidence to go on" and that it showed that "the nurse cares whether you walk again." Of the five subjects who did not see this as a positive nursing intervention, three stated that the nurse was only giving "moral" support and that it would have been of greater help if the nurse had held the patient's arm. They also stated that they would not like to have a nurse's arm around their back. All subjects stressed the importance of proper support to a patient beginning to walk again.

Slide six. Slide six shows a male nurse bending over a middle-aged woman. He is holding her hand and smiling at her. She is looking at him and also smiling. This situation was seen as positive by the majority of both medical and surgical subjects. All saw the patient as being depressed and lonely and saw the nurse's action as an attempt to cheer her. Following were some of the comments made:

He is letting her know that he is aware she is a human being and that he too is human.

He is reassuring her that she is in friendly surroundings.

Giving her security.

Showing her he thinks she's special.

She sees him as a supportive person.

All subjects stated that the nurse and patient were enjoying themselves and that this was good in most circumstances.

The four subjects (two medical and two

surgical) who saw this action as inappropriate stated that the nurse was unprofessional, was too close to the patient, was going beyond his capacity as a nurse, and was not being genuine. Jourard comments that, "Each person lives as if with an invisible fence around his body, a fence that keeps others at that distance which one feels most safe and comfortable."[11]

A 63-year-old man said that this interaction might be inappropriate but that, as long as the patient was not in pain or distress, it would probably be a supportive measure. He stated that, "Generally, in the medical world people feel that they must be damned impersonal" and further that "All people like some form of pat on the back, verbal or otherwise." A 54-year-old woman stated that she would not like the nurse to be that close to her. Possibly the close physical contact between the nurse and the patient in this picture was seen as an invasion of personal space, thus was perceived as a threat to the "self" by these four subjects.

Slide seven. Slide seven depicts a middle-aged female patient and a female nurse. The nurse has one hand on the patient's forehead and the other hand on the woman's arm. The nurse is not looking at the patient.

The action depicted in the seventh situation was acceptable to only two medical and three surgical subjects. These five made statements such as "She, the nurse, is probably looking at a monitor," and "She is reassuring the patient while something else is going on." The other twelve subjects made similar statements, but all qualified them by saying such things as the following:

If she is sincere and really trying to comfort the patient, she would be looking at her.

She could console better if she were looking at her—probably why woman isn't accepting her—could not accept this either.

Nurse should be looking at her.

May feel she is being ignored—take care of one person at a time—don't ignore verbally.

Actions must be appropriate with words.

Patient doesn't look happy.

Patient looks scared.

Nurse is talking to someone else—not thinking too much about what she is doing.

Two women commented that they would not like a nurse's hand on their heads. They did not see this as a comforting gesture. It appears from the comments made by these subjects that physical contact, unless coupled with visual contact, is not seen in a positive light. Thus it can be assumed that most of the subjects expect and want the nurses to give congruent verbal and nonverbal communication. It is not enough just to touch the patient; the nurse must, by both verbal and nonverbal behavior, communicate to the patient that attention is totally his for that moment in time.

Slide eight. Slide eight shows two nurses, one male and one female, with a young woman. The male nurse has one hand on the patient's head while holding one of her hands. The female nurse is holding the patient's other hand. Both nurses are looking at the patient.

Seven surgical and four medical patients gave favorable responses to slide eight. These subjects all saw this patient-nurse intervention as therapeutic, especially if the patient were very ill, in a great deal of pain, or in critical condition. In spite of their interpretation of this intervention as desirable, the same subjects thought that the situation was unrealistic and that "You never actually see two nurses with a patient for the sole purpose of offering comfort and support." The subjects who did not interpret this intervention as desirable said that the nurses were giving too much attention and that it would be overwhelming and frightening to the patient.

ADDITIONAL FINDINGS

Such factors as age, seriousness of present illness, number of previous hospital admissions, relationships with significant others, and the patient-nurse relationship were found to be related to how subjects perceived the use of touch as a nursing intervention. Age appears to affect the patient's perception of touch. On the one hand, subjects in the 20- to 30-year-old age group saw the use of touch as a positive aspect of nursing care, which should be used in everyday contact with the patient. On the other hand, older subjects claimed that touch should be used only for specific conditions such as pain, depression, and loneliness.

All subjects agreed that the use of touch was most important in caring for the very elderly patient. They stated that elderly patients need to reach out to someone and that touch conveys interest and caring. Davis quotes anthropologist Byers, who speculates as follows:

It's actually the old who suffer most in our society. They are touched perhaps less than anyone—in fact, it sometimes seems as if people are afraid old age might be contagious—and this literal loss of contact must add greatly to the old person's sense of isolation.*

Seemingly the younger subjects are more tolerant of the use of touch than those in the older age groups. Perhaps the recent popularity of encounter groups and the increasing sexual permissiveness among the youth of today accounts for the younger age group's lack of concern for the social taboos related to body touching. The responses from younger subjects indicated openness and frankness in dealing with interpersonal relationships. They show a willingness to admit that individuals need the support, comfort, and caring that the use of touch may transmit. The older age group, in whom social taboos are more firmly fixed, expressed a need for a reason to be touched. Their responses indicated a willingness to accept the warmth and compassion that touch may convey only if there is a physiological reason such as pain or an acceptable psychological reason such as depression or loneliness.

The seriousness of the subject's illness had a positive effect on the perception of touch in all age groups, as did the number of previous hospital admissions. Those subjects who had life-threatening diseases all saw touch as a sign that the nurse "cared," "was reaching out," and "was interested." All subjects stated the importance to them, in times of stress or severe illness, of the nurse's taking time to be with them. As one subject, a 52-year-old man with a diagnosis of acute leukemia, stated, "A touch of the hand gives you some feeling of comfort."

Also, patients who had a number of previous hospital admissions perceived the use of touch as a positive nursing intervention.

---

*From Davis, F.: Touching and smelling, Glamour Magazine, p. 151, Jan., 1972.

Eleven of the seventeen subjects in the sample had previous hospital admissions for the same or other conditions. One subject, a 27-year-old woman with a history of seven previous hospital admissions for recurring pancreatitis, was vocal regarding her need for the emotional support that she received from being touched by the nurses. She stated that the nurse, by touching her, was "reaching out to help me." Perhaps patients become more sensitive to their own emotional needs after a number of hospitalizations and are more willing to admit that they require the reassurance and comfort that may be given by the nurse through touch.

Significant others in the subjects' lives had an inverse effect on the subjects' perception of the need for touch, that is, in all age groups, subjects who had good family relationships and whose family and friends visited frequently stated that they had little need for the nurse to use this form of communication. They claimed that they received all the love, comfort, and support that they required from their families. However, all subjects agreed that if they did not have a family or friends who visited, they would then want the nurse to be able to fulfill these needs.

Nearly all subjects stressed the importance of the development of a good patient-nurse relationship as a basis for using touch as a nursing intervention. They claimed that they needed to get to know "their" nurse before the touch would provide the support and comfort that they required. A number of subjects also mentioned that frequently there was just one nurse whom they felt especially close to and perceived as genuinely interested in them. Usually this nurse had interests similar to theirs or came from a similar background. Thus subjects expressed a need for a common base on which to build their relationship.

The subjects all differentiated between what they generally called "moral" support and the type given when carrying out routine physical care. In the two pictures that showed a nurse walking the patient, the touch gesture was seen as "offering support," "giving courage," and "preventing falls." This physical contact was seen as something normal, desired, and expected. Many of the subjects commented on the best way to hold onto a patient to enable him to feel secure.

In the pictures that involved no apparent physical need for touch, the subjects were more varied in their responses. The 20- to 30-year age group saw the use of touch as a supportive, comforting measure that should be used by the nursing staff. The older age groups agreed that the touch gesture signified that the nurse was interested in their welfare, but they further stated that it should be used only if the patient were apprehensive, in pain, or depressed and lonely.

Apparently, from the sample studied, some difference exists between medical and surgical patients in how they perceive the use of touch. The surgical subjects saw the use of touch more positively and had less qualifications for its use than did medical subjects. However, this difference may be more apparent than real. The majority of the medical subjects, with an average age of 47.7 years, were older than the surgical ones, whose average age was 27.6 years. Thus this difference may be attributed to age difference, rather than to their particular illness and its treatment. The data obtained from the two surgical subjects over the age of 30 years in the sample substantiates this idea, since their responses were similar to those of the medical subjects.

From the sample studied, seemingly the male nurse is perceived more realistically by male than by female patients. The men had little comment regarding the situations involving the male nurse but did describe him consistently as a nurse. The female subjects, on the other hand, just as consistently described the male nurse as a doctor or attendant and, even when corrected, persisted in doing so. However, comments by the majority of subjects such as, "He is reassuring her," "She sees him as a supportive person," and "He is trying to cheer her up," would indicate that, for this group of subjects, sex did not have a bearing on the patients' acceptance of touch.

The expectation was that the subjects would perceive the use of touch as a positive nursing intervention. For the most part, this assumption was borne out by the responses of the sample population. Only two subjects were critical of this mode of interaction, but even then they qualified their statements so that they were not entirely negative. One, a 27-year-old former nurse, stated that she had often used touch in caring for patients and fully believed in its potentialities for communicating her interest in and concern for her patients. She said, however, that she herself had never cared to be touched by anyone whom she did not know well and that her family fulfilled these needs for her. The other subject, a 44-year-old woman, said that she realized the value of this form of nonverbal communication, especially for older people, but to her it was "mauling," and she did not like it.

Two male medical patients had divergent opinions regarding nurses. One subject, a 54-year-old man with a diagnosis of myocardial infarction, compared nurses to politicians. He stated that both groups were insincere and that both were just paid to do a job. He also stated that they should do their work as perfectly as possible but, apart from that, he did not expect anything from them. He did not see the nurse as being able to give him anything but routine physical care and made it clear that, in his opinion, that was all that was required. A second subject, a 32-year-old patient with a diagnosis of heart and kidney problems, asked, "Nurses aren't supposed to have any feelings toward their patients, are they?" He then went on to say, "Patients need love and care—that's what nurses are for." This patient, in contrast to the former one, admitted his need for something more than routine care.

CONCLUSION

Although the study was limited and involved only a small sample of subjects, some implications for nursing can be drawn from the study findings. First, the nurse should be aware that age may be a factor in the way a patient perceives the use of touch as a nursing intervention. Although touch is more likely to be acceptable to younger patients, the older ones may need reasons such as pain, fear, anxiety, or depression, before its use becomes acceptable to them. The exception to this may be the aged. The use of touch for the elderly can help to provide them with a sense of their own identity in a busy, impersonal hospital. It also serves as a method for providing reality orientation, as well as reassurance and support to the patient.

Second, the nurse should be aware of the importance of developing a good patient-nurse relationship before trying to use this method of nursing intervention. Nearly all subjects studied stated that they needed to know "their" nurse to derive the greatest support and comfort from touch. They also stressed the relationship as being a prerequisite to being comfortable with the nurse's use of touch.

Third, the nurse must be aware of the many different interpretations that may be placed on actions by different patients. All will perceive and interpret actions, such as touch, in the light of their own past experience. Consequently, the nurse's behavior may be viewed as inappropriate by the patient, or he may respond in a way that the nurse considers inappropriate.

The results obtained from this small, subjective exploratory study indicate many areas for future study. The limitations of the testing instrument necessitate the development of a more refined tool. Perhaps a movie of patients and nurses using the touch gesture in interaction would be more realistic, thus elicit more comment from subjects. Larger sample populations should be used to increase the likelihood of valid results.

Although this study was limited, it does serve to delineate variables such as age, seriousness of the illness, and previous hospital admissions that might influence a patient's perception of the nurse's use of touch. In future studies, such variables could be controlled to clarify their effects on the patients' perception of touch as a mode of nursing intervention.

One area for further study would be to investigate further the apparent differences between medical and surgical patients in their perception of the use of touch. For example, both younger patients (20 to 30 years of age) and older ones (31 to 55 years of age) in both specialties should be studied

independently, so that the age factor may be eliminated. Other areas for investigation would be the differences in perception of touch between male and female patients, in utilization of the touch gesture as a mode of nursing intervention between male and female nurses, and in acceptance of the touch gesture between male and female patients when utilized by both male and female nurses. Finally, investigation could be made into the patient's perception of what is *personal* as opposed to *professional* contact and under what circumstances one is seen more positively than the other.

The results of the study indicate that touch as a form of nonverbal communication apparently has great value as a method of demonstrating to the patients "their" nurse's interest and concern when it is used appropriately and when both patient and nurse are comfortable with its use.

References

1. Angrist, S.: Nursing care; the dream and the reality. In Lewis, E. P., editor: Changing patterns of nursing practice, New York, 1971, American Journal of Nursing Co., p. 144.
2. Aydelotte, M. K.: The use of patient welfare as a criterion measure, Nurs. Res. 11:10, 1962.
3. Burton, A., and Heller, L. G.: The touching of the body, Psychoanal. Rev. 5:126, 1964.
4. Davis, F.: Touching and smelling, Glamour Magazine, p. 83, Jan., 1972.
5. Dominian, J.: The psychological significance of touch, Nurs. Times 67:896, 1971.
6. Farrah, S.: The nurse's reported use of touch, unpublished masters thesis, 1969, University of Illinois, p. 6.
7. Farrah, S.: The nurse—the patient—and touch. In Duffey, M., Anderson, E. H., Bergersen, B. S., Lohr, M., and Rose, M. H., editors: Current concepts in clinical nursing, St. Louis, 1971, The C. V. Mosby Co., pp. 247, 252.
8. Frank, L. K.: Tactile communication, Genet. Psychol. Monogr. 56:209, 1957.
9. Goshen, C. E.: Your automated future, Am. J. Nurs. 72:62, 1972.
10. Johnson, B. S.: The meaning of touch in nursing, Nurs. Outlook 13:59, Feb., 1965.
11. Jourard, S.: Disclosing man to himself, New York, 1968, D. Van Nostrand Co., Inc., pp. 136, 137.
12. Lewis, G. K.: Nurse-patient communication, Dubuque, Iowa, 1962, W. C. Brown Co., p. 42.
13. Lockerby, F. K.: Communication for nurses, St. Louis, 1963, The C. V. Mosby Co., pp. 106-108.
14. Mercer, L. S.: Touch; comfort or threat? Perspect. Psychiat. Care 4:20, May-June, 1966.
15. Montagu, A.: Touching; the human significance of the skin, New York, 1971, Columbia University Press, pp. 97, 164.

16. Olson, E. V.: Needed; a shake-up in the status quo, Amer. J. Nurs. **68:**1491, 1968.
17. Peplau, H. E.: Interpersonal relations in nursing, New York, 1952, G. P. Putnam's Sons, pp. 289, 304-307.
18. Pluckham, M.: Space; the silent language, Nurs. Forum **7:**386, 1968.
19. Ruesch, J.: Disturbed communication, New York, 1957, W. W. Norton & Co., Inc., Publishers, p. 90.
20. Saunders, L.: Permanence and change. In Lewis, E. P., editor: Changing patterns of nursing practice, New York, 1971, American Journal of Nursing Co., p. 6.
21. Travelbee, J.: Interpersonal aspects of nursing, Philadelphia, 1968, F. A. Davis Co., pp. 96-97.

Bibliography

Books

Bellak, L.: The T.A.T. and C.A.T. in clinical use, New York, 1971, Grune & Stratton, Inc.
Davitz, L. J.: Interpersonal processes in nursing; case histories, New York, 1970, Springer Publishing Co., Inc.
Hall, E. T.: The silent language, New York, 1959, Doubleday & Co., Inc.
Hayes, W. J., and Gazaway, R.: Human relations in nursing, Philadelphia, 1964, W. B. Saunders Co.
Jourard, S. M.: The transparent self, New York, 1971, Van Nostrand-Reinhold Co.
Morris, D.: Intimate behavior, New York, 1971, Random House, Inc.

Periodicals

Bosanquet, C.: Getting in touch, J. Anal. Psychol. **15:**42, 1970.
Copp, L. C.: A projective cartoon investigation of nurse-patient psychodramatic role perception and expectation, Nurs. Res. **28:**100, March-April, 1971.
Daly, M. M., and Carr, J.: Tactile contact: a measure of therapeutic progress, Nurs. Res. **16:** 16, winter, 1967.
Dethomaso, M. T.: "Touch power" and the screen of loneliness, Perspect. Psychiatr. Care **9** (3):112, 1971.
Durr, C. A.: Hands that help—but how? Nurs. Forum **10:**392, 1971.
Gibson, J.: Observation on active touch, Psychol. Rev. **69:**477, 1962.
Harlow, H.: The nature of love, Am. Psychol. **13:** 673, 1958.
Hoffman, A.: A dialogue of touch, Ment. Hyg. **5:**24, 1967.
Hollender, M. H.: The need or wish to be held, Arch. Gen. Psychiat. **22:**445, 1970.
Peplau, H. E.: Professional closeness, Nurs. Forum **8:**342, 1969.
Rubin, R.: Maternal touch, Nurs. Outlook **11:**828, 1963.

Unpublished work

Farrah, S.: Effect of deliberative nursing intervention involving touch upon the alleviation of pain in selected female patients, unpublished independent study, 1968, University of Illinois.

29

Immediate nursing care following cervical cord injury

Jeanne N. Quesenbury
Sara Hammes

The nursing care of patients with severe cervical injury is based on the general problems that one would expect to encounter, the medical therapy prescribed, and measures necessary to prevent complications from occurring. The care given during the first forty-eight hours or so after hospitalization will be the focus of this chapter.

BRIEF REVIEW OF THE GENERAL MANAGEMENT

The initial hospital care involves establishing a diagnosis concerning the level and extent of the injury. X-ray examinations are made, and surgical laminectomies are sometimes necessary for purposes of decompressing the cord or reducing a fracture and dislocation of the osseous structure of the cervical spine. To relieve pressure on the cord and maintain reduction, skeletal tongs are usually applied in the emergency or operating room in preparation for the later application of skeletal traction. In our hospital skeletal traction is usually initiated with the idea of employing it for a period of approximately six weeks. Periodic portable x-ray examinations determine alignment of the cervical spine.

PROBLEMS THE PATIENTS ARE LIKELY TO EXPERIENCE

A period of spinal shock occurs after most severe cord injuries and always after those at the cervical level. For a period of a few days or weeks the central nervous system, particularly the autonomic section, becomes temporarily nonfunctional, probably due to the sudden loss of connections between the higher centers and the cord.

Some of the dysfunctions patients experience during this period of time include the following: The muscles below the level of injury become temporarily flaccid, with sensory loss below this level as well. There is paralysis of the intercostal muscles, which can greatly impair respiratory function even though diaphragmatic function does account for some 80% of the breathing effort. Paralytic ileus occurs because there is temporary interference of the parasympathetic impulses to the gastrointestinal tract. The latter condition produces stomach and bowel distention, which forces the diaphragm to rise into the lung space and further aggravates respiration. If shock is present, there will be a reduction in the amount of urine formed because of decreased kidney perfusion. Urine is retained in the bladder because of sphincter paralysis, and bladder distention is no longer signaling the brain of the need for emptying. Voluntary bowel control is also lost because of lack of sphincter signal to the brain. Mentally the patient experiences shock, disbelief, and feelings of unreality—that all this is happening to someone other than himself.

The nursing problems associated with the care of patients with severe cord injury are related to the patients' presenting conditions and, equally as important, to the prevention of those complications which frequently impede their programs of rehabilitation and cause them great discomfort and inconvenience. Fear, airway problems caused by the inability to handle secretions, breathing difficulties, and vomiting attributable to gastric distention are among the most frequent immediate problems. Pulmonary emboli, infection—especially of the urinary tract and respiratory systems—decubitus ulcers, and mental despondency are the complications most commonly identified with severe cord injuries. Some of the nursing practices we have used in caring for these patients in our hospital will be discussed at greater length here.

NURSING CARE

The nursing unit needs some time in which to prepare for the admission of the patient to the unit. Usually an orthopedic turning frame is made available, but the choice of a frame appropriate to the size of the patient, as well as suitable padding, will have to be made. If a regular bed is used, it has to be adapted so that the traction apparatus can be attached. Two mattresses with a bedboard between them for firmness will raise the level, so that the pulley can be placed over the headboard and the angle of pull made correct. After certain types of injury the patients are not permitted to be turned for one or two days. This, together with the fact that patients will be lying on their backs for considerable lengths of time if a regular bed is used, calls for some type of device for preventing pressure areas from occurring. To facilitate care of the patient while he is on his back, the bed can be made using two large cotton draw sheets, one of which is placed from the head of the bed to the patient's buttocks and the second from the buttocks to the foot of the bed.

For patients with cervical injury there seems to be a particular arrangement on the ward that is less frightening. The restriction of movement caused by the paralysis and traction apparatus is terrifying; when personnel can be seen and heard, the patients seem to be less afraid. For this reason, we try to provide rooms near the desk and have the beds or frames placed near the doors so that contact with other persons is maintained.

When the patient is first brought to the nursing unit, manual traction will be necessary to transfer him from the stretcher to the frame. The patient's head must be closely supported in neutral position, that is, in alignment with the back and without flexion or extension. To move the patient

as a unit we have found it necessary to recruit at least five persons to lift him from the stretcher onto the bed, which has been placed perpendicular to it. One person maintains the manual traction, and four persons carry the patient. The four who carry the patient are all on the same side, having their arms alternate with those of persons standing next to them so that evenness and smoothness is maintained throughout the transfer. After the patient has been transferred onto the frame or bed, the appropriate amount of weight is gently attached to the weight holder by the physician. Usually a greater amount of weight is used for reduction of the fracture, and a lesser amount is employed thereafter.

Maintaining proper traction is not usually a difficult problem, but constant attention is necessary. When the ropes run over the pulley, the weight carrier hangs free, and the patient is not touching the head of the bed, traction is correct. Occasionally we need to remind a team member that the weight carrier must not be caught on the bed when the patient is moved, and that the traction should not be interrupted by lifting the weight carrier while changing the patient's position. The mechanics of traction presuppose that the patient's body will serve as countertraction, so that when many pounds of weight are required, the head of the bed may have to be elevated to supply the countertraction. An advantage of the orthopedic turning frame is that the patient can be turned to both prone and supine positions and the traction will be maintained.

Most patients with cervical fractures tolerate the prone position for only short periods of time because of their breathing problems. This means that orders to turn a patient every two hours have to be adjusted to meet the needs of the individual. We find little to worry about concerning tongs slipping from their position in the outer skull. However, we do check for this and for the condition of the skin at the site of tong insertion. As a precautionary measure, we frequently cleanse the skin surface with a bactericidal solution. Clipping and washing the hair is necessary mainly for the patient's comfort.

Five persons are called on to help the

first few times to turn an adult in skeletal traction who is in a regular bed. One person stands at the head and places his hands on each side of the patient's face, and two persons stand on each side. A turning sheet is used, or all the nurses place their arms under the patient to support him from shoulder to hips. A pillow is placed between the patient's legs so that the uppermost leg will not fall when he is turned. Alignment is maintained when the nurse at the head guides the head and shoulders and the nurses at the side of the patient from which he is being turned pull him toward themselves while those on the other side guide and assist with the move. A neck support of sponge rubber is generally used when the patient is turned prone or to one side; pillows are used to support the uppermost leg and foot. We have found that patients soon become used to lying supine, and, when it is necessary to turn them to one side for the first time, a brief explanation is in order. To provide guidance and reassurance to the patient on this and similar occasions, the nurse must have great self-assurance and technical competence.

Helping the patient to breathe adequately is a major nursing activity. Some patients require a tracheostomy to assist them to breathe and to facilitate removal of their tracheal and bronchial secretions. The need for oxygen therapy is determined by arterial blood gas (oxygen, carbon dioxide) levels. We encourage the patient to cough as best he is able and to expectorate secretions, and then we assist him with the use of mechanical suction if necessary. In the past our technique for suctioning was not so aseptically strict as it is at present. Greater precaution is taken to prevent introducing microorganisms into the respiratory tract, which means that sterile gloves and suction catheter are used each time that suctioning is required. We are also now more aware of the status of the patient's oxygen reserve and use care not to remove vital amounts of inspired oxygen along with the secretions. Eight- to ten-second intervals are the maximum amounts of time in which the suction power is used without allowing the patient to breathe. We have found that after a patient is turned, the lung secretions loosen somewhat and begin to move into the main

stem bronchus, thus making it somewhat easier for the patient himself to cough up the secretions; therefore after turning we use cup clapping and encourage the patient to try to cough.

Nurses soon learn in listening to these patients that fright, loneliness, and disbelief are among the predominate feelings they experience during their waking hours. One young man said he was afraid that he might "forget to breathe" and explained how it frightened him to realize that he could not breathe well. To a patient such as this, we explain what is going on in terms he can understand. We tell him that he is experiencing what it feels like to use only the diaphragm for breathing, since his intercostal muscles are not responding. We keep in mind that he may also be saying that he is afraid of what might happen to him when he is alone; therefore we try to arrange for someone— a nurse, relative, or friend—to remain with him. When the patient is first admitted to the hospital, he is literally surrounded by people who can help him. After some hours there is less demand for the services of these persons, and they leave, so that he could be alone for seemingly long periods of time unless other arrangements have been made. He cannot move, does not have enough breath to yell, and may become very apprehensive. Even a sensitive call light such as the type that requires only minimal palm pressure may not be operable for him, depending on the level of his lesion.

In the effort to prevent skin breakdown due to pressure, we see turning and avoiding prolonged pressure as the key factors. In addition, we protect those areas of skin which are directly above bony prominences with synthetic sheepskin or similar felt padding and, of course, stimulate circulation to them by rubbing. A careful examination of all skin surfaces has become part of the bathing routine and is carried out whenever else it is necessary. Whenever medication is introduced into paralyzed muscle, special precautions are necessary. The injection site must be carefully chosen, the medication injected slowly, and the muscle massaged gently after the injection to facilitate absorption of the medication. Poor circulation and reduced body metabolism predispose the site of injection to abscess formation, which is another reason why frequent skin and muscle inspection is necessary.

The bath time is one of the good times in which assessment of the patient's neurological status can be carried out without it being made unduly obvious to him. We have learned that frequent periods of questioning and examination in which the patient perceives his inability to function normally are very depressing to him. One can observe his motor powers in his breathing and by the position his extremities assume. His ability to appreciate sensation can be learned by using the pinprick and, beginning with stimulation of the toes, working upward, asking him to tell when he perceives pain. The nurse must try to be prepared for his feelings of shock and disappointment. "My hands, my arms, I can't move them!" and statements of a similar nature are not unusual.

Patients on an orthopedic turning frame or in a regular bed with two mattresses have difficulty communicating because they are not able to look directly at those with whom they are speaking. When the staff and the family members use a footstool to stand above the patient, this problem is alleviated somewhat. One patient on a very low frame confessed that his problem was of a different nature: he was tired of "looking at the roofs of mouths" of people. For him we sat at his side so that he could see us better.

Although a urinary tract infection will not usually show up in a healthy young person for a couple of days after the injury, every precaution is taken to avoid common and severe complication. In the past continuous indwelling catheters have been used in our hospital as the means of preventing bladder distention. Recently, however, attempts have been made to reduce the number of urinary tract infections by using the intermittent method of catheterization. In the latter method the patient is catheter free except for those times when the bladder is full. The urine is drained and the catheter removed after each catheterization, so that one avenue by which microorganisms might enter the urinary system is removed. Another advantage of this procedure is said to be its ability to maintain bladder tone. Other hospitals have been using intermittent catheterization longer than we have, and references to their experiences are included in the bibliography at the end of the chapter.

When it becomes necessary to use an indwelling catheter, we take the precaution of maintaining a closed system. The irrigating solution is injected into the tubing itself (by means of a needle and syringe) rather than interrupting the tubing at its connection. We cleanse the periurethral area with a bactericidal agent twice daily, making sure to rinse the area well to prevent further irritation from the soap solution. In the male patient who has an indwelling catheter, it is well to tape the catheter to the abdomen and maintain the penis in retroflexion to prevent ulceration of the urethral floor at the penoscrotal angle (Fig. 29-1). The entire urinary drainage system requires frequent checking, which almost becomes routine each time one enters a patient's room. Is the indwelling catheter in the bladder, does it have a dependent loop to facilitate drainage and prevent pull on the meatus, and is it taped to the skin? Is the collecting tubing free from the weight of the patient and without kinks (Fig. 29-2)? Concerning the urine itself, what are its color and consistency?

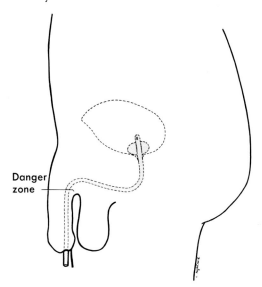

Fig. 29-1. Diagram illustrating how ulceration at the penoscrotal angle can occur when the catheter is taped to the leg.

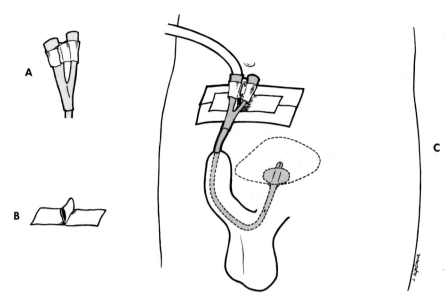

Fig. 29-2. A, The catheter tips are taped together to prevent the tubing from turning on itself. **B,** The tape is prepared to place onto abdominal tape strips. **C,** When the catheter is taped to the abdomen a continuous "circle" is maintained, which helps prevent ulceration.

Without normal peristaltic activity the stomach contents accumulate, creating the danger of vomiting and aspirating. Frequently, gastric intubation with continuous stomach decompression is used. When the patient is not intubated, we are even more alert to early signs of gastrointestinal distention. Supplemental intravenous therapy is administered until bowel function returns. When bowel sounds are heard and the patient is permitted to have food and fluids, he needs to be observed for signs of distention, since some degree of reduction of peristalsis will persist.

Although these patients will usually be insensitive to pain over large portions of their bodies, some pain and discomfort have been experienced by the patients with whom we have been associated. The most common source of pain is the area of the injury. Also, some patients do feel pain in the parts of their bodies below the level of the lesion when their lesions are incomplete ones. Comfort measures, such as the adjustment of a pad, pillow, or article of clothing, may be all that are required to help them feel better. But if the pain is severe, analgesics may be necessary. Morphine is not used because of the respiratory depressant action this medication is known to have.

We have mentioned some of the problems and fears of patients with severe cord injuries and have reviewed in greater depth the aspects of care that seem to cause the most difficulty for them. We would like to conclude by saying that we realize that nurses faced with the situation of caring for patients with severe spinal injuries have fears also. Recognition of these fears and striving to diminish them by attaining knowledge that will enable the nurse to perform the nursing activities necessary for the care of these patients should result in a positive interaction between nurse and patient.

Bibliography

Abramson, A. S.: Advances in the management of the neurogenic bladder, Arch. Phys. Med. Rehabil. **52:**143, April, 1971.

Betson, C.: Blood gases, Am. J. Nurs. **68:**1010, 1968.

Comarr, A. E.: Practical management of the patient with traumatic cord bladder, Arch. Phys. Med. Rehabil. **48:**122, March, 1967.

Licht, S., editor: Rehabilitation and medicine, Baltimore, 1968, Waverly Press, Inc.

O'Connor, J. R., and Leitner, L. A.: Traumatic quadriplegia: A comprehensive review, J. Rehabil. **37:**14, May-June, 1971.

Skinner, G.: Head traction and the Stryker frame, Am. J. Nurs. **52:**694, 1952.

30

Nursing care of the thermally injured patient

Lois A. Johns
Paul Silverstein
Katherine F. Galloway
Betty G. McGranahan

An individual can sustain no more immediate, devasting trauma than that caused by an extensive burn. He usually has no chance to prepare himself. In a matter of moments, an independent, self-sufficient man or woman can be reduced to a state of complete dependency.

Anyone who has worked in a burn unit cannot help but be impressed by the number of thermal injuries that could have been avoided by the use of elementary safety precautions. Approximately 2 million persons are burned in the United States each year. In 1968, 75,000 individuals were hospitalized for burns, and 12,200 died from fire-related injuries.

Obviously the initial act in burn care should be to extinguish the flame. The person on fire is likely to panic and run. This fans the fire and causes more severe injury. It is better to lie on the ground and roll, to smother the blaze. Water is the natural enemy of fire. If none is available, a coat or blanket can be used to extinguish the fire. Only as a last resort should earth be used to quench a fire, since it will further contaminate the wound.

Chemical burns should be washed and liberally diluted with water immediately. Smouldering clothes should be quickly removed from the victim's body. When possible, the burned area should be covered with some clean material, such as a sheet, during transportation to a hospital where definitive care is available. The patient should be driven at a safe speed to the care center. Useless haste only further endangers lives and increases the victim's fear and apprehension.

Today the person with extensive burns has a better survival potential than he did fifteen years ago. This improvement is due to a better understanding of the physiological sequelae of such injuries, control of burn wound sepsis, improved skin-grafting procedures, better patient monitoring through the use of intensive care units, and improved laboratory methods.

The four phases in the treatment of burns are (1) acute resuscitative phase (zero to seventy-two hours), (2) wound care including eschar separation and preparation for autografting (seventy-two hours to four weeks), (3) skin grafting and reconstructive phase (weeks to years), and (4) rehabilitation.

The objectives of the nursing personnel in a burn unit are to provide superior specialized nursing care for all patients following a therapeutic and individualized plan; to work closely with the physician to provide optimum care for patients; to recognize and meet the physical and emotional needs of the patient and to involve these individuals in their recovery process; to provide the patient's family with support and instruction so that they will be of maximum help to the patient throughout his illness and rehabilitation; to implement medical orders and to provide the physician with accurate and meaningful information about the physical and psychological condition of the patient; to work closely with allied medical personnel and chaplains toward the common goal of returning the injured individual to society as a useful and intact person as possible; and to provide these services efficiently and effectively with kindness and compassion.

RESUSCITATIVE PHASE

An experienced medical team consisting of a physician and nurse or technician may be used to transport the patient to a burn center. Movement of a patient with severe burns over a long distance requires good judgment and preparation. The chances for survival of patients with extensive burns are better if transfer is effected within forty-eight hours of injury to a center where facilities and trained personnel are available. If fluid losses are anticipated and replaced skillfully with appropriate intravenous therapy, thermally injured patients usually remain alert and cooperative for the first seventy-two hours. Bulky absorbent dressings provide the most comfort during movement from hospital to hospital.

The *Rule of Nines* is a useful guide in assessing the extent of thermal injury. This rule divides the body into surfaces areas of approximately 9% or multiples of 9%, as demonstrated in Fig. 30-1. A more detailed evaluation of the extent of the burn may be made and diagramed after admission (Fig. 30-2).

Judging the depth of the burn can be difficult and requires an experienced physician. First-degree burns present a dry reddened appearance and are painful: a sunburn is the best example of this type of burn. Second-degree burns usually are red, mottled, and frequently characterized by the appearance of blisters. This burn is ordinarily moist and exudes a plasmalike fluid. The wound is painful and sensitive to air and touch. Third-degree burns involve full-thickness skin destruction. The wound is dry and has a gray-white to to charred black color. Thrombosed veins may be visible through the parchmentlike skin. A third-degree burn is not usually very painful because the cutaneous nerve endings have been destroyed.

The quantity of intravenous fluid required to replace loss from the vascular system through thermally injured vessels may be estimated by any of several avail-

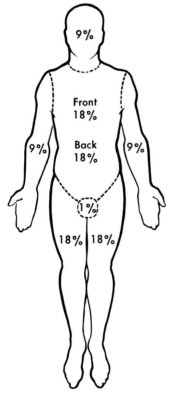

Fig. 30-1. Rule of nines.

BURN ESTIMATE AND DIAGRAM
AGE vs. AREA

Area	Birth 1 yr.	1-4 yr.	5-9 yr.	10-14 yr.	15 yr.	Adult	2°	3°	Total	Donor Areas
Head	19	17	13	11	9	7				
Neck	2	2	2	2	2	2		1.5	1.5	
Ant. Trunk	13	13	13	13	13	13		13	13.0	
Post. Trunk	13	13	13	13	13	13	7.5		7.5	
R. Buttock	2½	2½	2½	2½	2½	2½				
L. Buttock	2½	2½	2½	2½	2½	2½				
Genitalia	1	1	1	1	1	1				
R.U. Arm	4	4	4	4	4	4	2	2	4.0	
L.U. Arm	4	4	4	4	4	4				
R.L. Arm	3	3	3	3	3	3	3		3.0	
L.L. Arm	3	3	3	3	3	3				
R. Hand	2½	2½	2½	2½	2½	2½				
L. Hand	2½	2½	2½	2½	2½	2½				
R. Thigh	5½	6½	8	8½	9	9½				
L. Thigh	5½	6½	8	8½	9	9½				
R. Leg	5	5	5½	6	6½	7				
L. Leg	5	5	5½	6	6½	7				
R. Foot	3½	3½	3½	3½	3½	3½				
L. Foot	3½	3½	3½	3½	3½	3½				
TOTAL							12.5	16.5	29.0	

BURN DIAGRAM

AGE   15

SEX Female

WEIGHT 50 Kg

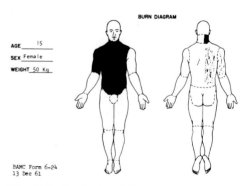

BAMC Form 6-24
13 Dec 61

Fig. 30-2. Example of burn estimate and diagram. Black area indicates third-degree burns; gray area indicates second-degree burns.

able formulas. The Brooke formula is one that is often used to estimate fluid loss (Fig. 30-3). All formulas are estimates subject to constant revision as determined by the patient's general condition, clinical signs, and laboratory data. A 50% burn is the recommended maximum burn size for calculations. This recommendation is made to avoid fluid overload, in full recognition of the fact that patients with larger burns will require more fluid. One half of the estimated fluid requirements for the first twenty-four hours is customarily given in the first eight hours postburn. One fourth of the calculated fluids is administered in the second eight hours postburn and the remainder in the last eight hours. One half of the first day's required colloids and electrolytes is usually needed during the second twenty-four–hour postburn period, and the water requirement for this period is estimated by the physician.

Admission

The patient with burns is generally brought directly to the burn unit. The following equipment must be readily available:

1. Cardiopulmonary resuscitating equipment and an ECG machine
2. Tracheostomy tray with appropriate tubes and humidifying equipment
3. Thermometer and blood pressure cuff
4. Masks, gown, and gloves; materials for dressings; and sterile basins
5. Assorted syringes and laboratory blood tubes
6. I.V. standards, tourniquets, alcohol sponges, I.V. sets, assorted I.V. catheters, and anticipated fluids
7. Venous cutdown tray and venous pressure manometer
8. Urinary catheter tray and closed drainage setup with accurate measuring device
9. Suction apparatus with soft catheters
10. Oxygen or compressed air
11. Turning frame of choice (Circ-Olectric bed, Stryker frame)
12. Nasogastric tubes and suction
13. Bed cradle and footboard
14. Tetanus toxoid and antibiotics and other emergency medications such as mannitol, aminophylline, and cardiotonic drugs

Initial care

The patient who has sustained fresh burns is usually mentally alert and apprehensive in the immediate postburn period. Much work needs to be done during this time, but the burn team must not become so technique centered that they fail to recognize the victim's psychological and emotional needs. The patient is in great need of support and reassurance. All procedures must be carefully explained to the sick individual to help allay his fear and apprehension.

At the time of admission, the following steps are taken.

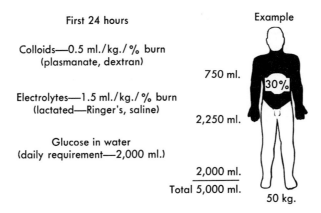

First 24 hours

Colloids—0.5 ml./kg./% burn
(plasmanate, dextran)

750 ml.

Electrolytes—1.5 ml./kg./% burn
(lactated—Ringer's, saline)

2,250 ml.

Glucose in water
(daily requirement—2,000 ml.)

2,000 ml.
Total 5,000 ml.

50 kg.

Example

30%

Fig. 30-3. Estimation of fluid needs by use of Brooke fluid formula.

1. The patient is examined carefully for evidence of any associated injuries, and the airway patency is checked.

2. A large-bore (14- or 16-gauge) I.V. lifeline is established under aseptic conditions. Fluid replacement is essential and receives priority. An accurate record of intake and output is necessary and is a nursing responsibility. The nurse must work closely with the physician to ensure that all orders for fluid replacement are clearly understood and implemented. The rate of fluid administration is directed by the physician, to maintain a urine output of 30 to 50 ml./hr. in the adult and 10 to 30 ml./hr. in children, according to their size. Constant nursing surveillance is needed to keep I.V. infusions on time. Each bottle of solution is clearly labeled with the patient's name, bottle number, medications added, and date and time. In children, I.V. solutions should not be hung in excess of 500 ml., and pediatric control units of 100 ml. should be used in children under 6 years of age. All I.V. sites must be kept as clean as possible and observed closely for signs of infection. The I.V., or cutdown, site is cleansed daily and an occlusive dressing applied. I.V. tubing should be changed at least every twenty-four hours. Solutions should be mixed just prior to administration and not several hours in advance, to minimize the possibility of contamination.

3. A Foley catheter is inserted to monitor the hourly urine output and specific gravity. Any decrease in urinary output below 25 to 30 ml./hr. in the adult or below 10 ml./hr. in the child should be brought to the physician's attention.

As long as the catheter remains in place, the genitalia should be washed carefully twice daily and bacitracin or some similar antibiotic ointment placed around the urethral meatus. The catheter should be taped to the abdomen to relieve traction on the catheter. If the catheter has to be disconnected from the drainage tubing, the free ends should be covered with sterile catheter plugs. Urinary drainage equipment should be changed once a week, unless the drainage tubing becomes contaminated. The urinary catheter is always removed as soon as possible in the postburn course to eliminate a possible source of infection.

4. An analgesic is administered intravenously in amounts specified by the physician, whenever necessary in the immediate postburn period.

5. A brief history of the accident's etiology should be obtained. Whether the fire occurred within an enclosed space should be especially noted, to alert one to the increased possibility of inhalation injury.

6. Blood and urine samples and a culture of the burn wound should be obtained.

7. Temperature, pulse, and respiration rates should be taken every two hours. Blood and venous pressures should be recorded as ordered by the physician. A subnormal temperature can be as significant in a patient with burns as a fever. All temperatures consistently less than 97° F. or above 102° F. should be reported to the physician. A consistently subnormal temperature may herald a lethal gram-negative or fungal infection.

8. Tetanus prophylaxis is given when the patient is admitted. One pattern of treatment is to administer penicillin during the initial burn period to control streptococcal infections. Thereafter antibiotics are ordered as deemed necessary by the physician to control specific infections, indicated by wound culture and sensitivity studies. Initially, all parenteral medications should be administered intravenously, if possible, because of unpredictable absorption from peripheral subcutaneous or intramuscular sites in the acute postburn period.

9. Patients should be weighed on admission. In the initial postburn period, daily weights can be a check on the accuracy of intake and output records, and may be used to predict fluid overloading or deficiency. In the later stages of burn wound healing, weekly body weights will aid the physician and the nurse in assessing the patient's general state of nutrition.

10. A nasogastric tube is inserted and gastric suction maintained if there is any indication of paralytic ileus. All patients suffering burns in excess of 20% of total body surface (TBS) should have a prophylactic nasogastric tube inserted for one to

two days, especially if the patient is a child. Ileus is so predictable that oral fluids should be avoided for at least forty-eight hours in these patients to prevent gastric dilatation and the possibility of vomiting and aspiration of stomach contents. Any solution used to irrigate the nasogastric tube must be measured, recorded, and deducted from the total gastric drainage.

11. After careful medical evaluation, the patient may be taken to a Hubbard tank and gently immersed on a litter into warm tap water (102° F.). The wounds are carefully cleansed with a small amount of surgical soap and debrided of necrotic tissue. The burned area is shaved. This skin preparation should extend at least 2 inches beyond the margin of the wound. With the patient exposed, the physician carefully reexamines the depth and extent of the burn injury and plots his estimates on a diagram. This diagram becomes a useful tool in planning the nursing care and positioning of the patient. The patient is then lifted from the tank and placed in bed, where he will usually complain of feeling cold. This discomfort can be alleviated by the discreet use of heat lamps. If only the lower extremities are burned, a

bed cradle with a sheet and small gooseneck lamps will maintain sufficient warmth.

In patients with circumferential third-degree burns of a limb, the distal circulation to unburned viable tissue may be impaired by rapidly forming edema under burned skin that has lost its elasticity. Frequently the physician will order elevation of the affected limb and passive exercise. Should color not return to normal or sensation remain diminished, escharotomy may be done (Fig. 30-4). It is a simple, effective procedure that can ordinarily be done on the ward by the physician without the use of an anesthetic, since it usually involves areas of insensitive third-degree burns. The use of a portable Doppler flowmeter, if available, has been most helpful in determining when escharotomy is indicated. The surgeon makes an incision through the eschar and subadjacent tissue to allow expansion of the eschar. Emphasis is placed on an adequate release of the eschar over involved joints. The open escharotomy wound can be protected from invasive sepsis by application of the same topical agent used to treat the burn wound.

Mafenide acetate (Sulfamylon) is one of the principal topical forms of chemother-

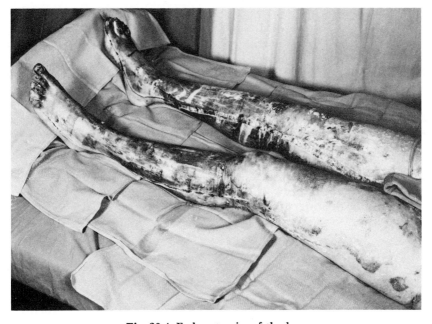

Fig. 30-4. Escharotomies of the legs.

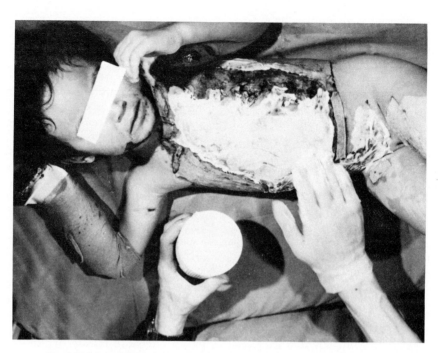

Fig. 30-5. Application of mafenide acetate using sterile gloved hand.

apy employed in the care of the burn patient. It has been found to be most efficacious in reducing the bacterial population of the burn wound between the time of injury and separation of the eschar. The water-soluble, nonstaining medication requires no dressings, thus simplifying nursing care. The cream is gently applied with a sterile gloved hand after initial debridement (Fig. 30-5). Other topical treatments in current use are 0.5% aqueous silver nitrate solution, gentamycin cream, and silver sulfadiazine cream.

12. After the patient is made as comfortable as possible, he should be allowed to see his family. The family should be fully prepared for this visit and accompanied by the patient's physician and nurse. The chaplain should be called to lend support at this difficult time. The medical social worker is also a valuable ally.

PHASE OF ESCHAR SEPARATION

Mafenide acetate (Sulfamylon cream) is applied to the burn wound twice daily and is cleansed from the wound every day. This procedure is usually carried out in the Hubbard tank or by bed bath. The physician inspects the wounds on a daily basis. Debridement is done without anesthesia to the point of bleeding or pain. More frequent application of mafenide acetate may be necessary in an active child or in case of much exudate from the wound. Patients with partial thickness burns often experience pain when this medication is applied and need nursing support. An analgesic may be given prior to application of the cream if necessary. The pain asociated with the hygroscopicity and acid pH of the medication subsides in twenty to thirty minutes. It is advisable for the nurse to stay with the patient during this period of discomfort to explain to him why this medication is necessary and to reassure him. The presence of a member of the family or a nurse is especially comforting to a small child.

Modified isolation procedure

A modified form of reverse isolation may be used in the care of the burn patient. All nursing personnel wear scrub dresses or scrub suits. Personnel assigned to the intensive care area wear masks while in the

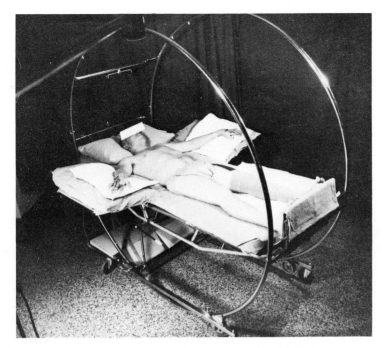

Fig. 30-6. Patient positioned on CircOlectric bed.

area and should change them each time they leave and reenter. Personnel working in the intensive care area must wear clean gowns over their scrub clothes when they leave the area for any length of time, such as for coffee breaks. Individuals working in the ward put on gowns and masks when they enter the intensive care area. These are discarded as soon as they leave the area.

All personnel wash their hands thoroughly with a surgical detergent and water when they enter and leave the intensive care area and between patients. Personnel use sterile disposable gloves when working with the burned patient. Any time that secretions, exudates, or any type of drainage may be contacted, personnel wear gloves. When rectal temperatures are taken, soiled dressings removed, or contaminated areas cleaned, gloves are worn as a protective measure both for personnel and patients.

Linen need not be sterilized, although this is done at many hospitals treating burn patients. Bacteriological studies have shown no pathological organisms present in clean linen returned from the hospital laundry. The linen is brought in a cart and stored in the linen room. It is not refolded, and handling is kept to a minimum. All used linen and waste material are placed in heavy bags and processed as contaminated articles. A number of burn units use sterile linen, total patient isolation, laminar air-flow units, and special foot coverings, but the value of such procedures remains uncertain.

Moving and positioning the patient

Ideally the burn wound should be left exposed after mafenide acetate is applied, but, when the burns are extensive, the patient must necessarily be turned on the wound area for limited periods of time. Turning frames provide the gentlest means of moving a patient frequently. The CircOlectric bed has a wider posterior frame and a slow-controlled turn that is not frightening to the patient or devastating to his vital signs (Fig. 30-6). It also places the patient on the same level as other patients in hospital beds and is probably the most comfortable frame on which to spend long periods of time.

When fractures and other orthopedic problems complicate the care of the pa-

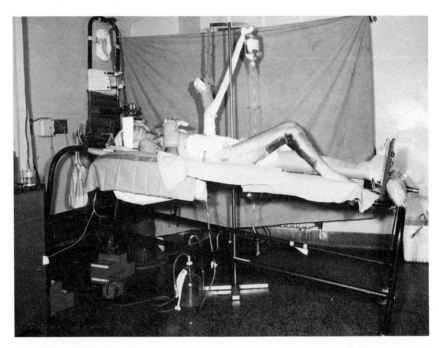

Fig. 30-7. Burned individual with concomitant injuries as positioned on a Foster frame.

tient with burns, the Foster or Stryker frames offer other advantages, since it is possible to maintain traction on fractures in these frames (Fig. 30-7). There is little difference in nursing time involved in turning patients on these frames; they are all heavy and cumbersome. The frame should be shown to the patient before he is placed on it, and the method of turning should be explained to him before it is done.

Because of the patient discomfort involved, all movement should be planned and purposeful. The patient's daily bath can be completed in the Hubbard or similar tank, and a shampoo can be given with minimal discomfort of movement. Nursing care must be planned around treatment and turn schedules. Linen is changed at the time of turning from the posterior to the anterior frame (i.e., from prone to supine). The patient must be checked for patency of his airway each time that he is turned to a prone position.

A sterile paper-backed pad with an absorbent cotton filling and a fine mesh gauze covering is placed under the patient's wounds. These pads absorb the wound exudate, and the fine-mesh gauze covering prevents painful adherence of the surface of the pads to the wound. A hole must be cut in the pad at the buttocks area and the patient positioned carefully over this aperture to allow evacuation of stool and urine with minimal contamination of the wound. Perineal care should be provided whenever needed.

When the patient is lifted, adequate personnel must be assembled to perform this task gently and with minimal discomfort. If a patient is able to cooperate, he should be instructed to hold himself as stiff as possible. In this position, he can be lifted at the shoulders or occiput and the feet and avoid painful pressure on his burned skin. Another means of minimizing discomfort is to have several persons lift the patient with the pads in place protecting the wounds.

Patients with burns are subject to all the respiratory problems that can complicate any bedridden surgical patient's recovery. In spite of the painful and impaired movement that results from extensive burns, patients must be ambulated as soon as possible. It is the nurse's responsibility to teach patients to cough and deep breathe and to change their position in bed. If the patient does not cough well after proper instruction and encouragement, the physician should be notified, and intermittent positive-pressure breathing may have to be initiated. When ambulation is not feasible, the patient can at least be lifted into a wheelchair so that he may sit up for meals. This improves his state of well-being and his ventilation. The heavy wooden old-fashioned wheelchair, with legs that can be elevated and a reclining back, is the most comfortable chair for the person with burns. Patients with burns of the lower extremity should have their legs elevated at all times, with equal pressure along the entire length of the limb. Burned upper extremities should be elevated above heart level, with the hands supported in a position of function. If a patient has sustained burns of the neck, a pillow should not be used. Contractures develop easily with neck burns, and the head should be hyperextended as much as possible while the wounds are healing.

Eye care

The eye itself is not usually damaged during a thermal accident. An individual instinctively shuts his eyes when confronted with flame. The lids, however, are very susceptible to thermal injury. Routine eye care is important when a patient has sustained facial burns. In the initial postburn period, he may not be able to open his eyes because of extensive edema (Fig. 30-8). This person must be reassured, after examination, that his blindness is temporary and will clear up when the swelling subsides. In the event that the patient cannot completely close his eyes, the physician will order eye irrigations with normal saline and the instillation of a protective ophthalmic ointment to prevent corneal ulcerations.

It is a nursing responsibility to provide eye care. Nursing personnel must be taught to speak to the sightless patient before they touch him. Patients who have a vision loss in one eye should not be placed in a bed with their functioning eye toward the wall. The ward orientation and training should be from a fixed location. If some corrective procedure on the eyelids is necessary, such

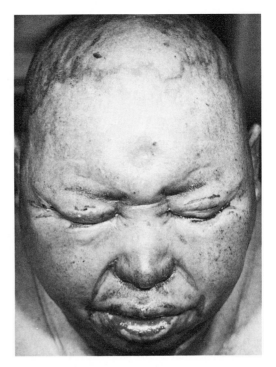

Fig. 30-8. Facial edema in the early postburn phase.

as tarsorrhaphy, the patient should be informed that the procedure is to be done and that any resultant impairment in vision is temporary.

Ear care

The skin of the external ear is very thin, and burns in this area require special nursing attention. If a chondritis develops in the burned ear, incision and removal of the necrotic cartilage is necessary.

The ears are not submerged during routine immersion in the Hubbard tank. It is the nurse's responsibility to inspect the ears and to clean them carefully. The external canal must be cleansed gently with applicators, and topical medications or physiological dressings should be applied. Pillows should not be placed under the head of a patient who has ear burns. A sponge pad or a rolled towel at the occiput will provide comfortable support without being a source of irritation to the wound itself. Enclosure of the ears in occlusive dressings is not advised because of the incidence of bacterial proliferation and the resulting possibility of infection.

Tracheostomy care

The three basic reasons for performing a tracheostomy are (1) to prevent or treat mechanical airway obstruction, (2) to provide efficient tracheobronchial toilet by removing secretions, and (3) to prevent the aspiration of swallowed substances in patients who are unable to protect their own airways. A principal indication for tracheostomy has been the prolonged need for ventilator support (more that three days). The patient with thermal injury must be monitored closely and the indications for such a procedure anticipated and carried out under optimum conditions of safety by a physician with adequate nursing support.

Each time the nasopharynx or trachea is suctioned, a new, sterile, soft rubber catheter is inserted. After each catheter is used, it is discarded. Personnel wear sterile, disposable gloves when performing tracheostomy care and oral or nasal suctioning (Fig. 30-9). Suctioning of the trachea requires skill and care on the part of the nurse, technician, or physician. Suctioning must be carefully and gently performed to prevent traumatizing the trachea. The patient is never to be suctioned for longer than ten to fifteen seconds at any one time. Patients must have confidence in the personnel. After insertion of the catheter into the trachea, one should not maintain a continuous flow of air but should intermittently lift the finger on the open end of the Y-connection so as not to deplete the patient of oxygen or suck up tracheal mucosa into the catheter. Overly enthusiastic suctioning may be as harmful to the patient as neglect. If the patient becomes restless or agitated, one should check the patency of the airway at once; the patient may be hypoxic. The inner cannula should be removed, and, if the outer cannula has an air cuff on it, the cuff should be deflated; then aspiration should be tried again. If there is any question of cannula patency, the physician must be called immediately.

Nursing personnel must be familiar with ventilatory equipment and the significance of blood gas determinations. The air cuff on the outer cannula should be deflated at regular intervals for a set period of time to minimize trauma and the possibility of ischemic necrosis of the trachea.

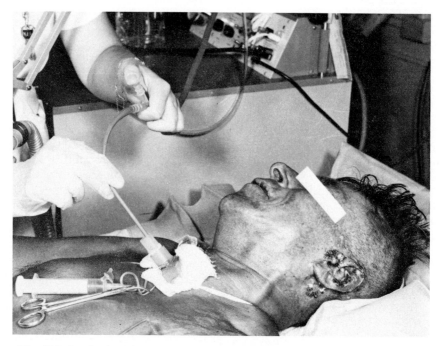

Fig. 30-9. Suctioning of a tracheostomy, showing use of sterile disposable gloves.

Dressings

The gentle application of a comfortable dressing is an essential nursing skill in the care of patients with burn wounds. The dressing material should be prepared in advance, using sterile technique, and carried on a tray or table to the patient's bedside or used in a special dressing room. It is important that the nurse or technician think ahead and assemble all needed material before donning sterile gloves and a mask to apply the dressing. Abandoning a patient halfway through a dressing change to retrieve forgotten equipment can be an unnecessary cause of discomfort.

After the bulk of the eschar has separated, frequently changed wet dressings may be employed to promote further debridement of the wound and prepare the recipient site for grafting. Coarse-mesh gauze is applied next to the wound defect when debridement is desired. These dressings *must* be changed every four to six hours and should not be applied to more than 20% of the body surface at any one time (Fig. 30-10).

Dressings can be gently removed and reapplied without causing undue pain and discomfort. It is important that the dressings be thoroughly wet down before they are removed. A dry dressing, carelessly pulled off an open wound, causes severe and unnecessary pain. Nursing personnel should explain the procedure to the patient in terms that he can understand. An informed patient is more cooperative and comfortable. The physician may be asked to order an appropriate analgesic if it is anticipated that a particular dressing change will cause excessive pain.

Fine-mesh gauze is employed in dressing new graft sites. A single layer is applied once around the circumference of an arm or leg and cut. (Continuous circumferential wrapping is avoided.) This procedure is repeated until the wound is covered. Gauze applied in this manner does not restrict circulation, causes less shearing effect on movement of the extremity and is easily removed. A gauze dressing, 16 inches wide, is applied over the fine-mesh gauze.

Circumferential outer Curlex or gauze rolls are started at the distal part of extremities and advanced proximally. Undue pressure is to be avoided over joints. A snug, comfortable covering that will re-

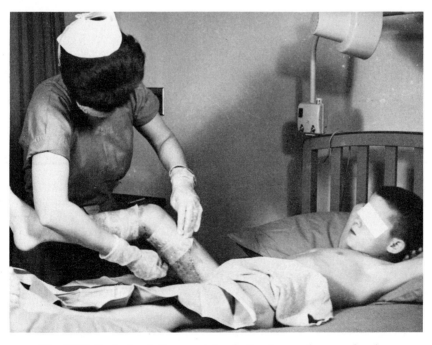

Fig. 30-10. Patient assisting nurse in placing fine-mesh gauze dressing.

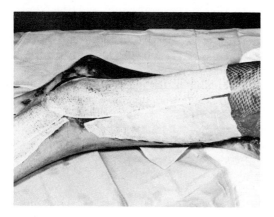

Fig. 30-11. Placement of porcine xenografts next to mesh autograft.

main in place without restricting circulation is the goal of a well-applied dressing.

The nurse, through study and observation, must develop a knowledge of the pathophysiology of the burn wound and report any suspicious areas of discoloration, hemorrhage, unusual exudate, or swelling to the physician immediately. Frequent biopsies of suspect areas will aid in the early histological diagnosis of bacterial, fungal, or viral invasion.

Viable skin grafts obtained under aseptic conditions from human cadavers or animals (usually porcine) and used as temporary physiological dressings control bacterial growth in the burn wound and appear to encourage development of granulation tissue after separation of the eschar. These temporary skin coverings are changed every two to four days or more frequently if there is an accumulation of purulent exudate under the graft (Fig. 30-11).

These temporary grafts help further debride the burn and reduce pain and heat losses from the wound, while preparing the area for autografting.

RECONSTRUCTION

Expeditious closure with autograft is the final goal in burn wound care. Patients anticipate the surgery and should be psychologically prepared for the event. In addition to counseling the patient and his family, the nurse must know what donor sites will be used and what portions of the wound will be grafted. In light of this information, an appropriate recovery bed must be selected and prepared and special splints, or immobilization devices, fabricated by the occupational therapist.

After grafting procedures, such as utilizing the back for the donor area, the patient will of necessity remain prone for a prolonged period, usually about ten to fourteen days, until the donor area is healed. This position is sustained best on the anterior frame of a circular electric bed. The patient should be informed that he will be in this position before he goes to surgery and, if possible, shown the bed. The prevention of decubitus ulcers during this recovery period is of utmost importance. Antidecubitus pads are useful beneath the chest area and under other pressure points —the knees, shoulders, and especially the iliac crests.

The patient must be carefully positioned over the aperture in the frame to provide for elimination of excreta. When it is necessary for the patient to defecate in this position, bed protectors and gauze can be placed between the thighs to keep the perineum clean. This unusual exposure of a private function causes the patient some embarrassment, and he must be reassured that he will not soil himself and that this method will meet his needs. The bed curtains should be drawn and the patient provided as much privacy as possible.

A mesh bed constructed from nylon netting and affixed to a modified Bradford frame is used occasionally for patients with both dorsal and ventral burn wounds (Fig. 30-12). This allows air to reach the burn and donor sites for drying purposes and allows better wound drainage. The bed is of value in caring for patients who have incurred fractures in addition to their burns, since it can be placed over the Hubbard tank and the patient gently immersed while still in traction. It is important that exposed surfaces, such as the elbow, be protected from abrasion on netting.

The air-fluidized bed has proved to be useful in the care of patients being prepared for or undergoing autografting or both (Fig. 30-13). It permits the patient's being placed in a position of comfort when the donor sites are on his back and the

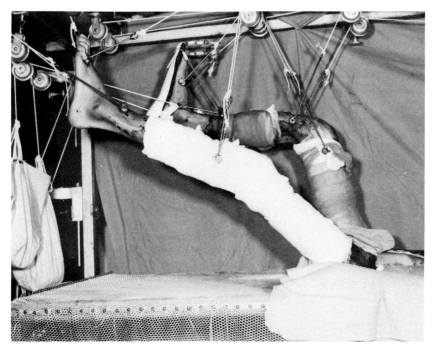

Fig. 30-12. Burned individual in balanced traction on mesh bed.

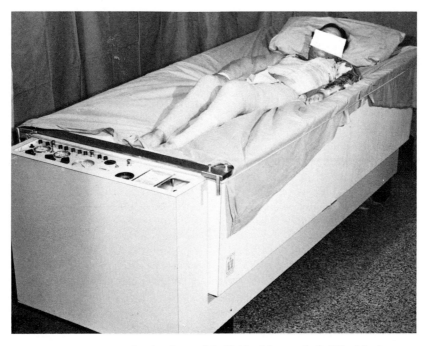

Fig. 30-13. Convalescing burned individual in an air-fluidized bed.

recipient areas are on the chest or abdomen, yet avoids wound maceration.

Small children may be placed in the prone position in their cribs on pediatric mattresses that fit over the ordinary mattresses. They are constructed with a central hole to provide for elimination. This hole can be covered with plastic if desired. A disposable paper container is inserted to fit closely into this space. The child must be placed carefully over this aperature and gently but firmly restrained if necessary. Young children are especially agile in escaping from restraints. One scratch can damage a donor area or tear a graft. It is imperative that children be watched closely, since, even with the best supervision, they invariably shear off more skin than an adult. Soft, quilted ankle and wrist restraints are used when necessary. Children do not require a turning frame. One or two persons can easily lift a small child in the prone position to provide needed hygiene and nursing care.

Care of donor sites is important, since it may be necessary to recrop the area a second time to provide skin for coverage of several areas of the burn wound. The donor site is covered in the operating room with fine-mesh gauze and is allowed to dry, with the help of infrared heat lamps. Once the sites are dry, the patient's discomfort diminishes. Gradual reepithelialization takes place beneath the fine-gauze until, at the end of approximately fourteen days, new skin is in place. The fine-mesh gauze must not be prematurely removed.

Nutrition

Nutritional needs of the burn patient must be carefully monitored. The burned individual has an increased metabolic rate and greatly increased caloric requirements. Balance studies have indicated a need for two to three times daily average food requirements (4,000-6,000 calories a day for adults). The usual diet fed to the burned patient is high in calories, protein, and carbohydrate. Emphasis must be placed on the role of nursing personnel in encouraging between-meal snacks such as fruit juices, milk shakes, and high-calorie protein supplements mixed with milk and chocolate syrup to augment routine caloric intake.

Weight loss in the burn patient may be as high as one third or more of body weight. If he does not consume the required number of calories daily, I.V. hyperalimentation may be required to achieve caloric balance. After a central venous catheter has been surgically inserted and determined, by x-ray film, to be properly placed, hyperalimentation mixtures may be administered. The usual schedule is to administer 1,500 calories a day and increase by increments of 500 calories a day until adequate calories are received daily by the patient. Many patients are able to tolerate no more than 2,500 calories a day and have problems when this amount is exceeded. Urine specimens should be tested for sugar and acetone at least four times a day. Physicians will order frequent determinations of blood glucose and serum electrolyte levels if hyperglycemia or dehydration or both are suspected. Insulin may be administered if needed, as well as trace elements not commonly supplied in standard I.V. solutions.

The administration of hypertonic glucose solutions requires careful nursing care regarding the site of administration and the venous catheter used for administration. A large, long catheter is percutaneously inserted into a brachial external jugular or subclavian vein and is directed into the superior vena cava. Infrequently the catheter may be inserted into the femoral vein and directed toward the inferior vena cava. The nursing staff is responsible for proper skin care around the entrance site of the catheter. The area of insertion is checked frequently by the physician for erythema and local infection and the site changed at his discretion, generally every two to three days.

Nasogastric tube feedings may be ordered by a patient's physician as a substitute for or supplement to routine oral feedings. The usual tube feeding preparation provides 1 calorie per ml. of solution. Administration of tube feedings varies according to patient needs. A size 8 or 10 French feeding catheter is preferred, to minimize irritation of the nasopharynx and esophagus. Prior to each feeding, the stomach is aspirated. If 50 to 100 ml. of fluid are aspirated before two consecutive feedings, the physician must be notified to rule out the danger of paralytic ileus and gastric distention. The feedings are removed from the refrigerator and administered within the time limit set by the patient's physician. Feedings are given by syringe, Murphy drip method, or Baron pump. The nasogastric tube is rinsed with 30 to 50 ml. of tap water after each feeding.

THE PATIENT AS A PERSON

The nurse must familiarize herself with the patient, as well as the burn injury and the protocols of therapy, even though maintaining a professional detachment. Initially, the person is often confused and uncooperative. During this time, the nurse must remember that restraints are a tool, not the solution. Anyone who has worked at the side of a confused patient has learned that reassurance and the knowledge that someone is there calms the disoriented far more than do restraints. However, at times an attendant cannot be constantly at the bedside. Therefore bedrails and other appropriate restraints are needed to keep the burned, confused person from harm. Causes of confusion should be documented to rule out serious physiological system failure due to sepsis, shock, and hypoxia.

Certainly, if the person has periods of lucidity, finding himself shackled must come as a shock if not an insult. Therefore the nurse must be nearby to explain the use of restraints. Whenever possible, restraints should be released when the patient seems oriented and someone can be present to help him. Reality must be reinforced. Tell the sick person where he is and what happened to him, and assure him that he is being cared for. Let him know if his family is nearby. Nursing personnel must never treat the comatose or semicomatose patient as an inanimate object or a disease entity. It is impossible to know what the sick person hears and understands or misunderstands. The entire staff must consistently speak and act as though each patient were coherent and conscious. The time spent with a patient carrying out nursing tasks can be doubly therapeutic if the nurse works at establishing rapport with the person that she is tending. An awareness of the person's feelings and apprehensions and an appropriate response to these needs are the marks of a professional nurse.

Sensory deprivation

Persons caring for burned patients have noted that the latter may show signs of sensory deprivation. There are two facets to this problem: the patient is isolated because of the nature and extent of his injury and the loss of tactile sensation in areas of third-degree burns. In extensive second-degree burns, the patient is apparently overwhelmed by incoming sensations, due to a lack of protective integument. Excessive neural stimulation and resultant fatigue may cause inability to respond in a normal pattern. In the face of overwhelming stimulus-response requirements, a form of protection may be developed within the central nervous system, and stimuli may not be interpreted as such.

Many burn patients experience periods of disorientation. In those who have severe injuries, such disorientation might be the result of diminished sensory input. Another pattern of hallucinatory response may result from a combination of sensory deprivation or acute sensory stimulation and toxicity resulting from infection. A patient who becomes disoriented will be carefully evaluated by the physician to determine the cause of his hallucinations.

Frequently patients who have had no serious disorientation will develop difficulties when they are "isolated" through the application of facial dressings or wraps. Disoriented patients need to be brought back to reality. One of the nurse's primary responsibilities is to help the patient maintain his contact with his environment. Telling the patient the day of the week and the date of the month each morning at first greeting is one method of keeping the patient time oriented. Individuals have the shared need of face-to-face contact with other persons, whether or not they have been injured. This need must be met by nursing personnel and members of the patient's family. When a person has facial dressings, individuals talking to him should stand directly in his line of vision. When he is in a prone position, people should place themselves within his visual perimeters. Families can sit on low stools while visiting, and burn unit personnel may bend or kneel so that the patient is able to see their faces. A mirror may be attached to the turning frame so that the patient may use it as a periscope to see what is going on around him. Prism glasses are also useful in bending the line of vision.

Patients with burns have a loss of tactile sensations resulting in misinterpretation of the size and position of objects. Nursing personnel should work closely with burn-care physicians in explaining such phenomena. Patients should be informed that the lost sensations will return over time, although some changes may be inevitable. Tactile losses play a role in patient hallucination. These losses must be considered by the nursing staff when the patient complains of uncertainty concerning physical sensations.

Teaching the burn patient how to wear and use a prosthetic device may be difficult when the amputation site has been the site of burns. Amputees are dependent, to some degree, on stump sensations for aid in placing and using prosthetic devices, and the burned amputee therefore faces additional problems of adjustment. The stump may require autografting and delay shaping and prosthetic fitting.

Sociological patterns

Nurses often are concerned with a patient's life patterns. It is important to discover from a patient's family what type of personality he had prior to his burn injury. For example, what foods does he prefer? Is he normally withdrawn or outgoing? Is he usually sedentary or active? Nursing personnel caring for long-term patients should know the answers to such questions to be better able to plan nursing care and rehabilitation. Although the foregoing does not play a major role in the physical care of burn patients, it contributes to a better understanding of sociological patterns and allows the nurse to assist the patient in adjusting to his disabilities.

Mutual aid

Burn patients appear to progress more rapidly when they are near other patients with burns than when isolated from other patients. They may be placed in four-bed cubicles on relatively open wards. They show pleasure as they progress from the acute-care areas of a burn unit to the convalescent parts of it. They aid one another in many ways, both physical and psychological. Mutual aid is given particularly when patients are preparing for discharge; they seem to bind themselves together in common interests and problems.

The physical closeness of the patients seems to serve as a form of mutual support. Burn patients do not care to be alone when they leave the ward to go to the cafeteria or barber shop or for a walk. Husbands and wives may leave together to visit such areas; however, they are frequently accompanied by another burn patient. When members of a patient's family are not present, two or three patients will accompany each other. Patients have stated that they do not feel "too different" from other hospital patients when several of them are together. When alone for any reason, such as flying home, patients have stated that their "aloneness" upsets them at times. This is particularly true when individuals, especially children, stare at them or make remarks concerning their burn deformities. With family assistance, patients think that they will be able to overcome the majority of these difficulties in interpersonal relations.

Family

The role of the burn patient's family is extremely important. The individual's perception of his family's acceptance of his altered appearance has an effect on the patient's motivation and attitude toward his injuries. Patients should be given a mirror when they ask for it. The actual changes in their physiognomy might not be so bad as they had imagined. Changes seen in himself by the patient and his family's expectations in view of his injuries develop the new patient-family relationship.

Studies carried out in Great Britain have revealed the feelings of a number of parents toward their burned children. Some of the parents were shown to have been unaccepting of their children's disfigurements. In several instances, divorce followed the burn injuries of a child. Marital problems that existed prior to the accident precipitated insoluble situations.

Parents of burned children frequently demonstrate guilt feelings that persist after the burns have healed or especially if the child has died. The mother tends to blame herself for the child's accident, and, on occasion, this feeling is reinforced by the attitude of her husband. Possibly guilt feelings play a part in the unwillingness of parents to wait until burn scars have matured to begin reconstructive surgery. Personnel caring for burned children need to recognize these guilt feelings and the hostilities that may emanate from them.

A similar situation develops when one marital partner has been burned and the other is unwilling or unable to accept the injury. Discussions with social workers have revealed that divorce usually follows for those who had marital problems prior to occurrence of the burn. The injury and resultant changes precipitate but do not appear to be the underlying cause of divorce in these patients. For many couples, injury to one marital partner appears to lead to a closer relationship and better understanding.

Family assistance in helping the patient face his injuries cannot be overemphasized in his rehabilitation. The attitude of the family influences the patient's outlook. If the family indicates withdrawal and inability to accept the injuries, so does the patient. Reassurance of a man by his wife that she expects him to resume his prior role is beneficial. The person who is wanted and needed works to return to his family.

Extraunit personnel

Social worker. The well-trained social worker involved with burn patients and their families assists them in many ways. Members of a family may be interviewed on an individual basis in an effort to work out potential problem areas between patients and their families. Weekly meetings of social-service personnel, family members, and invited burn unit staff may be of value to these families. In these sessions, families may ventilate hostilities, aggressions, fears, and general anxieties. Material discussed in such meetings often has been discussed within the families prior to these sessions. Discussions in an open meeting led by a sympathetic impartial counselor often lead to beneficial catharsis and acceptance of a previously unacceptable decision concerning their relatives. Attendance by unit staff members enables families to ask generalized questions concerning care being given, and association with relatives of other patients undergoing the same psychological turmoil creates an atmosphere of mutual support. Group meetings of social workers and convalescing burn patients can bring out common fears of these patients. Methods of coping with anticipated difficulties, such as departure from the hospital, can be explored in such meetings.

The chaplain. The clinically prepared chaplain working with burn patients receives many calls for assistance and counseling from patients, families, and burn unit personnel. Patients must be encouraged to discuss their feelings regarding their injuries and their concept of other reactions. A patient's relationship with the chaplain should be a secure one.

The clergyman meets the spiritual needs of the burn patient in many ways. He solaces the patient and is ready to pray with him should the need arise. He understands the patient's feelings of guilt and interprets his frustrations.

The chaplain should be capable of helping the patient to help himself in accepting his injuries and anticipated disabilities. He must work with the patient's family as they learn to accept the situation, and he must be able to relate to burn unit personnel, so that they in turn can rely on him as an individual with common goals and interests.

Allied medical services

Three therapeutic disciplines, in addition to medicine and nursing, play major roles in burn therapy: diet, physical, and occupational therapy. The practitioners of each apply training in a special area and add their expertise to the overall care of burn patients.

Diet therapy. Nutrition, as mentioned previously, plays an important role in the healing of the burn wound. In addition to diet management, the dietitian copes with the common problem of anorexia. Malaise, fatigue, and discomfort contribute to lack of appetite. When they are able, patients must be encouraged to eat and feed themselves to achieve independence, maintain motion, and minimize contractures.

A dietitian assigned to a burn unit serves in several capacities. When working with burn patients, her primary responsibilities are to provide palatable food, calorie counts, tube feedings, and assistance in metabolic studies. Calorie counts are monitored on specific patients at the request of the physician. By this means, an effort is made to define and treat subtle metabolic problems reflected by the kinds and amounts of food consumed by these patients.

Physical therapy. Physical therapists perform an extremely important function in a burn center. They assist physicians in debridement and range-of-motion exercises, when the patient is in the hydrotherapy tank. Therapists can also assist by cleansing the patient while he is in the tank. He has little additional discomfort when this is done carefully.

The aim of physical therapy is to prevent loss of motion, preserve joint function, and minimize contractures. Physical therapy should commence when a patient is admitted to the unit and continue until the time of discharge. Therapy is discontinued for forty-eight hours after the application of autografts. Unit therapists keep careful records concerning joint mobility and loss of motion and sensation. Those patients with second-degree burns involving any given joint should lose no motion if they exercise as directed.

Occupational therapy. Occupational therapists similarly are concerned with the prevention of loss of motion and with facilitating the burn patient's ability to carry out the various activities of daily living. Whenever feasible, these personnel begin the training that will be needed by amputees as they learn to use prosthetic devices.

An active program of positioning and splinting, dynamic and static, is enforced in an effort to minimize deformities. Efforts are made to help the burned patient

help himself, through the use of feeding blocks, plate guards, and smoking tubes, or "smokers" (Fig. 30-14). Self-sufficiency is encouraged. After discharge from a burn unit, the occupational therapist more fully enters into the rehabilitative phase of postburn care.

Consulting specialties. Burned patients often require medical assistance beyond that given in the care of their burn wounds. General medical problems, fractures, or amputations must be treated simultaneously with the burns. One or both hands may be burned and require special efforts to maintain function. Orthopedic surgeons often are called for consultations concerning complicated fracture reductions, the application of skeletal traction, and the positioning of limbs.

The burned patient often develops cosmetic problems related to scarring of the face, head, and hands that lead to difficulty in interpersonal relations. Facial scars, like other burn scars, ordinarily require a period of maturation prior to revision. Patients whose ears have been destroyed by third-degree burns or chondritis may require prosthetic ears prior to or instead of reconstruction. They should be taught how to color, position, and affix such prostheses.

Patients with scalp burns frequently have irregular hair patterns due to scarring or grafting and may require hairpieces that can be procured through a hospital purchasing agent or individually. Patients

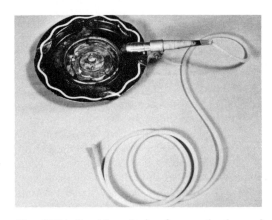

Fig. 30-14. Smoking device for use by burned individuals.

state that they are more comfortable in public with the hairpiece, and every effort should be made to provide an adequate wig or toupee prior to hospital discharge.

Returning home

Leaving the hospital is looked forward to by all but a few burn patients. Plans for reunion with family and friends are an important morale booster. Some degree of anxiety is involved with preparation for this leave-taking: the patient wonders how he will be received by the persons he loves and how he will react to strangers who stare.

The burned individual poses many questions about himself that he alone will be able to answer in the future. Many of the questions are rhetorical, but common to all burned patients. How will the general public accept him? Will the disfigurements that he has be accepted by his family and friends? Will he and his wife be able to resume married life as they knew it, or, if not, what changes will be required?

The patient's physical appearance after a period of convalescence away from the hospital is indicative of his desire to help himself and overcome his handicaps. Patients who are well motivated toward recovery will return to the unit with improved or static ranges of motion of involved joints if they have continued to use night splints and exercise as directed. A patient may return with flexion contractures because he did not exercise or wear splints as directed. He may return with abraded areas on his wounds because he failed to cleanse himself, therefore delaying his eventual discharge from the hospital. The usual burn patient uses his periods away from the hospital to prepare for a constructive and prosperous life in society. Many hours of counseling and guidance may be required as he works through his problems and seeks reestablishment in the wider world in preference to prolonged hospitalization. Be aware of the malingerer who inflicts factitious wounds on himself to delay expulsion from the protective hospital environment.

Nurses who care for burn patients find that they must sharpen all their skills. Nursing observations aid in treatment pre-scribed by the physician. The nurse must be able to respond quickly to rapidly changing conditions. The nurse carries more responsibility in the care of burn patients, necessitating decisions and direction of others in accomplishing needed care.

The team relationship among physicians, nurses, and technicians should be stressed. Physicians are dependent on nurses and technicians for assistance and observations. Nurses are dependent on physicians for translation of these observations into therapeutic plans. The technicians are skilled individuals who are able to perform many nursing-related tasks to maintain patient care at a constant level of excellence.

Personnel caring for burned individuals must recognize the high-stress situation in which they find themselves. The complexity of burn intensive care requires constant spans of attention and quick reaction. Fatigue leading to depression may undermine function in emergency situations. The morale of burn unit personnel thrives on the knowledge that each individual can depend on other unit members. There is a mutual sence of trust, and each person feels that the work load is evenly shared.

Care of the burned individual is challenging but may be traumatic to the young inexperienced nurse. Yet the satisfaction derived from total involvement in patient care, from admission to final recovery, allows the nurse to mature quickly and to thrive on the intense relationships and challenges presented in a burn center.

Bibliography

Andreasen, N. J. C., Norris, A. S., and Hartford, C. E.: Incidence of long-term psychiatric complications in severely burned adults, Ann. Surg. **174:**785, 1971.

Andreasen, N. J. C., Noyes, R. J., Hartford, C. E., Brodland, G., and Proctor, S.: Management of emotional reactions in seriously burned patients, N. Engl. J. Med. **286:**65, 1972.

Artz, C. P., and Hargest, T. S., editors: Air fluidized bed clinical and research symposium, Charleston, 1971, Medical University of South Carolina.

Artz, C. P., and Moncrief, J. A.: The treatment of burns, ed. 2, New York, 1969, W. B. Saunders Co.

Boswick, J. A., and Stone, N. H.: Profiles of burn management. II. Emergency and intermediate treatment, and adaptations for definitive care in a general hospital, Ind. Med. Surg. 37:665, 1968.

Bromberg, B. E.: Burn wound management with

biologic dressings, N. Y. State J. Med. **70:**1645, 1970.

Bruck, H. M., Asch, M. J., and Pruitt, B. A., Jr.: Burns in children; a 10-year experience with 412 children, J. Trauma **10:**658, 1970.

Sister Mary Claudia: TLC and sulfamylon for burned children, Am. J. Nurs. **69:**755, 1969.

Curreri, P. W., and Pruitt, B. A., Jr.: Evaluation and treatment of the burned patient, Am. J. Occup. Ther. **24** (7):1, 1970.

DiVincenti, F. C., Moncrief, J. A., and Pruitt, B. A., Jr.: Electrical injuries; a review of 65 cases, J. Trauma **9:**492, 1969.

Foley, F. D.: The burn autopsy; fatal complications of burns, Am. J. Clin. Pathol. **52:**1, 1969.

Henley, N. L.: Sulfamylon for burns, Am. J. Nurs. **69:**2122, 1969.

Hoshal, V. L., Jr., Ause, R. G., and Hoskins, P. A.: Fibrin sleeve formation on indwelling subclavian central venous catheters, Arch. Surg. **102:**353, 1971.

Hummel, R. P., MacMillan, B. G., and Altemeier, W. A.: Topical and systemic antibacterial agents in the treatment of burns, Ann. Surg. **172:**370, 1970.

Hummel, R. P., MacMillan, B. G., Maley, M., and Altemeier, W. A.: Reverse isolation in the treatment of burns, J. Trauma **10:**450, 1970.

Lamb, F. S., Silvan, Y., Jr., and Walt, A. J.: Thomas Blizard Curling—the man and the ulcer, Surgery **64:**646, 1971.

MacMillan, B. G., Hummel, R. P., and Altemeier, W. A.: The influence of controlled environment on the management of burn patients. In Matter, P., Barday, T. L., and Konickova, Z., editors: Research in burns, Bern, Switzerland, 1970, Hans Huber, pp. 248-251.

Minckley, B. B.: Expert nursing care of burned patients, Am. J. Nurs. **70:**1888, 1970.

Monafo, W. W.: The treatment of burns; principles and practice, St. Louis, 1971, W. H. Green, Inc.

Moncrief, J. A., Rose, L. R., and Switzer, W. E.: Burn therapy—a requirement for team effort, South. Med. J. **56:**1063, 1963.

Moyer, C. A.: Burns and cold injury. In Moyer, C. A., editor: Surgery, principles and practice, ed. 3, Philadelphia, 1964, J. B. Lippincott Co.

Moylan, J. A., Jr., Inge, W. W., Jr., and Pruitt, B. A., Jr.: Circulatory changes following circumferential extremity burns evaluated by the ultrasonic flowmeter; an analysis of 60 thermally injured limbs, J. Trauma **11:**763, 1971.

Munster, A. M., DiVincenti, F. C., Foley, F. D., and Pruitt, B. A., Jr.: Cardiac infections in burns, Am. J. Surg. **122:**524, 1971.

Munster, A. M., and Pruitt, B. A., Jr.: Recent advances in the management of burns, Med. J. Aust. **1:**484, 1971.

Nash, G., Foley, F. D., Goodwin, M. N., Jr., Bruck, H. M., Greenwald, K. M., and Pruitt, B. A., Jr.: Fungal burn wound infections, J.A.M.A. **215:**1664, 1971.

Ollstein, R. N., Cukelair, G. F., Symonds, F. C., and Corliss, S.: The burn center concept, Hosp. Manage. **3** (1):22, 1971.

Order, S. E., and Moncrief, J. A.: The burn wound, Springfield, Ill., 1965, Charles C Thomas, Publisher.

Pruitt, B. A., Jr.: Current treatment of thermal injury, South. Med. J. **64:**657, 1971.

Pruitt, B. A., Jr., and Curreri, P. W.: The burn wound and its care, Arch. Surg. **103:**461, 1971.

Pruitt, B. A., Jr., and Silverstein, P.: Methods of resurfacing denuded skin areas, Transplantation Proc. **3:**1537, 1971.

Reckler, J., and Mason, A. D., Jr.: A critical evaluation of fluid resuscitation in the burned patient, Ann. Surg. **174:**115, 1971.

Shuck, J. M., Pruitt, B. A., Jr., and Moncrief, J. A.: Homograft skin for wound coverage; a study in versatility, Arch. Surg. **98:**472, 1969.

Silverstein, P., and Dressler, D. P.: Effect of current therapy on burn mortality, Ann. Surg. **171:**124, 1970.

Smets, H., Friedman, L. R.: Prolonged venous catheterization as a cause of sepsis, N. Engl. J. Med. **276:**1229, 1967.

Snyder, W. H., Bowles, B. M., and MacMillan, B. G.: The use of expansion meshed grafts in the acute and reconstructive management of the thermal injury; a clinical evaluation, J. Trauma **10:**740, 1970.

Stein, J. M., and Pruitt, B. A., Jr.: Suppurative thrombophlebitis, N. Engl. J. Med. **282:**1452, 1970.

White, M. G., and Asch, M. J.: Acid-base effects of topical mafenide acetate in the burned patient, N. Engl. J. Med. **284:**1281, 1971.

Williams, B. P.: Life styles of severely burned men. In ANA Clinical Conferences, 1969, Minneapolis/Atlanta, New York, 1970, Appleton-Century-Crofts, pp. 242-252.

Wilmore, D. W.: The future of intravenous therapy, Am. J. Nurs. **71:**2334, 1971.

Wilmore, D. W., Curreri, P. W., Spitzer, K. W., Spitzer, M. E., and Pruitt, B. A., Jr.: Supranormal dietary intake in thermally injured hypermetabolic patients, Surg. Gynecol. Obstet. **132:**881, 1971.

Woodward, J. M.: The burnt child and his family; the impact on the family, Proc. R. Soc. Med. **61:**1087, 1968.

Zawacki, B. E., DiVincenti, F. C., and Moncrief, J. A.: The effect of topical sulfamylon on the insensible weight loss of burned patients, Ann. Surg. **169:**259, 1969.

31

A perspective on chronic obstructive pulmonary disease

Patsy A. Perry

Currently, chronic obstructive pulmonary disease (COPD) is a major health problem, constituting the foremost cause of disability under Social Security and a death rate that is increasing annually at more than 20%.[1] Societal focus on air pollution, coupled with the need to provide more effective care for individuals with COPD, has stimulated the birth of emergency respiratory care centers. However, the incidence of COPD continues to rise. This rise in incidence is due to multiple factors, of which complex psychological and physiological stresses play a major role.

The individual with COPD is one who, for undetermined or questionable reasons, has developed a decrease in pulmonary function that poses a threat to life and productivity. Once this decrease in function becomes apparent, the individual attempts to adjust his behavior to the failing system. Gradually the individual realizes that little of definite value can be done for him and, with this realization, come emotional problems, which continually increase in severity. Subsequently, the individual may become angry and self-destructive, or he may feel overwhelmed by the seeming hopelessness of the situation and succumb to depression. Regardless of his response, however, he pays a psychological and physiological price.[2]

Breathlessness is an inherent component of the progression of pulmonary disease. Therefore the patient's response to breathlessness seems to be a critical variable, and a consideration of breathlessness necessitates an in-depth analysis of the meaning of the concept of breath. From earliest biblical times, when God breathed the breath of life into Adam's nostrils; in the prehistoric period, during which magical and invisible powers were ascribed to breath; and during the Egyptian, Indian, Chinese, Greek, and Roman Empires, breath was considered, recorded, and explored in writing. Its symbolic interpretation, that is, that breath is life, has remained relatively unchanged, even amidst our vast technological and scientific advances. Implicit in this concept are a multiplicity of symbolic interpretations that are rarely verbalized but invariably influence one's response to breathlessness. In addition to the symbolic aspects of the concept of breath, the biological, sociological, ecological, and psychological perspectives are important considerations; only then is one made cogently aware of the significant implications of breathlessness. Man actually lives simultaneously in two environments: the natural environment, which consists of all the things that are actually present, and a symbolic environment, in which man has reconstructed his surroundings.[3]

Documentation of the relationship between the experience of breathlessness and the ensuing psychological and physiological stresses is immediately met with difficulty, since highly sensitive instruments have not been developed to measure accurately psychological or physiological stress or the pathophysiological progression of chronic obstructive lung disease. However, in the literature there are reports of studies that lend support to this relational concept.

Although the etiology of COPD involves many questionable factors, the pathophysiological progression of the disease is associated with the individual's inability to cope with or modify his experience with the psychological and physiological stresses that he encounters. As lung function, either real or perceived, decreases, the individual's respiratory system seems to be less and less able to respond accurately or adequately to environmental input. Therefore disability is now produced by a variety of factors that previously had little or no effect. It becomes apparent then that the pathophysiological progression of this particular disease process could be explained as a feedback mechanism (Fig. 31-1).

The degree of physiological and psychological change would depend on the significance, severity, and duration of the stress encountered or the degree to which the stress is experienced. Experiencing the initiating stress is complicated by the physiological changes that ensue, which, in turn, are further complicated by psychological response. The latter may either ac-

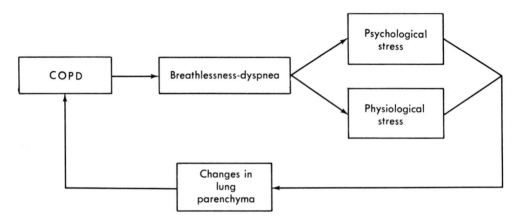

Fig. 31-1. Proposed feedback mechanism in COPD.

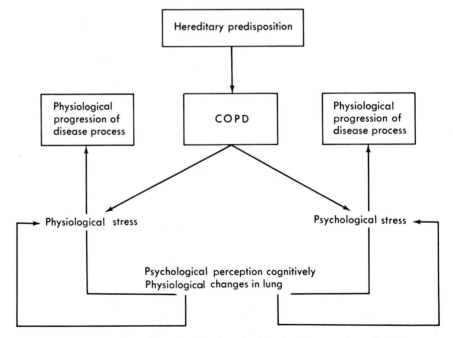

Fig. 31-2. Proposed explanation for the physiological progression of COPD.

centuate or minimize further physiological and psychological change. However, in the experiencing of breathlessness by an individual with COPD, the complicating psychological response is seen as accentuating both the physiological and psychological changes that occur. (See Fig. 31-2.)

Another important component to consider is the individual's attitude toward or reaction to environmental inputs such as noxious substances in environmental air, overcrowding in a bus, a smoke-filled room, friction within the family constellation, and other circumstances that initiate a response involving the respiratory system. The attitude that gradually develops is intimately related to the function of the physiological process with which it is associated. Consistency in attitude (i.e., poor attitude) is important in keeping the disease process active.[4] For example, a poor attitude is associated with poor pulmonary function; a change in attitude facilitates change in pulmonary function.

Physiological adjustments of the respiratory system, which take place appropriately in some circumstances, (i.e., in the event of psychological or physiological stress) are, in the presence of COPD, inappropriate and serve to further the pathophysiological progression of the disease process. One example that would serve to enhance understanding of this is the reaction of the respiratory system to what the individual perceives as noxious or irritating. The respiratory system reacts by trying to exclude the agent through the swelling of mucous membranes and hypersecretion. Although these responses are considered essential to the healthy respiratory system, in the presence of COPD they seem to enhance the disease process.

Although the respiratory system is capable of responding in a variety of ways to sensory input, one must keep in mind that individuals with COPD seem to respond to environmental stimuli with psychological and physiological changes that lead to further disability. The majority of individuals with COPD who fail to respond to treatment are seen as having few psychosocial and physiological assets with which to defend themselves against noxious environmental inputs.[2] Therefore these individuals adopt a life style that they believe will insulate and protect them from environmental stimuli. As time passes, their life style becomes constricted—avoidance of social gatherings and places where large numbers of people may congregate, denial, dependency, and isolation. Also of interest is the fact that individuals with COPD[5] have an increased incidence of peptic ulcer. Thus the picture of the individual with COPD emerges as a vicious cycle that, if allowed to continue uninterrupted, will lead to further disability, loss of productivity, psychological disturbances, and eventual death.

Individuals respond to stressful situations in a variety of ways; however, the way that one responds is largely dependent on the reactions that the situation evokes as a result of past symbolizations of experience. Since man is, in reality, an integrated entity, all these forces operate simultaneously in every event of his life. Therefore the individual with COPD must find alternate methods of responding to environmental inputs that are perceived as stressful. Now more than ever before in Western culture, there is growing interest in the study of man's learning willfully to control his body and cognitive forces.

Psychologists, in conjunction with physicians in the cardiovascular, pulmonary, and gastroenterological areas, throughout the United States are presently involved in research with biofeedback techniques, establishing significantly that, in many cases, by force of mental discipline alone, heart rates may be slowed and regulated, blood pressure lowered, intestinal tract contractions regulated, and breathing controlled. In New Delhi, experiments were recently conducted with individuals who practice yoga. One individual who had practiced it for thirty-five years was placed in an airtight container, and his respiratory rate and oxygen consumption were monitored from outside. It was clearly demonstrated that through mind control he was able to reduce his oxygen consumption to one third of the amount normally needed for basic metabolism. It still remains to be seen to what extent an individual with COPD can gain precise and reliable control over the things that he fears—such as breathlessness.

Each time that the individual with COPD responds in a manner that leads to further disability, energy is lost from the system. The more energy one expends or loses due to stress or conflict, the less is available for restoration and recovery. The attempted restoration of this energy is the task of the nurse. This restoration can best be accomplished through the use of measures that will facilitate the reduction of psychological or physiological stresses or both or the interruption of the feedback loop that is part of the fear cycle demonstrated in Fig. 31-1. By teaching and assisting patients to control their minds and thus their attitudes and responses, nurses may be able to provide the individual with COPD the means by which he can control unpleasant and unproductive stress. This is based on the premise that conflict due to psychological or physiological encounter with the environment generates stress, which in turn is associated with energy production and loss.

The feeling of loss of control is a primary factor in the advancement of the psychological component of this disease process. The individual with COPD often thinks that he has little control over anything, even his ability to breathe. Therefore, if he can learn how to control his response to stressful situations through conscious, concentrated mental processes, his sense of self-determination could be renewed dramatically and at will. Biofeedback techniques are seen as having potential for learning mind control. Biofeedback would seemingly accomplish two important goals: (1) the patient would develop a sense of control over his responses to stressful situations and (2) this sense of control would help to alleviate the feelings of powerlessness and hopelessness that these individuals experience.

A critical appraisal of current methods of treatment in COPD is warranted. Primary considerations include (1) pulmonary physiotherapy that includes bronchial hygiene, postural drainage, and breathing exercises; (2) intermittent positive-pressure breathing; and (3) oxygen therapy, including portable oxygen units and bronchodilators, along with other pharmacological agents. These measures have served effectively to reduce actual time and frequency of hospitalization. The time has come, however, for therapy of more definitive value to be accessible to these patients, that is, to provide them with the means through which an optimum level of productivity, enhancement of self-esteem and satisfaction, and renewal of control can be realized. This, coupled with current modalities of treatment, would provide this individual with the internal and external resources needed for his optimum level of functioning.

The nurse is in a unique position to work with these patients in a meaningful way. The developmental model shown in Fig. 31-3 provides for an end state and the process of becoming, as well as the optimal level of achievement for each individual. The model also provides direction and a well-defined form of progression. One must keep in mind, however, that forces may affect this progression at any stage in development.

The nurse may enter at any developmental stage and aid in improving the feedback process, which would then allow for self-steering or corrective action to be taken by the patient. Realizing that individual potentiality, as well as the ability to master internal and external forces, is different for each patient, any stage in the developmental model may be the terminal stage for a particular patient. The model also provides for the possibility of regression to an earlier stage of development.

The model is not exhaustive at this time in regard to the choices available to the individual at each developmental stage. However, it is hoped that, through additional exploration in this area, a more comprehensive model will emerge. One must also keep in mind that a model is not of value unless it is useful and used.

Initially, activities for the nurse referred to in the model require a concerted use of time and effort. Gradually, however, the patient assumes more and more responsibility for directing his progression toward his own optimal functioning.

Implications for nursing, both in relation to the psychological and physiological interrelations and the developmental model, reach beyond the particular dis-

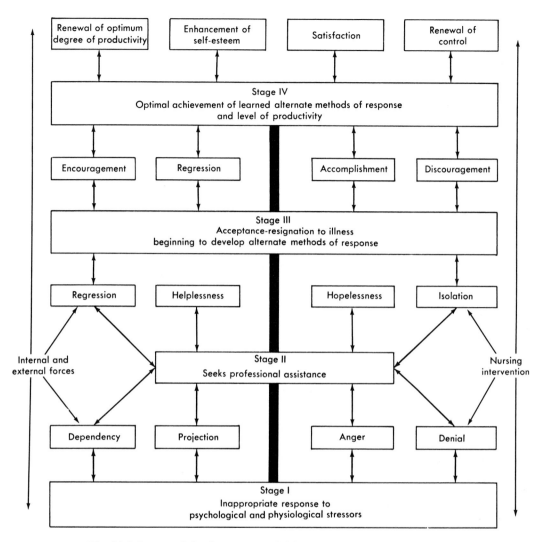

Fig. 31-3. Proposed development model for the individual with COPD.

ease process focused on here. Considerable evidence is currently being investigated concerning the interrelationship between physiological and psychological factors and the pathophysiological progression of other diseases. Therefore, it seems imperative that the nurse become increasingly cognizant of the dynamic effects and far-reaching implications of a knowledge base including the concepts explored in this chapter.

References

1. Dudley, D. L., Martin, C. J., Masuda, M., Ripley, H. S., and Holmes, T. H.: Psychophysiology of respiration in health and disease, New York, 1969, Appleton-Century-Crofts.
2. Grace, W. J., and Graham, D. T.: Relationship of specific attitudes and emotions to certain bodily diseases, Psychosom. Med. **14:**243, 1952.
3. Petty, T. L., and Nett, L. M.: For those who live and breathe with emphysema and chronic bronchitis, Springfield, Ill., 1967, Charles C Thomas, Publisher.
4. Public Health Service Publications 1529 and 1802, Chronic respiratory diseases control program, Arlington, Va., 1968, National Center for Chronic Diseases Control.
5. Shibutani, T.: Society and personality: an interactionist approach to social psychology, Englewood Cliffs, N. J., 1961, Prentice-Hall, Inc.

32

Trauma—skiing and nursing

James E. Bock

Man has long been faced with the problems of existence in a hostile world. That he has survived these problems is a tribute not only to his adaptive capabilities but to his ingenuity and determination as well. By various techniques he has overcome the natural hazards of his environment and transformed it into a relatively suitable habitat. Clothes and housing have counteracted the deleterious effects of weather. Improved modes of transportation and communication have negated the effects of time and distance. Industrial and agricultural advancements have ensured the availability of substances essential for comfort, security, and nutrition, and newly developing energy sources promise added support to these resources. Yet perhaps the most important and far-reaching of man's adaptive developments has been in the area of medicine. If man had been unable to control the adverse consequences of disease and trauma, many of his other advancements would have been impossible. It is the purpose of this chapter to explore one aspect of medicine—trauma—and more specifically to relate this concept to an area of clinical interest and significance for nursing.

To simplify the presentation and clarify the topic the various components of the concept will be discussed individually, and then their relationships will be formulated. After development of this conceptual framework has been completed, it will be applied to those athletic injuries resulting from snow skiing.

TRAUMA

In spite of the extensive literature on the etiology and management of trauma, relatively little has been done to conceptualize some of the factors resulting in trauma. An attempt will be made here to

do so. However, to facilitate the subsequent discussion, some discussion of the definition of this term should first be made. Trauma can be divided into two general classifications, psychological disruption and physical disruption. Physiological disruption would be a third category appearing primarily as a subclassification under each of the first two headings. This chapter will deal primarily with the physically defined aspect, since this is the more common connotation of trauma. Also, causal factors in physical trauma are more readily identifiable.

A recent article by Schilling[33] identified trauma as one of five major disease entities, including traumatic, congenital, inflammatory, neoplastic, and metabolic disorders. He pointed out that, although trauma, which he defined simply as bodily injury, was the fourth leading cause of death among the previously mentioned categories, it was the primary cause of loss in productive life years. Thus the importance of study into any one of the many aspects of trauma will become obvious. Schilling dealt primarily with the physical aspects of trauma, as can be seen in his mention of those factors resulting in injury: "Trauma is caused almost invariably by a force which is decelerated by the human body, or where the moving body or one of its parts is decelerated against a relatively stationary object."*

Perhaps the definition of trauma most suited to this chapter is the following: trauma is that sudden alteration of the physiological, anatomical, or psychological status of the individual when exposed to external force. Several facets of trauma are implicit in this definition. First, suddenness

---

*From Schilling, J. A.: Trauma, J. Okla. State Med. Assoc. **61**:499, 1968.

of onset is one identifiable characteristic of trauma. This serves to separate trauma from other health problems more insidious in nature. Certainly other illnesses, although insidious in their development, may also be rapid in onset of overt symptoms. However, the second characteristic of trauma serves to differentiate between the two. That second characteristic is the presence of an identifiable external force as the causal factor in change of status. Third, the pattern of alteration, whether physiological, anatomical, or psychological, is usually one that is sufficiently different in nature from other disease processes to indicate its origins. These three factors—sudden onset, causation by an identifiable external force, and characteristic pattern of alteration—when taken together usually are sufficient to identify trauma.

Force

As has already been mentioned, trauma is produced by the application of force, an obvious oversimplification. Degrees of force differ, as do levels of trauma. Generally speaking, externally induced trauma cannot occur without a sufficient level of force, implying that force is a strength, or energy, level. However, numerous energy sources at work in the environment do not cause harm. Sunlight, wind, and temperature are all forms of energy that normally do not cause injury. What then can be classified as an injurious force?

The answer to the preceding question can be found if force is viewed as a continuum, running from very low to very high energy levels. That force which causes injury is usually confined to the upper levels of this spectrum, although there are exceptions, which will be discussed later. Those forces which produce injury can generally be classified as excessive, unnatural, or misapplied. Excessive force is the presence of unnatural levels of natural energy. Wind is a good example of this category. Although wind in normal amounts is harmless and usually somewhat pleasant and useful, it can become dangerous and destructive at the level of a hurricane. Unnatural force is that which is not normally encountered and therefore not compensable by the individual's actions or physical

makeup. An example of this would be a sudden blow to the head, as by a thrown object. Closely allied to this force is misapplied force. That same unnatural force, a blow, if applied to the side of the knee, would result in injury. This might not be due to the strength of the blow but to the site of application. The knee is structurally designed to compensate for even an unnatural blow (through the action of the joint, muscles, and ligaments), so long as that force is applied either frontally or anteriorly. However, application from a lateral angle circumvents the natural defensive action of the knee and often leads to trauma. This relationship will be dealt with in the following section.

Resistive capacity

Just as there are levels of trauma and force, there are also levels of resistance. Resistance level could probably best be defined as the simultaneous presence of several factors leading to the accumulation of potentially harmful energy stores or the depletion of resistive reserves or both and their ratio. This concurrent accumulation of injury-producing effects or depletion of injury-resisting effects or both could be termed *resistance* or *susceptibility*, depending on which effect is greater. Following are the factors that determine this ratio:

1. Biomechanical factors include those stresses produced by environmental obstacles such as trees, walls, and other persons and/or self-induced magnification of physical laws, such as the following:

    a. Momentum: Mass times velocity (of either the injuring force or the individual himself). Increasing momentum generally decreases resistive capacity.

    b. Strength, or elasticity: Force-absorbing capability of an object to recover without damage. Studies have shown the relationship between the compensatory action of body structures (e.g., bones) and the degree of injury that they receive.[14,24,30] An increase in strength, or elasticity, of the affected tissue decreases susceptibility to injury.

c. Inertia: Tendency of a stationary object to remain stationary when force is applied or for a moving object to continue. The inert object may be a natural obstacle such as the individual himself; he may collide with an obstacle or an object may collide with him. In either case the result will be the same. Inertia is largely uncontrollable.

d. Deceleration: Function of the squared velocity divided by twice the stopping distance (the square of stopping time divided by the rate of deceleration). This is closely related to inertia and is measured in g.'s (a measure correlated with gravitational pull effects).[33] Obviously, an increase in rate of deceleration (faster stopping time) can have advantageous as well as deleterious effects. The sudden stop of a collision could injure, whereas stopping suddenly might also prevent a collision.

e. Torsion: Rotation about an axis. Here the example of a twisting injury to an extremity, such as a sprain, is applicable. Torsion is a natural body phenomenon (e.g., rotation of the forearm or neck) but, when applied abnormally, generally will cause injury.

f. Leverage: Creation of a product moment, enhancement of force by mechanical means. Leverage is also prone to cause injury if applied in excessive amounts to weakened areas (e.g., most skiing accidents occur due to the leverage action of the ski).

Many other physical laws could play a role in resistive capacity, but the foregoing are the major contributors. The overall influence of biomechanical factors can be positive or negative. A decrease in some factors such as momentum, torsion, and inertia might be beneficial, as might an increase in others such as strength, rate of deceleration, and leverage. This relationship is largely dependent on the context of ac-

tivity. Likewise, environmental hazards are not independent of the activity being performed but are usually predictably associated with it.

2. Physiological factors encompass those innate characteristics of human organisms that can act either to increase or decrease innate resistive reserves. In this context, these characteristics are largely components of fatigue. Definitions of the latter are as numerous as are articles on the subject. Pathak[31] defined *fatigue* as ". . . a decrement in response coming as a result of activity." He assigned a combination of psychological, physical, and mental characteristics to it. Bartley[3,4] states, however, that fatigue and impairment of performance are not the same—that fatigue has much more complex physical, biochemical, physiological, homeostatic, and sensory cognitive levels that can exist independent of measurable performance decline. The latter case is undoubtedly true when higher psychological mechanisms intervene (e.g., highly repetitive tasks requiring concentrated mental effort). However, within the area of athletic endeavors the former definition retains a large degree of credibility. In terms of purely physical endeavor (such as athletics) the physical components of fatigue seem to be most important in their effects on resistive capacity.

Many causal factors for fatigue have been identified. Selye[34] theorized that stress, either physical or psychological, prompted physical biochemical changes that produced a sensation of fatigue. Grandjean[16] related fatigue to performance levels and stated that those levels are controlled by the degree of activity of the brain's inhibitory system and the activating stimulus of the reticular formation. Another theory encompassing both biochemical and neurological aspects was that of del Castillo and Katz.[10] They claimed that fatigue was due to a decrease in acetylcholine in nerve fiber synapses to below the level necessary to allow impulse conduction and uniform muscle contraction. Several studies have implicated tissue hypoxia, such as that occurring in excessive muscular effort, as a main limitational factor in activity. Blake's[5] study showed that both acclimatized and unacclimatized individuals are subject to fatigue at high altitudes, where aerobic performance was decreased. Anoxia is generally believed to lead to the accumulation of lactic acid and hydrogen ions that act to cause local as well as systemic muscle changes leading to fatigue. Perhaps one of the best explanations of the phenomenon of fatigue was presented by Pathak:

> The energy expenditure of most of the tissues under normal conditions is such that there is a considerable reserve for increasing the activity, within limits, without induction of fatigue. However, this is not quite true for skeletal muscles which may be called upon to perform very strenuous exertions within a short time. The energy requirement under such conditions could be so exacting that the reserve is rapidly crossed and with all the available circulatory and respiratory resources, the muscles cannot continue to work to their full capacity. The work performance fails till no work is possible at all. This is pure physical fatigue. Physical work involves a combined neuromuscular action. Either the neural elements or the muscular elements or both could be the site of fatigue. Transmission of nerve impulses across synapses involves special processes. The synapses in the central nervous system or at the periphery could also be the site of fatigue. Frequently a feeling of discomfort during and after exertion exists partly because of dyspnea and partly due to the action of sensory impulses arising in the active muscles. Actual muscle pain and cramps may also develop. The feeling of discomfort and disinclination to repeat the work soon after exertion have both psychological and physical bases. The development of the psychological feeling to avoid work, also implies a link between physical and psychological fatigue. However, the physiochemical changes in the muscle seem to form the main basis of physical fatigue.*

Simonson[35] has classified the causal factors of fatigue under two headings: the first is accumulation of fatigue-producing substances such as lactate, hydrogen ions, and pyruvate, and the second includes depletion of those substances essential for activity, including body fuels (e.g., proteins, carbohydrates, fats, potassium), hormones (e.g., adrenaline, ACTH, insulin, thyroxin), and tissue oxygen levels.

Although the relationship between fatigue and resistive potential might seem ambiguous, a close relationship between the two is involved. The presence of fatigue usually results in a decreased potential for controlled muscular activity; the fatigued organism responds less readily to potentially hazardous stress situations. Under the right circumstances and relative to other factors affecting the resistance potential, this may result in susceptibility of the organism to trauma. If fatigue can be eliminated or its effects controlled, the resistance potential will be increased.

3. Psychosocial factors include one's self-concept of adequacy in dealing with stress-producing situations (i.e., obviously dangerous performance tasks) and will largely determine the course that is followed and the adequacy of that choice. The self-concept is in turn dependent on past experience (success in meeting similar situations) and social pressures. These psychosocial factors may override the effects of both the biomechanical and physiological factors. Social pressure may lead one to take unnecessary risks despite recognition of the potential hazards; it might also lead to temporary disregard for physical laws (e.g., taking a "dare" to race on a winding mountain road). And certain physiological alterations are known to take place due to the emotions. Weiss[41] found that fear induced decreased performance ability, although perceptual ability remained largely unchanged. Crawford[9] called this psychological alteration in physical responsiveness *stress fatigue*. He demonstrated that a stress situation first results in oversensitive behavior and overreaction, but that later the trend is toward decreased reactivity to environmental stimuli.[19] Muscular tension, anxiety (fear and apprehension), and emotional stress were all held responsible for a deterioration in con-

---

*From Pathak, C. L.: Muscular work and fatigue, Indian J. Physiol. Pharmacol. 13:87, 1969.

trol nervous system standards of performance by McFarland.[26]

It should be obvious that the psychosocial aspects of resistance are vastly important, since they exert strong effects not only on resistance potential but also on those other categories of factors previously mentioned.

COMPONENT RELATIONSHIPS

Excessive, unnatural, or misapplied force may act to produce trauma in any personally or environmentally produced stressful situation of adequate dimensions. That it does not do so more often can be related to certain of the components already discussed. For force to produce trauma, it must first act through and be mediated by the resistance potential of the individual. This resistance potential is the product of biomechanical, physiological, and psychosocial factors, which determine the susceptibility state of the individual. The relationship between the force component and the resistance component determines the probability and extent of trauma that is likely to occur.

A sudden increase in force magnitude with an unchanged resistance potential is one type of relationship that may often lead to trauma. A pedestrian struck by a passing automobile or a falling brick is a good example of this relationship. Here the resistance potential of the individual remains constant; yet, because of this sudden application of excessive, unnatural force, there is no compensation, and injury occurs. The rapidity of force onset is a factor here. If the rate of application were slowed, the individual might be able to perceive the impending danger and alter his resistance potential to compensate. This is a second type of possible relationship. If the individual is able to recognize the signs of impending force, he is, as it were, able to get ready for it. In the previous examples, an individual who saw a speeding automobile approaching might have time to relax just before being hit (lessening the force of inertia and therefore the force of impact as well), or, in the case of the falling brick, if the individual saw it falling or a bystander warned him, he might either

raise a protective arm or move quickly to avoid a collison. In either of these cases, a relatively slowed rate of application has allowed the resistance potential to be increased in response to the increase in force application. Avoidance of or decrease in extent of trauma would therefore occur. Still a third possible relationship exists. If, for some reason, the resistance potential were to be decreased significantly, a state might be reached wherein the individual could be highly susceptible to relatively normal or harmless levels of force. This is when those factors contributing to the resistance potential become so important.

As previously mentioned, the resistance potential is the product of biomechanical, physiological, or psychosocial factors. These three factors must be viewed in terms of quality and overall contribution to the resistance potential. In any given situation they would not be equally important and certainly not be equally distributed. Desirable levels and importance of each vary. Generally speaking, however, a trend toward highly desirable levels of all three factors would lead to a high resistance potential. A low-quality level of one or more might not have adverse effects, depending on the given situation. Perhaps examples of the positive and negative effects of each factor would be beneficial. An individual driving an automobile at excessive speed on a crowded freeway would be greatly magnifying the negative effects of the biomechanical factor. Not only is he lessening his resistance potential by exposing himself to large numbers of environmental hazards (other automobiles), but he is also greatly magnifying the potential effects of any force application (such as a blowout) by exaggerating certain physical laws, including momentum, deceleration, and inertia. He has thus opened the way for potential trauma from force levels that otherwise would not be sufficient to produce injury. Conversely, proper application of physical laws in the foregoing situation might serve to increase resistance potential. The same individual, by the use of seat belts, could increase his resistance potential by lessening the effects of the physical laws of deceleration and inertia. The effects of the physiological factor may be illustrated using the same example. A driver suffering from fatigue, whether mental or physical, would be less able to adjust to sudden environmental changes. Unexpected movement by another vehicle, an unforeseen road hazard, or a mechanical malfunction might lead to loss of control and occurrence of an accident. However, a mentally fresh and alert individual would be more able to compensate. The psychosocial factor could be manifested in the previous situations in any number of ways. Even though the individual might recognize the potential hazards of driving at high speed on a crowded freeway while fatigued, he might violate his better judgment. Perhaps social pressure to arrive at his destination on time might cause this, or the psychological pressure of an important decision might lead to a temporary mental lapse, or preoccupation. A psychosocial drive to "prove" himself to those about him or to fortify his own ego might prompt his speeding. Whatever the cause, an increase in the negative sum of his resistance potential would occur. The happy, self-confident individual would not face these problems, and his psychosocial status would contribute to an increase in his resistance potential.

From the foregoing examples, it should be obvious that the biomechanical, physiological, and psychosocial factors are not independent of one another. Physiological fatigue might not be so important if the physical factor of speed were decreased. The psychosocial need to "show off" by speeding might not be so dangerous if the individual were mentally alert and reactive. Obviously the possible variations in the force-resistance-trauma cycle are many. Only a thorough examination of each individual situation would reveal the forces at work.

IMPLICATIONS FOR NURSING

Nurses have always been associated with trauma intervention. Unfortunately this intervention always seems to occur at the trauma end of the force-resistance-trauma sequence. That is, nurses usually find their role to be that of repairing and rehabilitating traumatized individuals. This is a vital role, but is it the highest possible one for nurses? If there are three levels of the trauma sequence, why not three levels of possible intervention?

Care after injury should be regarded as the lowest, or least desirable, level of intervention. Nurses have been content to function too long at this level. The primary goal of nursing should be prevention of illness and injury, not perfection of myriad and beautiful techniques for "after the fact" care. In this context the highest intervention would be at the level of force. The ideal situation would be to eliminate all excessive, unnatural, or misapplied forceful elements from our world. This is not only extremely unlikely but might even be unwelcome. Humans seem to thrive on a certain level of threat, or danger—so much so that they often go out of their way to seek experiences in which the element of risk is present. Such experiences seem to enliven the daily monotony of living and make it more enjoyable. Concussions, fractures, and amputations, however, are not so enjoyable; few would argue this point. Intervention at the first level might lie in better public education regarding certain harmful practices. If more nurses were able and/or willing to fill this gap, much could be done by way of preventive medicine. Many persons expose themselves to potentially harmful situations from ignorance of the dangers involved; others create harmful situations from otherwise innocent ones through ignorance. Many areas of illness and injury could be included under this category.

The second level of nursing intervention takes into account the inevitability of exposure to force and attempts to compensate for it. Here nursing should strive to increase the resistance potential by increasing or decreasing those factors of which it is composed, to produce an adequately protected individual. Research is vital to effectiveness at this level. Knowledge of the biomechanical factors associated with resistance potential could be utilized in such areas as preexposure training (especially in most areas of athletics), proper equipping (development of protective equipment and devices), and activity-area planning and coordination to decrease environmental hazards. Special exercise programs might lead to a positive contribution by the physiological factor. Programs serving to increase strength and endurance and lessen fatigability are good examples. Benefits from knowledge in these first two areas would assist in controlling the psychosocial factor. Not only would better knowledge, training, and preparation contribute to self-concepts of adequacy in meeting stress situations, but they would also lead to more mature, knowledgeable judgment and emotional control, thus lessening susceptibility to social pressure.

Certainly one cannot rule out the need for intervention at the third level. Despite one's best efforts, there will always be individuals at this level. The conventional role could be greatly expanded, however. What better time than during treatment and rehabilitation of a traumatized individual could one find for education that might have been missed regarding the first two levels? Certainly the need for such knowledge will be glaringly apparent to the patient at this time. A nurse certainly could take advantage of such a "captive" audience.

APPLICATION TO A CLINICAL AREA

Many statements in this section are applicable generally to many athletic areas. However, snow skiing has been singled out for discussion because of its high level of personal interest.

Few sports so graphically demonstrate the force-resistance-trauma relationship as well as this type of skiing. Tremendous stress is placed on the individual engaged in this sport. High speeds, uneven and irregular terrain, great mechanical leverage, profound physical exertion, and psychosocial influences (from self and peers) all are present. These factors, coupled with a phenomenal rise in skiing popularity and availability in the last twenty years, has turned skiing into a major medical problem. National skiing injury rates range from four per thousand skier days to greater than ten per thousand skier days. Although this is a relatively low incidence rate, the sheer numbers of skiers and the serious nature of their injuries make skiing a serious health problem among the various sports.

Current studies

Due to the widespread popularity and growth of skiing, many studies have been carried out in different locales of the incidence and etiology of skiing injuries. Many variables contributing to skiing injuries have been identified, including snow conditions, skiing equipment (e.g., boots, bindings, and skis), and the competence, age, fatigue, technique, and speed of the skier.

Spademan[36] analyzed 428 lower-extremity skiing injuries at Squaw Valley, California. He found the mean population age to be 23 years; yet over 50% of those injured were under 21 years old. Also he found a higher rate of incidence among women, (more of whom were in the "beginner" classification). The peak injury occurrence time was between 11 A.M. and 2 P.M. (implying a possible fatigue factor). He claims that loss of control and malfunction of safety bindings were the major causes of these injuries.

A five-year study at Syracuse, New York, showed fractures of the lower leg and sprains of the knee and ankle to be the most common injuries. Overconfidence, poor conditioning and control, and, again, improper bindings were cited as the main causes of injury.[18]

Major injuries in the Mount Telemark, Wisconsin, study were equally divided between ligamentous injuries of the knee and ankle and bone damage to the tibia and fibula. The most common bone injury was a fracture of the shaft of the tibia or fibula or both. The most common ligamentous injury was a sprain of the medial collateral ligament of the knee. Most injuries occurred after lunch and toward the end of the skiing day (again implicating fatigue as a possible factor). The investigators claim that, in this instance, skiing conditions were a major cause of injuries. Children were also shown to have fewer ligamentous injuries but more fractures (indicating a possible difference in physical makeup).[37]

The ankle, knee, and lower leg again contributed the majority of injuries in a study of the Anchorage, Alaska, area. Of the injuries reported, 47% were sprains and 33%, fractures. A major variation in injury rate was seen according to age (highest in males under 20 years of age) and experience level (higher in beginners). Fatigue was again implicated as a causal factor, since the highest percentage of injuries occurred later in the day, one hour after peak skiing time.[25] Almost identical results were obtained in a study done at the St. Marguerite ski area in Quebec. In this case, the researchers divided the causes as follows: loss of control (due to poor physical conditioning, inexperience, fatigue, and speed), dangerous skiing conditions (hazards and snow quality), weather conditions (temperature, light, and visibility), and faulty equipment (improper bindings, lack of safety straps, and other factors). They were also able to correlate skiing speed and type of accident with the location and severity of the injury.[28]

Two different analyses of injuries occurring at Mt. Snow, Vermont, were made in 1962. One dealing with injury distributions found that sprains (primarily of the knee and ankle) accounted for 43% of the total injuries, whereas fractures (primarily ankle and tibial-fibular) totaled 35% of all injuries. Young skiers were found to have more tibial fractures, whereas older skiers had more ankle injuries. They stated that this difference was due to developmental bone weakness in the younger skiers' long bones.[12] The second study dealt primarily with causal factors for the same group of injuries. Their major findings were of the injury-reducing value of release bindings (more so for men, due to their greater weight) and increased experience, as manifested in skiing technique. Those skiers who could manage only the "snowplow" technique had nearly three times as high an injury incidence as those using more advanced techniques.[17]

Results of a large study done at Sun Valley, Idaho, showed many similarities to these other studies. Of the total injuries, 43% consisted of ligamentous damage (again primarily ankle and knee), and 22% were fractures of the tibia or fibula. Most of these injuries also occurred in the afternoon but were primarily during the second hour of skiing, thus not so conclusively demonstrating a fatigue-injury relationship. They were able to find little evidence of the effectiveness of release bindings.[11] A National Ski Patrol survey (of national scope), completed at approximately the

same time, showed 47% sprains and 30% fractures (with the knee, ankle, and lower leg again the primary locations). These statistics showed the primary injury group to be persons between 13 and 30 years old. They found little relationship to snow conditions and injury but state that lack of control was a factor in 70% of the injuries.[22]

An earlier study done at Sun Valley found a 4:1 relationship between sprains and fractures in torsional lower extremity injuries. Peak injury periods were found to be noon and 4 P.M., or after three hours of skiing. Beginners and those with two to five years' experience were the most frequently injured groups. Fatigue, safety bindings, and previous instruction were claimed to affect the probability of injury. Around 70% of the total injuries were directly related to the leverage effect of the skis used.[29]

Erskine's[13] study (1959) showed a fracture-sprain incidence and distribution similar to later studies. He found definite evidence of causal relationships between injury rate and skier age and experience level.

A recent study by a physician, although on a smaller scale, obtained results similar to those conducted elsewhere, indicating geographical factors may not much alter the validity of comparisons made between this area and other skiing locations throughout the country.[27] A recent study at Vail, Colorado, illustrated the desirability of ski instruction as a means of reducing injuries.[15]

Several foreign articles in English have been written on research into skiing injuries. Studies of the incidence of injury in Australia, Scotland, and Germany show a close resemblance to American findings.[6,21,40] Another foreign author has shown that a definite reduction in ski injuries occurs with the use of proper ski bindings.[20]

Two enlightening articles have been written on the mechanical changes (forceful rotation and sudden forward flexion) that bring about lower extremity injuries.[7,38] Leidholt[24] has written an excellent article on the biomechanics of skiing and the force-resistant properties of bone. These works help to formulate a basis for the study of any type of skiing injury.

SKIING TRAUMA

From the foregoing review it is evident that skiing injuries have all the characteristics of trauma. Rapidity of onset and the presence of force cannot be argued. The forces encountered in skiing could all be classified as excessive, unnatural, or misapplied in one or another situation. That a characteristic pattern of disruption in skiing injuries occurs should be obvious from a comparison of findings in those studies already presented. There is a definite pattern of major injury types (fractures and ligamentous damage), as well as location of injury (ankle, knee, tibia, and fibula). A number of lesser injuries, such as contusions, lacerations, concussions, and dislocations, occur regularly, but in a far more irregular and infrequent pattern. These are often secondary to a more serious problem such as a sprain or fracture.

SKIING FORCE

The presence of force in skiing is so obvious that little will be said about it here. The levels of force can be seen in skiing injuries with the demonstrable change in injury patterns relative to skier speed and type of accident. Nature's forces are magnified to excessive levels in skiing, due to the speed and weather conditions involved. Unnatural forces are created by the very act of skiing (e.g., collision with another skier or with a tree). Many characteristic skiing injuries are the result of misapplied force. Ligamentous damage to the knee or ankle results from the leverage effect of the ski, causing an unnatural, forceful rotation. The "boot top" fracture results from the need for the leg to bend where no joint exists. More will be said about these relationships in the discussion of biomechanical factors associated with resistance potential.

RESISTIVE CAPACITY IN SKIING
Biomechanical factors

This category can be further subdivided in the case of skiing into environmental, equipment, and physical components. Environmental hazards are always present in skiing, whether from natural sources such as trees, steep slopes, and snow conditions or from unnatural sources such as other skiers, "sitzmarks" (indentations where other skiers have fallen), "moguls" (hills of snow created by repeated turns), lift towers, signs, and buildings. Many ski areas try to eliminate most of these hazards in an effort to make their facilities safer. However, there is a limit to how many hazards can be removed without destroying the elements of danger or beauty or both that make skiing so attractive.

The equipment produces several of the biomechanical stresses involved in skiing. Ski boots have been designed to allow greater control of and "feel for" the skis, in addition to providing greater ankle protection. Unfortunately the rigid immobilization this requires can often result in a tibial fracture when the skier is forcibly flung forward, as in a sudden stop. This is what is referred to as a "boot top" fracture. Fortunately, another recent innovation in equipment, the "forward release" binding, is greatly reducing this type of injury. This binding, which permits the heel to be released when under sufficient forward strain, is now often combined with the older "lateral" or "rotational" release binding. The latter releases when sufficient torque is applied by the weight of the skier. Unfortunately the presence of such devices does not always ensure against injury. Bindings are adjustable and therefore subject to maladjustment. Often a skier will tighten them to such a degree (through ignorance or poor judgment) that the level of force required to effect release is greater than that needed to produce a lower-leg fracture; the bone breaks instead of the binding. Also bindings may be so loose that they release during normal skiing maneuvers, which can be fully as hazardous as the opposite extreme. Ski poles contribute to injury as well. A rare fracture of the metacarpals occurs almost solely from the leverage effect of the ski pole in a fall.[8] Skis themselves are perhaps the single most important equipment factor in skiing injuries. They are so closely allied with most of the physical laws at work in skiing that the two must be viewed together.

Most of the major injuries occurring in skiing (e.g., sprains and fractures of the lower extremities) can be linked to the magnification of physical laws that skis produce. Erskine[13] explained the forces resulting in skiing injuries by stating that ". . .[if] force is exerted in such a way that the skis act as levers, a moment is created, and the force is increased several times." Cletcher and Gamble[7] related this increase in force to the location and severity of skiing injuries. Leidholt,[24] in his work with biomechanics and stress-absorbing capabilities of bone, noted the increase in stress when ski leverage is combined with momentum. The injuring force in lower extremity skiing injuries has been defined as ". . .momentum multiplied by the distance from the boot to the ski tip."[23] Harwood[18] defined the same stress in terms of "torsional force" and Moritz[29] cited it as being the primary factor in lower extremity injuries. Logically, then, one could assume that a primary factor in the production of force sufficient to cause injury would be the length of this torsion-producing lever:

> The long lever of the fore part of the ski acts on a fulcrum at the ankle, and it has been shown experimentally that a load of 7 kg. applied laterally to the tip of the ski, one meter from the ski boot, will result in a torque of 700 kg. cm., which could be expected to produce a fracture (of the tibia) in 60 per cent of cases.*

From such observations one can see that the skis themselves play a vital part in the creation of all the previously mentioned physical laws: momentum, strength, inertia, deceleration, torsion, and leverage. Momentum, inertia, and deceleration are closely related, since they all pertain to speed. Often the speed that a skier can attain is dependent on several factors operating simultaneously: the slope grade, snow conditions, skier weight and technique, and gliding characteristics of the given skis. The latter is largely a function of length and weight per square inch of surface area. Strength, torsion, and leverage interact, since any given level of physical strength may be overcome if force is magnified by torsion and leverage combined. Unfortunately, most of the biomechanical factors in

skiing seem to be force contributive rather than force resistive.

Physiological factors

Physiological factors are less concisely applicable to skiing than are biomechanical factors. Most researchers tend to agree that fatigue can be a primary factor in the etiology of ski injury. Due to the difficulty in finding suitable measures for fatigue levels, this theory remains largely unproved. From a review of the work that has been done in studying fatigue, the theory would seem to be plausible. The hypothesized relationship of tissue hypoxia and lactic acid formation in strenuous exertion seems to be the one most applicable to athletic activities such as skiing. Certainly the profound muscular effort and tension required in skiing could contribute to fatigue. Interestingly the results of the previously mentioned study show the increased fatigability of all persons at high altitudes, where most skiing areas are located. In skiing the psychosocial factors affecting attitudes and fatigue are so closely allied with the physiological that they are difficult to differentiate.

Psychosocial factors

Reading the previous section under this same heading one may easily apply the findings of Crawford,[9] Weiss,[41] and McFarland[26] to skiing. Fear, anxiety, and other emotional stresses are present in skiing to a large degree. Anxiety can be produced not only by a fear of bodily injury but of loss of self- and peer-esteem as well. Skiing is a social sport (at least in its most popular form), which can place demands, real and imaginary, on the individual. Social pressures, such as those to "keep up" or to "show off," are all too frequently encountered in skiing. This activity lacks the limitations that are present in other sports on participation by the unskilled beginner. Often this lack of controls can lead to serious consequences if the individual is challenged beyond his ability, either intentionally or by accident:

> . . .The second [injury-causing] factor is fear, a purely psychological one, and about which we have little objective data. A skier who is relaxed and happy rarely gets hurt. When frightened, he

---

*From Frankel, V. H., and Burstein, A. H.: Load capacity of tubular bone. In Kenedi, R. M., editor: Biomechanics and related bio-engineering topics, Oxford, England, 1965, Pergamon Press, Ltd., p. 394.

becomes tense, the legs lose their suppleness and the reaction time slows up—a good set-up for an accident. The cause of the fright is usually a situation which the skier is not trained to handle: the slope may be steeper than expected, getting up too much speed, etc.*

Previous experience apparently affects injury potential in skiing. Experience certainly affects self-concepts of adequacy in dealing with stress and therefore no doubt interacts with the stress-fear-tension sequence. Above all, the psychosocial factors can have an overriding influence on both biomechanical and physiological factors in determining susceptibility of a skier.

COMPONENT RELATIONSHIPS IN SKIING

The most common application of force to an individual in skiing is a fall. This fall does not necessarily occur at great speed, and the causes may vary. Loss of control is the most common cause. Collision with natural or unnatural hazards and equipment malfunction are less common causes. That trauma does not result more often from such falls is evidence of the force-resistance potential-trauma concept in action. When trauma does occur, it can often be traced to a weakness in the individual's resistance potential. Skiing incorporates all three of the previously mentioned force-resistance relationships: sudden increase in force without a concurrent increase in resistance potential, gradual increase in force with a gradual increase in resistance potential, or a marked decline in resistance potential relative to unchanged force levels.

The first of these relationships can be exemplified by a collision-type accident. Here force is increased so drastically and so rapidly that no amount of resistance could counteract it. In the second relationship, adequate time is allowed for the skier to respond to the impending stress situation by increasing his resistance potential. This might take the form of relaxing and going into a sideways fall to avoid gaining excessive speed on a steep slope. The third relationship might be demonstrated by an individual who sus-

tains a lower-leg fracture while slowly negotiating a snowplow turn. Here he has decreased his resistance potential by using long skis (probably with improperly adjusted release bindings), which can wedge themselves into the snow and magnify the force of momentum by their leverage; this results in injury.

The level of resistive potential is probably the most important link in the production or prevention of trauma. Unfortunately most of the factors associated with skiing can contribute to a negative (or injury-contributory) resistive potential. Biomechanical factors are particularly negative in nature. Environmental hazards are such largely by design. Equipment, with the exception of release bindings, poorly compensates for many of the forces encountered in skiing but is often a contributing factor to magnification of physical laws resulting in injury. For most individuals, the physiological aspects of resistance are negative in nature. Poor physical conditioning and preparation are the rule rather than the exception. Exhaustion and fatigue result from this poor conditioning and overexertion without enough rest. The psychosocial elements in resistance can contribute to susceptibility also. Fear, inexperience, poor self-concepts of adequacy, peer pressure, and other factors can lead to injury. Fortunately this aspect of resistance potential can exert strong overriding controls on the first two. Often the psychosocial influences are the ones that prevent injury in any potentially stressful situation. Common sense, good judgment, and the influence of friends who are good skiers may help the individual meet or circumvent these situations. Knowledge of the inherent dangers of the biomechanical and physiological factors present in skiing allows the individual to compensate for them in ways such as proper adjustment and selection of equipment, skiing within one's capabilities, and taking adequate rest periods, or "pacing" oneself. Such mechanisms must function in skiing; otherwise a much higher injury rate per number of falls than the present one would prevail.

Levels of trauma can be correlated with the mediating effects on stress of the force-resistive aspect of the resistance potential.

---

*From Erskine, L. A.: The mechanisms involved in skiing injuries, Am. J. Surg. **98:**669, 1959.

The differences between injuries sustained in identical falls result from these effects. Hopefully a thorough and detailed investigation and application of the relationships present in resistance potential will lead to a reduction in ski traumas.

NURSING IMPLICATIONS IN SKIING

As with many areas of trauma in athletics, nursing intervention occurs almost solely after the injury, taking the form of palliative care of the injured part and occasionally rehabilitative counseling. These roles are vital, but there is a wider role as well.

Intervention at the first level is difficult. Humans have a disinclination to listen to those things which they do not want to hear. However, a program of realistic public education on the hazards of skiing might encourage more people to examine skiing from a practical viewpoint and decide whether the risks present in skiing are outweighed by its benefits. From the present level of skiing popularity, the realistic assumption is that a large majority of those inclined toward skiing would think that such risks were reasonable in view of the rewards provided by the activity.

At the second plausible level of intervention the decision is made to accept an unalterable situation and prepare individuals mechanically, physically, and psychologically to meet the inevitable stresses encountered in skiing. The goal here is to decrease the harmful effects of force-contributive factors and increase the effects of force-resistive factors. The best possible method of obtaining this goal is through knowledge, which is best obtained through research.

Examination into the contribution of each individual factor in resistive potential could lead to numerous implications for increasing the safety of the skier. The biomechanical area needs utmost attention. Examination and analysis of ski equipment could lead to improved mechanical function, as well as recommendations for design changes that would make such items safer. An example of such investigation might be a study of the injury-reducing effects of the new shorter skis, which originated more for recreational purposes than for safety. In the early 1950s, a skiing instructor named Clif Taylor developed the idea when he began using sawed-off standard-length skis for his own use and for pupil instruction. From this limited beginning the short skis have grown to be a popular method of instruction for beginners, as well as a new experience for more advanced skiers. Karl Pfeiffer, also a skiing instructor, has developed a whole system of ski instruction using short skis. Now known as G.L.M. (for graduated length method), such schools are now operating in many major ski areas across the country.[1] "Shortie" skis range in length from 100 to 200 cm., whereas "standard" skis are usually between 170 and 205 cm. for most adults.[2,32] The implications that short skis present for trauma prevention are many. Primarily their shorter length should decrease the leverage effect that they produce, thus decreasing their injury-producing rotational torque. Short skis are also more controllable, due to their shorter length and improved handling characteristics. This additional control could serve to reduce injuries by lowering speed and allowing more rapid attainment of better skiing technique. Both of these alterations have been shown to reduce the likelihood and severity of injury.[39] A third possible benefit of short skis might be their tendency to decrease fatigue. This is due not only to improved control and relaxation but also to lessened muscular effort (resulting from the reduced "swing weight" of the smaller skis).[32] These benefits could lead to an improved emotional state resulting from the confidence produced by improved control and lessened tension. Investigations into other types of skiing equipment might be equally beneficial.

The physiological factors could be investigated in terms of ascertaining what factors contribute most to fatigue and its prevention. Exercise and preconditioning programs could be developed. Studies to determine the optimal frequency and duration of rest periods need to be made.

The psychosocial element could be evaluated, using psychological and sociological methodology. This is the area wherein much of the knowledge gained in other areas could be utilized in the form of public education. Preskiing schools should include contributions by health personnel on the safety aspects of skiing. The importance of skiing within one's limitations, developing good technique, assessing terrain, good slope manners, and good judgment in general could be included. Working with existing agencies and individuals such as ski schools and area operators might enhance their contributions in these areas, as well as those of the nursing profession.

Intervention on the third level, post-trauma care, is and always will be important. Here again the nurses' role could be expanded. Thorough investigation of the causal factors in skiing would be beneficial in the development of improved treatment methodologies. Rehabilitative counseling could be given new depth by such knowledge. The nurses' role could be further expanded by their working more closely with organizations such as the National Ski Patrol, trauma clinics, orthopedic care units, and other groups or interested individuals.

SUMMARY

The intent of this chapter has been to develop a concept of trauma that would be readily adaptable to most clinical areas. In the course of doing this, special consideration has been given to one particular area of interest—athletics—and more specifically to the sport of snow skiing. It is hoped that the ideas presented and the explanations and examples used are sufficiently forthright to allow meaningful application to other areas as well. If nursing is to continue its growth, such investigations and applications must be made into all areas of our daily life.

References

1. Addison, M.: The new way to learn to ski, Colorado 8:27, Nov.-Dec., 1970.
2. Auran, J. H.: All aboard the short-ski bandwagon, Skiing 25:85, Sept., 1972.
3. Bartley, S. H.: Fatigue: mechanism and management, Springfield, Ill., 1965, Charles C Thomas, Publisher, pp. 34-35.
4. Bartley, S. H., and Chute, E.: Fatigue and impairment in man, ed. 1, New York, 1947, McGraw-Hill Book Co., Inc., p. 53.
5. Blake, B.: Work capacity and its limiting factors at high altitudes. In Weihe, W. H., editor: Physiological effects of high altitude, Oxford, 1964, Pergamon Press, p. 233.
6. Brocklehurst, G.: A season's skiing, J. Royal Army Med. Corps 110:239, 1964.
7. Cletcher, J. O., Jr., and Gamble, W. E.: Management of ski injuries of the leg, G.P. 38:78, Nov., 1968.
8. Coventry, M. B., and Bianco, A. J.: Ski fracture of the metacarpals: one of the first sports injuries reported in the medical literature, Minn. Med. 47:1055, 1964.
9. Crawford, A.: Fatigue and driving, Ergonomics 4:143, April, 1961.
10. del Castillo, J., and Katz, B.: Changes in endplate activity produced by presynaptic polarization, J. Physiol. 124:586, 1954.
11. Earle, A. S., Moritz, J. R., Saviers, G. B., and Ball, J. D.: Ski injuries, J.A.M.A. 180:285, April 28, 1962.
12. Ellison, A. E., Carroll, R. E., Haddon, W., Jr., and Wolf, M.: Skiing injuries. Clinical study, Public Health Rep. 77:985, 1962.
13. Erskine, L. A.: The mechanisms involved in skiing injuries, Am. J. Surg. 97:667, 1959.
14. Evans, F. G.: Impact tolerance of human pelvis and long bones. In Gurdjian, E. S., editor: Impact injury and crash protection, Springfield, Ill., 1970, Charles C Thomas, Publisher, p. 402.
15. Garrick, J. G.: The epidemiology of ski injuries, Minn. Med. 54:17, 1971.
16. Grandjean, E.: Fatigue: its physiological and psychological significance, Ergonomics 11:427, 1968.
17. Haddon, W., Jr., Ellison, A. E., and Carroll, R. E.: Skiing injuries. Epidemiologic study, Public Health Rep. 77:975, 1962.
18. Harwood, M. R., and Strange, G. L.: Orthopedic aspects and safety factors in snow skiing, N. Y. State J. Med. 66:2899, 1966.
19. Heimstra, N. W.: The effects of "stress fatigue" on performance in a simulated driving situation, Ergonomics 13:209, March, 1970.
20. Heinkel, K.: Statistics on the safety binding, Congress Report at Davos Parsenn, 1958.
21. Hutchings, J.: A five-year survey of skiing fractures from Falls Creek, Victoria, Med. J. Aust. 2:174, July 26, 1969.
22. Judd, W. R., and Hendryson, I. E.: Sitzmarks or safety, Denver, 1960, National Ski Patrol System, Inc.
23. Leidholt, J. D.: Ski injuries, Lancet 1:1388, 1962.
24. Leidholt, J. D.: Biomechanics of ankle injuries in skiing as related to release bindings, Surg. Clin. North Am. 43:363, April, 1963.
25. McAlister, R., Brody, J. A., Hammes, L. M., et al: Epidemiology of ski injuries in the Anchorage area, Arch. Environ. Health 10:910, 1965.
26. McFarland, R. A.: Fatigue in industry: understanding fatigue in modern life, Ergonomics 14:1, 1971.
27. Magill, C. D.: Ski injuries and their prevention, Rocky Mt. Med. J. 65:47, Dec., 1968.
28. McIntyre, J. M.: Skiing injuries, Can. Med. Assoc. J. 88:602, 1963.
29. Moritz, J. R.: Ski injuries, Am. J. Surg. 98:493, Sept., 1959.

30. Nicholas, J. A.: Injuries to knee ligaments: relationship to looseness and tightness in football players, J.A.M.A. **212:**2236, 1970.
31. Pathak, C. L.: Muscular work and fatigue, Indian J. Physiol. Pharmacol. **13:**87, April, 1969.
32. Pfeiffer, D., and Maginn, M.: The Lilliputian revolution, Skiing **25:**120, Oct., 1972.
33. Schilling, J. A.: Trauma, J. Okla. Med. Assoc. **61:**499, Oct., 1968.
34. Selye, H.: Stress of life, New York, 1956, Mc-Graw-Hill Book Co., Inc.
35. Simonson, E., editor: Physiology of work capacity, Springfield, Ill., 1971, Charles C Thomas, Publisher.
36. Spademan, R.: Lower-extremity injuries as related to the use of ski safety bindings, J.A.M.A. **203:**445, 1968.
37. Sponsel, K. H.: Weekend ski injuries at Mt. Telemark, Cable, Wisconsin: 1965-1966 season, Ind. Med. Surg. **36:**35, 1967.
38. Van Der Linden, W.: The skiers' boot top fracture, rising incidence, characteristics, treatment, Acta Orthop. Scand. **40:**797, 1970.
39. Voorhees, R. L.: Injury prevention, Minn. Med. **54:**19, 1971.
40. Waldie, W.: Orthopaedic hazards of snow and ice, Practitioner **201:**892, Dec., 1968.
41. Weiss, B. W., Katkin, E. S., and Rubin, B. M.: Relationship between a factor analytically derived measure of a specific fear and performance after related fear induction, J. Abnorm. Psychol. **73:**461, Oct., 1968.

Bibliography

Frankel, V. H., and Burstein, A. H.: Load capacity of tubular bone. In Kenedi, R. M., editor: Biomechanics and related bio-engineering topics, Oxford, England, 1965, Pergamon Press.

Simonson, E.: Ski injuries, Lancet **1:**1388, 1962.

An excursion into the law of nursing practice

with an introduction by
Betty S. Bergersen
Margery Duffey

The study of law is the curriculum laggard of the nursing profession. Why does this situation exist at a time when nurse practitioners are advancing in knowledge and assuming responsibilities not known to nursing a decade ago, when every day the boundaries of practice are being extended, and when functions are continually being realigned between medicine and nursing? In this period of rapid change in the delivery of health care, legally sensitive words are commonly used in describing future roles for nurses such as, "primary health-care givers," "independent practitioners," and "expanded roles," to name just a few. These should cause the reader to pause and turn to the law for the support that is now available and that, when implemented, will add safety to health care and increase the confidence of the nurse who is providing the service.

For too long, the study of law has been limited to the search for answers to narrow questions of procedure or to concern over who would assume responsibility if the conduct of the nurse should be the cause of harm. This kind of discussion has been interspersed with liberal amounts of "anecdotal law." Without legal reasoning to support the decision, the discussions have been of little service in acquainting nurses with sound legal concepts and, in fact, have been psychologically disturbing in the overemphasis on the punitive aspects of the law. The chapters in this section present the law as a viable, constructive, and socially oriented discipline that has had insufficient attention on the part of planners of continuing education and associate, baccalaureate, and higher degree programs.

Chapter 33 sets the stage for a new approach to the study of the law of nursing practice that, in the future, may well become an integral part of the total body of the law of health sciences, wherein nursing will have a unique contribution. Chapter 34 melds ethical, moral, and legal issues in the nurse's increasing involvement in human experimentation. Chapter 35 follows a natural sequence in its focus on human rights and shows that consent for their invasion is far from a perfunctory exercise. Chapter 36 introduces the concept of the legal duty to foresee harm as a commonality in nursing practice and relates the depth and scope of the duty to foresee the potential for harm to the knowledge and skill that the nurse practitioner brings to the act.

The primary purpose of this section is to introduce, in selected areas, the conceptual framework of law necessary for decision making in nursing practice.

33

Nursing jurisprudence: the need for a conceptual framework

Irene Murchison

The degree to which a profession continually searches for the *why* of its practice is a measure of its viability as a profession. Knowledge of the law can make a meaningful contribution in guiding nursing practice and in improving the quality of patient care.

> Nurse educators are asking if law should be one component of the interdisciplinary base of nursing science.
>
> Nurse practitioners are asking for knowledge about legal sources of authority to guide the determination of boundaries of practice in the delivery of health services.

A major continuing objective of each volume of *Current Concepts in Clinical Nursing*[1] has been to bring the field of nursing into focus and to project guidelines for professional nursing practice by presenting a broad spectrum of new and current concerns and functions of nurse practitioners. Concern for nursing functions mounts as practice becomes increasingly complex because of the rapidly expanding knowledge of medical science and technology. At the same time, consumer demands for comprehensive health care are bringing about a need for a complete reorganization of the method of delivering health care. The nursing profession is found in the mainstream of this change and is addressing itself to the challenge by preparing practitioners to assume greater responsibilities and to exercise a hitherto unknown degree of independence, which is both exciting and awesome in its legal implications. A conceptual framework of law, such as that needed by the nurse clinician, could not be more timely or more directly related to these objectives.

Although nurses have been interested in learning about the legal implications of their practice, their concern has been chiefly for the procedural rather than the substantive content. They have been satisfied that the knowledge of law should evolve from problems that occur in daily nursing practice, whereas, with other sciences, they accepted the principle that the science foundation must precede and support the art of nursing. Historically, the physical and biological sciences of chemistry, physiology, and, to a lesser degree, physics received first attention by nurse educators. Since the field of knowledge was vast in each of these sciences, it was necessary to identify and select content that would best guide the nurse in understanding the patient's disease and the reasons for therapeutic intervention. This integration served to bring about a meaningful relationship between these sciences and the knowledge of nursing. It was a slow process, however, chiefly because nurses were not at that time prepared to bridge the gap between the content of the sciences and their syntheses into clinical nursing.

The introduction of the social and behavioral sciences into nursing curricula followed the biological and physical sciences but moved more rapidly, since nursing had long been a profession dedicated to caring for and about people. A conceptual framework of these sciences within nursing practice fell into place as a natural component of patient care. At this point, law might have been included as a logical part of the social and behavioral science sequence. Why it was not still remains an open question.

Law is only another study of human beings and their social interactions. Social and behavioral scientists and lawyers have traditionally recognized the interrelationships of their disciplines and how each influences the investigations and applications of the other. Sanctions imposed by law for deviant conduct are not unlike those imposed by family and religious life as studied in related disciplines.[4] Legal sanctions in general are intended to be positive, rather than punitive, in their influence on bringing about an orderly society. In fact, their deterrent effect promotes a socially healthful society, just as a program of preventive medicine aims for optimum health for all members of the community.

Law is so deeply rooted in the social fabric of our lives that some legal educators view law as another behavioral science, whereas others take a more conservative position but are willing to admit that it is behaviorally oriented. These shades of meaning, although interesting, should be left to the legal scholars for continued study. It is sufficient for nursing that the social components of patient care should include a body of knowledge drawn from the social and behavioral sciences as well as law. Each in its own way contributes to the rationale for human conduct, including that of nurse and patient.

It would be less than accurate to imply that the nursing profession has not had a genuine social-legal concern for safety in the delivery of health care. It has supported statutory laws that have provided for the creation of boards of nursing. These regulatory bodies have served a distinct social purpose by screening the competent from the incompetent practitioners through the licensing process. Boards of nursing have also significantly influenced the improvement of nurse preparation by their accrediting procedures.[4, p. 395] However, statutory control of practice is not the sole means of determining the source of authority for the conduct of the nurse practitioner. Two areas of law commingle in this determination, statutory[4, p. 12] and tort law.[3] Tort law deals with civil wrongs in which one person seeks redress for the interference with his person, property, or other tangible interests. These acts of interference are broad in scope; they may involve the man on the street, the shopkeeper, the artisan, or the professional practitioner.

Although the distinction between the origins of statutory and case law is known to many nurses, restatement may serve to emphasize the importance of each area as it relates to nursing practice. Statutory law is enacted by a state or federal legislative body. It is by statutory law that administrative agencies are created, such as boards of nursing, the Civil Aeronautics Board, and numerous other agencies. These agencies are formed in response to a social concern about the need for governmental control of some area of activity, whether business, industry, or professional practice.[4, p. 389] As opposed to the formal enactment of statutory law, tort law is judge-made law. It is written as an outgrowth of the settlement of a dispute in which someone is claimed to have harmed another through socially unacceptable conduct. Tort law sets a legal standard for determining fault, for fixing blame, and for measuring economic loss to the one injured.[4, p. 72] It may also serve as precedent for similar cases to be decided in the same way.

Numerous illustrations of the interrelationship of statutory and tort law can be found within nursing practice. For example, if a claim of negligence were made against a nurse, the judge would probably turn to the statutory definition of nursing practice to seek information regarding legally authorized nursing functions. If the statutory definition of nursing conduct were descriptive of current nursing practice, the judge might use this section of the law as a source of authority in the settlement of the dispute and write it into his decision (case law). Statutes may lag, however, and no longer reflect current practice. When this happens, the judge may then, at his discretion, write new law into his decision, as was done in the case of *Cooper v. National Motor Bearing Co.*,[2] in which a significant part of the decision deals with acts of diagnosing by nurses and sets forth their legal obligation to do so within the bounds of knowledge and skills expected of a professional nursing practitioner. Case law is an index to social thinking and is often a forerunner of needed changes in statutory law.

As is commonly known within the nursing profession, the role of the nurse is clouded by many ambiguities and shows signs of accelerated change. The social and professional forces bringing about this change are not within the scope of this article. Suffice it to say, however, that the forces for change are so intimately related to the demands for health care that a new type of nurse practitioner will emerge. Whether the nurse practices in an institutional or a community setting, the role will be that of a pathfinder skilled in independent decision making that will require a knowledge of law to support professional practice. Such knowledge will not only bring professional confidence but also will permit optimum utilization of knowledge and skill in the delivery of health services.

In summary, a curriculum lag has been noted in the present preparation of nurse practitioners. The need is evident for in-troduction of instruction in the broad field of law at the undergraduate, graduate, continuing, and in-service levels of nursing education. Its justifications, simply stated, are those of adding safety to patient care and increased confidence within nurse practitioners to permit expansion of nursing practice in response to the expectations of society.

References

1. Bergersen, B. S., Anderson, E. H., Duffey, M., Lohr, M., and Rose, M. H., editors: Current concepts in clinical nursing, vol. 2, St. Louis, 1969, The C. V. Mosby Co., p. ix.
2. *Cooper v. National Motor Bearing Co.,* 288 P.2d 581 (1955).
3. Murchison, I. A.: Role of law in the decision-making process in occupational health nursing, Occup. Health Nurs. 21:16, July, 1973.
4. Murchison, I. A., and Nichols, T. S.: Legal foundations of nursing practice, New York, 1970, The Macmillan Co.

34

Human experimentation in clinical nursing research: observations from a legal perspective

Thomas S. Nichols

THE PROBLEM AND ITS SETTING

Medical and nursing research provides the building material for advances in medical and nursing science. Objective, realistic, and insightful experimentation forms the basis for improvements, modifications, and, sometimes, spectacular breakthroughs in the continuing search for better care of human injury and disease. Through research comes the confidence that the use of new techniques, new drugs, and new procedures will further the ever-present objective of providing the highest quality of health care to the largest number of people.

Much attention has been given in recent years to the status, needs, and future of nursing research.[2] The need for properly conducted, properly controlled *clinical* research is repeatedly emphasized. Clinical research may take a myriad of forms and deal with a great spectrum of problems; it may mean research conducted in the hospital, in the home, in the clinic, or in other settings. Although the range of particular aspects of nursing care that may be dealt with is very wide, there is one element common to every study—it involves human beings. To state it another way, people are the subjects of the experiments, and it is their responses, attitudes, or conditions that are being watched, measured, and analyzed. Human reactions are being transformed into numbers, percentages, readings, and experimental results; for some period of their lives, such persons are the raw material of scientific experiments.

But humans are not experimental animals, and more than any other, the health professions seek to shelter and enhance the humanness of human beings. The very foundation of medicine and nursing is the respect for life and personality. As independent clinical nursing research expands in stature and in quantity and as clinical medical research grows, with nurses as active participants, it becomes imperative that the nursing profession continually focus on and confront the legal and ethical problems that inevitably exist whenever any experiment is designed and carried out utilizing human subjects.

On reflection, two broad lines of clinical research are evident. One is the search for effective therapy for a particular disease in a particular patient; the other is the search for knowledge that will advance medical knowledge and potentially aid future patients. Experimentation of the first kind occurs when new drugs or new techniques are tried in an effort to save an otherwise doomed patient. Here significant risks are perceived and accepted because the alternatives appear even more dangerous or unsatisfactory. At this point in time many organ transplants fall into this category.

Experimentation of the second kind appears in the strictly observational experiments and in those in which therapeutically neutral techniques may be carried out on some or all the participating subjects. In this kind of project advancement of the short-term interests of those undergoing study is not the goal; rather observations and data of patient reaction are collected and analyzed. It is through the overall analysis of these data that medical advances occur that are of potential use to future patients but not to the subjects themselves. Experiments in which the effects of placebos are compared with those of therapeutic drugs may fall in this category. Although there may be some overlap, the legal-ethical considerations that impinge on these two types may differ significantly.

In experimental studies with human subjects, the nurse may occupy the position of an independent investigator designing and carrying out research studies and accepting ultimate responsibility for all phases of experimentation. Alternatively, the nurse may directly participate in carrying out an experiment designed and led by others. But whichever role is adopted, it is important that the nurse reflect on the status of the human subjects involved and be aware in any experiment of the professional-legal-ethical implications of participation.

A threshold question is which experiments possess such implications? Certainly, any experiment that directly affects or may affect the physical condition of a patient raises the questions in their starkest form. None would doubt that direct or potential impact on the patient's mental or emotional state also presents squarely the same questions. At another step removed are the observational studies that publish data about patients in more or less summarized and anonymous form. Here, too, important patient rights are involved: the right to confidentiality and the right to privacy, rights protected by nursing ethics and the law alike. On consideration of these factors and situations, it is apparent that in virtually any investigation in which patients are the subjects, their rights must be carefully considered, and the difficult choices for the researcher that arise as a consequence must be confronted.

It is obvious that experimental studies are conducted precisely because the outcome is unknown; were it known, there would be no occasion for experimentation. This means that in every case there is an unknown and unpredictable element. Every experiment in changed technique involves the risk that the new technique may be less effective than the old, that is, that patients being subject to the new way may be worse off than had they been treated or handled in a time-tested way. This risk must always be recognized.

With these thoughts in mind, the primary conflicts in needs and values may be identified.

First, it is the right of the subject to avoid any risk, pain, discomfort, or exposure, which may conflict with the vital need for information to advance medical and nursing science for the benefit of future patients and generations, even at some cost in suffering.

Second, there is the right of the patient to full and complete disclosure of all aspects of any experiment, which may conflict with the real or imagined requirement that the experimental subject be kept ignorant of some aspects of the study to avoid biased results or the introduction of uncontrolled variables.

THE LAW'S VIEW OF EXPERIMENTATION ON HUMAN BEINGS

Legal considerations of experimentation on human subjects, that is, those which involve analysis of subjects' rights and nurses' duties in the context of litigation instituted against nurses, are inseparable from the general law that governs nursing practice as a whole. The definition and dimensions of the standard of care to which nurses are held in the practice of their profession and the delineation of the legal duties owed to those for whom they provide health care are fundamental and provide the framework for legal analysis. The basic principle is that a nurse, like every other professional, must conduct her practice in accordance with the level of professional competence prevailing in the medical community within which the work is carried out. The nurse's practice is based on specialized education and training, and the law demands that the nurse ably use these tools.[17, pp. 77-83] Furthermore, the nurse must conduct professional practice in such a way as to avoid, to the extent possible, injury or harm that is foreseeable to the eye of the professional practitioner.[17, pp. 120-131]

These generalizations have in many types of situations been the subject of judicial discussion and refinement; the courts have over the course of many years and numberless cases developed more precise standards. Matters such as the nurse's responsibility toward a delirious or disoriented patient[21] or the nurse's responsibilities when confronted with a patient with a deteriorating physical condition and an indifferent physician[23] have been analyzed from the legal point of view in many different cases. But, although the concern about the legal position of health researchers is a legitimate one, the fact is that there are virtually no decisions that have been rendered in cases arising from an alleged misuse of techniques in human experimentation. The few cases that tread close to the area deal with obvious charlatans or clear cases of malfeasance. The courts have not been confronted with the difficult borderline cases; therefore definitive law is lacking.

Nonetheless, the legal decisions that have been rendered impose strict limitations on medical research. The indications from the few cases are that no experimentation, of any kind, is proper without total disclosure to the patient of all risks and all facets of the experimental procedure. Furthermore, the amount and intensity of litigation centering around the duty of disclosure in ordinary medical and nursing treatment, coupled with the powerful propensity on the part of the courts to intervene to protect rights of individuals, compel the conclusion that, in all probability, the courts would not be sympathetic with medical or nursing researchers when physical injuries, emotional trauma, or invasion of privacy have occurred.

But it has to be recognized that the courts are not experts in medical or nursing practice. They cannot be certain, without guidelines from the professions themselves, what appropriate limitations there may be on the utilization of experimental subjects or what limitations the health professions themselves have defined for such situations. Therefore there is every reason to think that in an attempt to delineate the legal principles applicable to litigation involving research, the courts will turn to the ethical standards promulgated by the health professions. Although perhaps the courts would not convert all ethical standards into legal ones, the basic principles should be expected to be very persuasive and influential.

Accordingly, to measure the legal rights and duties that evolve on the nurse researcher, as independent investigator or participant, ethics must be the point of primary analysis. Nursing ethics are very likely to determine the legal standard of care for nursing researchers.

ETHICAL STATEMENTS REGARDING MEDICAL RESEARCH ON HUMANS

The ANA Guidelines on Ethical Values, the Nurse in Research,[4] establish professional ethics for nursing. The guidelines do not draw a distinction between therapeutic and nontherapeutic research but emphasize the distinction between the nurse as investigator and the nurse as practitioner. They do, however, clearly require that when any study involves a risk of injury, full disclosure must be made and an independent judgment must be made on whether to continue the experiment. These guidelines provide the following:

RIGHT TO FREEDOM FROM INTRINSIC RISK OF INJURY

In studies where the nature of the research design subjects the individual to risk of emotional or physical injury, the degree of risk must be measured against the amount of direct benefit the subject can expect from the procedures. Not only must the investigator afford the prospective subject full information about the proposed investigation, but he must also utilize the professional judgment of his peer group, such as members of the review committee, as well as his own in deciding whether or not to implement the research design.*

These guidelines also contemplate, however, that certain studies which are undoubtedly nontherapeutic in nature may be done without consent on the judgment of a peer group or public body. In this respect the guidelines provide the following:

Studies which must be done without the consent of the subjects, i.e., behavioral responses of ethnic groups to a selected event in the everyday world, require the considered judgment of a peer group or of a public body as to the social need of the study and the necessity for a study of nonconsenting subjects.*

Point 6 of the Code for Nurses adopted

---

*From ANA guidelines on ethical values, the nurse in research, Am. J. Nurs. **68:**1506, 1507, 1968.

by the American Nurses Association is also pertinent:

> The nurse participates in research activities when assured that the rights of individual subjects are protected.*

The interpretive comments to Point 6 also emphasize the nurse's duty to assure that disclosure has been made and consent obtained:

> The nurse practitioner is, first of all, responsible for rendering quality nursing to all patients entrusted to her care. Implicit in this care is the protection of the individual's rights as outlined in the above publication: privacy, self-determination, conservation of personal resources, freedom from arbitrary hurt and intrinsic risk of injury, and the special rights of minors and incompetent persons.*

Thus current ethical statements applicable to nurse involvement in human experimentation permit, under specific circumstances, the carrying out of certain kinds of studies without full disclosure to the patient/subject of the risks, purposes, and elements of the research program.[1]

Nursing research is part of the broad area of medical research. Its goals and techniques are comparable, and the same ethical considerations are present whether the research study is denominated "nursing" or "medicine." Nursing ethics, therefore, do not stand isolated or independent from other ethical statements. With the latitude and potential for abuse inherent in the carrying out of nonconsensual human research, it seems important to consider statements from other health agencies in analyzing the ethical position of nursing researchers.

There is a great body of literature recognizing and discussing the ethical questions arising in connection with experimentation on human beings, with every possible shading or viewpoint respresented. One author has assembled more than 500 authorities,[12] and numerous other studies have continued to appear.[15,16] With such deep and philosophical issues, it is perhaps not surprising that definitive statements and widespread agreement have yet to be reached.

One of the most authoritative and influential formulations of an ethical statement regarding human experimentation arose out of the trials at Nuremberg of more than twenty Nazi physicians and scientists, based on experiments they carried out on political prisoners. Against this tragic background, American physicians prepared a ten-point code, now known as the Nuremberg Code,[22] which set out the principles governing the use of human subjects in medical research. The code follows:

1. The voluntary consent of the human subject is absolutely essential.
2. The experiment should be such as to yield fruitful results for the good of society, unprocurable by other methods or means of study, and not random and unnecessary in nature.
3. The experiment should be so designed and based on the results of animal experimentation and a knowledge of the natural history of the disease or other problem under study that the anticipated results will justify the performance of the experiment.
4. The experiment should be so conducted as to avoid all unnecessary physical and mental suffering and injury.
5. No experiment should be conducted where there is an a priori reason to believe that death or disabling injury will occur; except, perhaps, in those experiments where the experimental physicians also serve as subjects.
6. The degree of risk to be taken should never exceed that determined by the humanitarian importance of the problem to be solved by the experiment.
7. Proper preparations should be made and adequate facilities provided to protect the experimental subject against even remote possibilities of injury, disability, or death.
8. The experiment should be conducted only by scientifically qualified persons. The highest degree of skill and care should be required through all stages of the experiment of those who conduct or engage in the experiment.
9. During the course of the experiment the human subject should be at liberty to bring the experiment to an end if he has reached the physical or mental state where continuation of the experiment seems to him to be impossible.
10. During the course of the experiment the scientist in charge must be prepared to terminate the experiment at any stage, if he has probable cause to believe, in the exercise of good faith, superior skill and careful judgment required of him that a continuation of the experiment is likely to result in injury, disability, or death to the experimental subject.*

*From Murchison, I., and Nichols, T.: Legal foundations of nursing practice, New York, 1970, The Macmillan Co., p. 468.

*From Trials of war criminals before Nuremberg military tribunals 2:181, 1950.

Note that the Nuremberg Code grants no leeway in the matter of consent; under its terms "the voluntary consent of the human subject is *absolutely essential*."

A second influential code of ethics is not so restrictive. In 1964 the World Medical Association, meeting in Finland, promulgated the Declaration of Helsinki,[9] as follows:

Recommendations Guiding Doctors in Clinical Research

INTRODUCTION

It is the mission of the doctor to safeguard the health of the people. His knowledge and conscience are dedicated to the fulfillment of this mission.

The Declaration of Geneva of The World Medical Association binds the doctor with the words, "The health of my patient will be my first consideration"; and the International Code of Medical Ethics which declares that "Any act or advice which could weaken physical or mental resistance of a human being may be used only in his interest."

Because it is essential that the results of laboratory experiments be applied to human beings to further scientific knowledge and to help suffering humanity, The World Medical Association has prepared the following recommendations as a guide to each doctor in clinical research. It must be stressed that the standards as drafted are only a guide to physicians all over the world. Doctors are not relieved from criminal, civil and ethical responsibilities under the laws of their own countries.

In the field of clinical research a fundamental distinction must be recognized between clinical research in which the aim is essentially therapeutic for a patient, and clinical research the essential object of which is purely scientific and without therapeutic value to the person subjected to the research.

I. BASIC PRINCIPLES

1. Clinical research must conform to the moral and scientific principles that justify medical research, and should be based on laboratory and animal experiments or other scientifically established facts.

2. Clinical research should be conducted only by scientifically qualified persons and under the supervision of a qualified medical man.

3. Clinical research cannot legitimately be carried out unless the importance of the objective is in proportion to the inherent risk to the subject.

4. Every clinical research project should be preceded by careful assessment of inherent risks in comparison to foreseeable benefits to the subject or to others.

5. Special caution should be exercised by the doctor in performing clinical research in which the personality of the subject is liable to be altered by drugs or experimental procedure.

II. CLINICAL RESEARCH COMBINED WITH PROFESSIONAL CARE

1. In the treatment of the sick person, the doctor must be free to use a new therapeutic measure if in his judgment it offers hope of saving life, reestablishing health, or alleviating suffering.

If at all possible, consistent with patient psychology, the doctor should obtain the patient's freely given consent after the patient has been given a full explanation. In case of legal incapacity consent should also be procured from the legal guardian; in case of physical incapacity the permission of the legal guardian replaces that of the patient.

2. The doctor can combine clinical research with professional care, the objective being the acquisition of new medical knowledge, only to the extent that clinical research is justified by its therapeutic value for the patient.

III. NON-THERAPEUTIC CLINICAL RESEARCH

1. In the purely scientific application of clinical research carried on a human being, it is the duty of the doctor to remain the protector of the life and health of that person on whom clinical research is being carried out.

2. The nature, the purpose and the risk of clinical research must be explained to the subject by the doctor.

3a. Clinical research on a human being cannot be undertaken without his free consent, after he has been fully informed; if he is legally incompetent, the consent of the legal guardian should be procured.

3b. The subject of clinical research should be in such a mental, physical and legal state as to be able to exercise fully his power of choice.

3c. Consent should, as a rule, be obtained in writing. However, the responsibility for clinical research always remains with the research worker; it never falls on the subject, even after consent is obtained.

4a. The investigator must respect the right of each individual to safeguard his personal integrity, especially if the subject is in a dependent relationship to the investigator.

4b. At any time during the course of clinical research the subject or his guardian should be free to withdraw permission for research to be continued. The investigator or the investigating team should discontinue the research if in his or their judgment, it may, if continued, be harmful to the individual.*

This statement was adopted by the American Medical Association in 1966.

The Helsinki statement of principle contemplates in Section II the possibility that the physician may, under certain limited

---

*From Declaration of Helsinki, Br. Med. J. 2:177, July-Sept., 1964.

circumstances, provide an experimental therapeutic treatment without full disclosure or consent. Like the Nuremberg Code, however, Section III of the Declaration of Helsinki requires full explanation and free consent for nontherapeutic clinical research.

From a comparison of these ethical statements it can be seen that there is a conflict between the statements of medical ethics and the statements of nursing ethics. This conflict is that nursing ethics appear to permit, under some circumstances, experimentation with human subjects without the consent of those involved. The Nuremberg Code and the Declaration of Helsinki positively reject any such research as unethical. Although there is no certainty that a strict application of the Nuremberg Code would be made in the courts, it must be remembered that this code arose out of trial proceedings conducted by American lawyers and judges and was authored by American medical practitioners. Therefore it can be expected that the American judiciary will strongly resist giving their stamp of approval to ethical standards in the health professions less rigid than those imposed by this code.

Generally speaking, the requirement that voluntary consent be obtained falls first on the investigator. But the nurse as participant in clinical research also has defined and significant duties. Point 6 of the Code for Nurses implies the same requirement imposed by the Nuremberg Code in its definition of "voluntary consent":

This means that the person involved should have legal capacity to give consent; should be so situated as to be able to exercise free power of choice, without the intervention of any element of force, fraud, deceit, duress, overreaching or other ulterior form of constraint or coercion; and should have sufficient knowledge and comprehension of the elements of the subject matter involved as to enable him to make an understanding and enlightened decision. This latter element requires that before the acceptance of an affirmative decision by the experimental subject there should be made known to him the nature, duration, and purpose of the experiment; the method and means by which it is to be conducted; all inconveniences and hazards reasonably to be expected; and the effects upon his health or person which may possibly come from his participation in the experiment. *The duty and responsibility for ascertaining the quality of the consent rests upon each individual who initiates, directs, or engages in the experiment* [italics mine]. It is a personal duty and responsibility which may not be delegated to another with impunity.*

Under the Nuremberg Code there is no distinction between the independent investigator and the participant. If such a standard were to be built into the law—and there is every reason to believe it would be—the nurse has an absolute duty to disclose all matters relating to the experiment, whether or not the physician has done so, and *whether or not the experimental design contemplates such consent.*

PROBLEM AREAS IN MEDICAL AND NURSING RESEARCH

The most highly publicized instance of legitimate research that became embroiled in controversy arose in the course of studies in Brooklyn, New York.[10] Two distinguished cancer researchers were testing some of their immunological hypotheses; live cancer cells were injected into twenty-two seriously ill patients. None of the patients was advised that the injections contained live cancer cells, and none was advised that the injections formed no part of their therapeutic regimen. None of the patients contracted cancer or experienced harmful effects of any kind.

The fact of the study emerged into public view, and a great furor arose about the propriety of the physicians' conduct.[13] After extended inquiry, the New York Board of Regents, the medical licensing authority in New York, held the conduct unethical and suspended the licenses of the physicians concerned.

Perhaps the most noteworthy aspects of this matter are that the physicians were acting in good faith, that they were pursuing a line of research regarded as highly promising and of great potential worth in the never-ending search for a cancer cure, that they were among the most distinguished in the field, and that no harm befell the patients. These factors neither individually nor collectively outweighed the elemental facts that patients are not to be viewed as experimental subjects and that these pa-

---

*From Trials of war criminals before Nuremburg military tribunals **2:**181, 1950.

tients had not been given a full and frank disclosure.

The absence of harm in the New York situation is in unfortunate contrast to a number of research studies described by Beecher.[6] Beecher lists twenty-two published studies in which questionable experimentation was clearly involved, with serious consequences, including death, ensuing for subjects of the studies. These included the administration of placebos in place of known effective treatment, the administration for study purposes of injurious drugs, the carrying out of physiological studies injurious to the patients, and the use of new techniques on normal patients. Each study may well have involved nurse participation and probably knowledge on the nurse's part of the possible outcomes. Each study was doubtless conducted in the name of science and for the presumed benefit of medical progress.

Review of nursing research literature does not produce a bounty of questionable practices, for which the research arm deserves the plaudits of the profession. Indeed, although a full search has by no means been undertaken, no research report has been found in which it can be inferred that harm was suffered. Nonetheless, the literature does contain instances that raise the problems under discussion.

Example 1. At a large urban hospital, concern developed over the delays in care of orthopedic patients in the emergency room.[7] Accordingly, it was decided at the hospital's highest level to permit emergency room triage nurses to order x-ray examinations. During a one-month period triage nurses, after an orientation phase, were permitted to order x-ray examinations in cases that they determined fell within the guidelines the hospital had established. Thereafter, the nurses' performance was compared with the physicians' performance over a comparable period. The results clearly established the competence of the nurses to make the decision as to the need for x-ray films and to carry out the associated operations. As a result, a significant improvement in patient care was achieved.

Nonetheless, in the absence of full disclosure such a study is subject to criticism for violation of the ethical principles regarding experimentation. While the study was being carried out, no one *knew* that nurses would demonstrate the proficiency that they actually did; there was a clear risk that some patients treated by the nurses would receive significantly inferior treatment compared to those treated by the physicians. Had that occurred, the conclusion is inescapable that those patients would have been the victims of experimentation, and those responsible would have been in an ethically and legally unjustified position.

The legal factor is one that must be reckoned with in the process of experimental design. All this is not to suggest that experimentation cannot occur. It does point up, however, the need to conceive and conduct experiments in such a way as to avoid ethical problems. For example, the experiment could have been conducted by dual and independent physician and nurse decisions on the same patients, followed by x-ray evaluation of each one's decision. Cumbersome, perhaps, but the existing ethical and legal standards and interpretations probably require no less.

Example 2. Recognition of the potential adverse impact of anxieties present in all types of patients is and has been the subject of considerable attention. To identify the factors associated with extreme anxiety and to determine whether generally accepted signs of anxiety could be consistently observed, a number of patients were studied through the mechanism of interviews, physiological tests, etc.[11] The approach taken was sophisticated, the objectives faultless. The report of the experiment, however, makes it perfectly clear that the purposes of the study were deliberately concealed from the patients, on the grounds that disclosure "could have introduced many types of discomfort, distortion and additional sources of bias into the data." This fact, coupled with the risk that the interview process itself could in some patients increase their anxieties, once again raises the ethical question of whether such research is within the bounds of medical and nursing ethics. Can a patient be subject to any risk, even a remote one, of having his emotional state rendered less healthy by means of misleading statements. Strict interpretation of the ethical guidelines already established would clearly answer this question with a definite "no."

Example 3. Almost any procedure that involves the use of a control group receiving no comparable care or a group receiving an alternative form of care can pose ethical problems because the efficacy of the procedure is by definition uncertain. Thus reported studies on methods in preoperative teaching,[14] behavior changes in mentally retarded children,[5] relaxation therapy in heart surgery patients,[3] physical activity in infants,[19] and stress during bedmaking[18] all could be subject to criticism on legal grounds if disclosure and consent were lacking. Once again, there is no need to curtail or abandon such research. It is a question of full disclosure and free and informed consent. No experiment in which there is any possibility, even remote, of a patient coming to harm or receiving a less efficacious treatment than normal can ethically be conducted without such disclosure.

In an experiment in which a new treatment is being tested against a standard one, it is essential that the data be continually monitored and that the experiment be terminated whenever the data *suggest* that the experimental treatment is less efficacious than the alternate. There is arguably a legal duty to terminate such an experiment even though it is not complete and even though the researcher knows that rigorous analysis of the data collected would not yield significant results. Self-discipline is required on the part of the researcher and those working with him. It may be costly in terms of effort and expense to call a halt to a promising study on the basis of meager information. The underlying principle is that the patient must not be exposed to risk; at the first indications that such exposure is occurring, the rights of the patient prevail over the needs of science.

Example 4. Another type of study involves essentially no risk or discomfort to the patient, but it raises questions about invasions of privacy and whether data can be collected and disseminated about a patient without his knowledge or consent. First, it must be clearly understood that if a patient's problems or condition is publi-

cized in such a way as to identify him and expose his affairs to public scrutiny, there is clear legal responsibility. Instances that have reached the courts include publication of photographs of deformed infants and body exposure to persons whose presence was medically unnecessary.[17, pp. 296-297]

Inclusion of anonymous statistics in a group of data such as in connection with studies of behavior of addicts,[8] studies of blood pressure techniques,[20] and the like probably do not present serious ethical or legal questions, although caution and a strict adherence to full disclosure principles dictate a complete explanation to the patients and the collection of data with the consent of the patients concerned.

SUMMARY AND CONCLUSIONS

This chapter has attempted to suggest once again ethical and legal problems inherent in nursing research. The discussions are, as the reader doubtless will have noted, notably lacking in solutions. From the sanctuaries of distance and nonresponsibility, it is all too easy to overlook or minimize the practical problems embodied in the necessity to obtain full consent and to make full disclosure under any and all circumstances. Nevertheless, as the standards and legal principles have been articulated up to now, nothing less is required. Nursing researchers, then, must build into their experimental design the making of full disclosure and the obtaining of voluntary consent. With full attention and concern to the problem, the fertile minds of those engaged in this challenging field will doubtless preserve the twin goals of nursing advances and individual integrity of the person and mind of the experimental subject.

References

1. Abdellah, F. G.: Approaches to protecting the rights of human subjects, Nurs. Res. **16**:316, Fall, 1967.
2. Abdellah, F. G.: Overview of nursing research 1955-1968. Part I, Nurs. Res. **19**:6, Jan.-Feb., 1970.
3. Aiken, L. H., and Hendrichs, T. F.: Systematic relaxation as a nursing intervention technique with open heart surgery patients, Nurs. Res. **20**:212, May-June, 1971.
4. ANA guidelines on ethical values, the nurse in research, Am. J. Nurs. **68**:1504, 1968.
5. Balthazar, E. E., English, G. E., and Sindberg,

R. M.: Behavior changes in mentally retarded children following the initiation of an experimental nursing program, Nurs. Res. **20**:69, Jan.-Feb., 1971.

6. Beecher, H. K.: Ethics and clinical research, N. Engl. J. Med. **274**:1354, 1936.
7. Bliss, A., Decker, L., and Southwick, W. D.: The emergency room nurse orders x-rays of distal limbs in orthopedic trauma, Nurs. Res. **20**:440, Sept.-Oct., 1971.
8. Brink, P. J.: Behavioral characteristics of heroin addicts on a short-term detoxification program, Nurs. Res. **21**:38, Jan.-Feb., 1972.
9. Declaration of Helsinki, Br. Med. J. **2**:177, July-Sept., 1964.
10. Fletcher, J.: Human experimentation: ethics in the consent situation, Law and Contemporary Problems **32**:620, 1967.
11. Graham, L. E., and Conley, E. M.: Evaluation of anxiety and fear in adult surgical patients, Nurs. Res. **20**:113, March-April, 1971.
12. Ladimer, I., and Neman, R.: Clinical investigation in medicine, Boston, 1963, Boston University, Law-Medicine Research Institute, p. 494.
13. Langer, E.: Human experimentation, New York verdict affirms patients' rights, Science **151**:663, 1966.
14. Lindeman, C. A., and Van Aernam, B.: Nursing intervention with the presurgical patient—the effects of structured and unstructured preoperative teaching, Nurs. Res. **20**:319, July-Aug., 1971.
15. Morse, H. N.: Legal implications of clinical investigations, Vanderbilt Law Review **20**:747, 1967.
16. Mulford, R. D.: Experimentation on human beings, Stanford Law Review **20**:99, Nov., 1967.
17. Murchison, I., and Nichols, T.: Legal foundations of nursing practice, New York, 1970, The Macmillan Co.
18. Palmer, E. M., and Griffith, E. W.: Effect of activity during bedmaking on heart rate and blood pressure, Nurs. Res. **20**:17, Jan.-Feb., 1971.
19. Porter, L. S.: The impact of physical-physiological activities on infants' growth and development, Nurs. Res. **21**:210, May-June, 1972.
20. Putt, A. M.: A comparison of blood pressure readings by auscultation and palpation, Nurs. Res. **15**:4, Fall, 1966.
21. *Spivey v. St. Thomas Hospital,* 31 Tenn. App. 12. 211 S.W. 2d 450 (1947).
22. Trials of war criminals before Nuremberg military tribunals **2**:181, 1950.
23. *Valentin v. La Societe Francaise,* 76 Cal. App. 2d 1, 172 P. 2d 359 (1946).

35

Patients' rights: consent for their invasion

Helen Huber
Irene Murchison

The intentional invasion of the legally protected rights of others is unavoidable in nursing and medical practice. Knowledge of the law clarifies these rights and alerts the nurse to conditions under which invasion is permissible. At the same time, it serves to emphasize that sensitivity to and responsibility for the rights of others is an essential part of nursing care.

Patient A has been confined to an institution for the mentally ill for several weeks. He has shown improvement in attitude and in cooperation with his plan of care. One day supervisor B notes that A is not at lunch. She goes to his room, where she finds him sullen and hostile. B tries to persuade him to come with her to lunch. When A persists in his refusal, B becomes firm and finally says, "If you continue to behave this way, we are going to have to start your shock treatments again." When B makes this statement, she knows that the patient is fearful of shock treatments and that the possibility of resuming them has not been discussed with him.

Does A have cause for legal action? Were the legally protected rights of A invaded? Having known the legal meaning of such conduct, how could the nurse have avoided liability? Suppose that A in further expression of his hostility should push B away from him with so much force that she falls over a chair, striking her head on the radiator and lacerating her scalp; if she provoked the situation, does she have cause for action?

The situation of patient A and supervisor B sometimes occurs in nursing practice. Nurses are often confronted with varying degrees of lack of patient cooperation. Questions arise concerning the nurse's authority for persuasion, threats, or even force to carry out the therapeutic regimen prescribed in the intended best interest of the patient. Legal answers are not easy. Here, as in many similar situations, the conduct of the nurse and the patient has cut across broad areas of the law dealing with the rights of the individual. Had B known the substance of the law, it is doubtful that a situation so fraught with potential legal liability would have been provoked.

For reasons discussed in other chapters in this section, there has been a lag in including substantive law as a part of the behavioral science strand of nursing science. It is true that, at this point, there has been some recognition of the need for preparation of the nurse practitioner in this area. However, it has been evidenced chiefly by concern for answers to questions of liability for malpractice or for authority needed to undertake certain procedures that have resulted from the transfer of functions from medical to nursing practice. In other words, the focus has been on the specific application of law to an immediate situation, rather than on developing the conceptual base from which the application should flow. Just as in many other applied disciplines, the professions of nursing and law use basic scientific knowledge to give a rationale for conduct unique to their fields. How logical it would be, when nursing conduct and law converge, for the nurse to turn to that area which would be of assistance in formulating a rationale for decision making.

The newly graduated nurse practitioner of the 1970s possesses a stronger and more comprehensive theoretical foundation of science on which to base nursing skills than in previous years. In basic preparation, the nurse has had the opportunity to apply this knowledge under supervision and to develop skills in a wide variety of community settings—hospital, homes, and clinics. In today's system of health care delivery the nurse must be competent to give a broad spectrum of health-related services. In so doing, the nurse is called on to identify client needs and resources, to assign priorities, to seek additional resources, and to refer the client to other health-care professionals. In this process the technical knowledge and skill of the nurse is used not only for physical care, but also in extending the professional role as a direct participant in the therapeutic process with patients and their families. Such mobility on the part of the nurse requires skill in independent problem solving and decision making. What the nurse does and where therapeutic interventions are carried out introduce innumerable legal variables. From the entire field of law, how does one select content to give the nurse a conceptual basis for conduct to enable the practitioner to move with safety and confidence in giving a more informed level of patient care?

One legal component always present in nursing practice is the law that deals with person-to-person interaction. In daily practice, the nurse takes into account a myriad of behavior patterns in individuals, in patients, in families, in various members of the community, and in colleagues. The nurse is aware that the law does not condone substandard practice or acts of inadvertence when another individual comes to harm because of that conduct. Legal responsibility does not end here, however. The law has set positive, constructive, and reasonable rules for controls on human conduct, even though it may be apart from any injury-producing situation.

To effect this control, the law has defined individual rights or interests that hold for all persons. It has also defined the manner in which these rights may be violated without incurring legal liability. Here is an opportunity for the nurse to build a conceptual framework of the law: the legal meaning of the interests protected, why they were established for mankind in general, and how these interests run counter to some daily nursing and medical practice. The law then states that, under certain circumstances, these protected rights may have to be invaded; when this is necessary, it sets forth methods of procedure to avoid legal liability. This broad under-standing of consent offers a new meaning to the legal procedures followed in treatment settings in which the nurse is making direct application in daily practice. The nurse, like any practitioner, can utilize such understanding in a typical or actual situation, instead of relying on a policy manual for the *do's* and *don't's.*

Key words under discussion in this area of the law are *protected interests* and *intent.* The word *interest,* in a broad sense, indicates the object of any human desire. Not all interests are given legal protection, or need they be. One may have a personal interest in the collection of fine paintings, rare coins, or beautiful clothes. With these the law would have no concern. Certain interests are considered socially important because they represent the basic fundamental rights or needs of individuals. These rights are then given legal protection and may not be infringed on by others. The law, in recognition of these needs, imposes sanctions on all persons or classes of persons to enjoin them from conduct that would threaten these interests.[8,pp.2-14] Those chosen for consideration in this chapter because of their bearing on nursing practice are interest in freedom from apprehension of harmful or offensive contact, interest in freedom from harmful bodily contact, and interest in freedom from confinement.

In some types of illness the patient's protected interests and needs come in direct conflict with each other. A person's right to freedom of movement may be a hazard if he is so intent on injuring himself that he turns an ordinary piece of household equipment into a weapon. The need for safety from harm is in direct conflict with the right to freedom from bodily contact or freedom from confinement. There is no legal choice other than to move counter to the patient's desires. The nurse would be obliged to interfere intentionally with the patient's freedom of movement if it contributed to his self-destruction.

Intent, as used legally, means a deliberate desire to bring about the consequences of an act and furthermore that the actor is substantially certain that the desired results will follow.[8,pp.15-18] The law does not judge one for evil intentions toward another or for a desire to bring about harm unless the desire is carried out. When harm does occur through deliberate intent, there seems to be a tendency for the courts to judge this form of misconduct more harshly than when the act is one of inadvertence.

On first thought, evil intentions, or a desire to harm another, would seem to have no relationship to nursing practice. Although this is true, the intentional invasion of the protected rights of another may give rise to a cause for action against a nurse even though the action may have been taken in consideration of the best interests of the patient, as was the case with supervisor B in the opening example. Although not so expressed, there seems to be little sympathy for one who deliberately invades the interest of another under the mistaken notion that he is doing no wrong. Society expects a professional person to know how to move with legal safety in bringing about desired results without offense to the client.

To be held liable for an intentional tort, one must deliberately undertake to bring about a probable foreseeable result. Troublesome legal problems arise when there is a thin line between intended acts and those of varying degrees of negligence. For example, C fires a gun into the air to frighten and disperse a crowd that is inciting a riot. The bullet ricochets and hits D. C intended to fire the gun but did not foresee the harm that took place. Such an incident might give rise to two legal questions: (1) was what happened due to intent, or (2) was it an act resulting from recklessness and poor judgment? A reasonably prudent nurse may intentionally limit the freedom of a patient by applying restraints to quiet a disturbed patient, failing to foresee that the patient might lacerate himself in his attempts to gain freedom. The charge against the nurse might be one of negligence for failure to foresee harm and eliminate a known risk or one of violating the patient's right of freedom of movement.

Intentional interference with the body of another, either through assault, battery, or limitation of freedom, is a recognized type of conduct for which legal redress

may be sought. What is the meaning of each?

Sometimes the terms *assault* and *battery* are used concurrently, since an assault may be so quickly followed by a battery that the act becomes one and the same. In other instances, the terms may be erroneously used interchangeably, the one as a synonym for the other. However, the law distinguishes between these two terms.

In an *assault,* the actor intends to create fear of bodily contact or apprehension of physically offensive conduct and has the potential ability to carry out his threat. Note that it is an act of intention and involves no body contact. Here the interest in freedom from damaging or embarrassing contact[8,pp.2-14] is invaded by means of *threat.*

R springs through an open door into the living room of X, points a gun, and says "I am going to kill you." The gun may not be loaded, but the fear of bodily harm, even to the point of death, is sufficient to constitute an assault.

Supervisor B (p. 335) did not touch the patient but verbally aroused fear of consequences to him if he persisted in not going to lunch; the patient may have believed that she had the authority to carry out the threat. B was guilty of an assault.

M, a male nurse, carrying medications to a ward, stopped beside patient L, a sexual deviant, and made an indecent proposal to her; he did not know that the patient was deaf. He was not guilty of an assault.

Nurse C, carrying a syringe of vitamin B solution, comes to the bedside of a well-adjusted postoperative patient and playfully says, "I am going to give you a shot, and you won't wake up for a week." The supervisor overhears the remark and quickly intervenes to reassure the patient, who had failed to perceive that the remark was made as a joke. C was nevertheless guilty of an assault. If one puts another in fear of apprehension, he is liable, even though the threat is not carried out.

The nurse or physician who uses threats or coercion to bring about patient cooperation renders himself liable for an assault.

A *battery* is an intrusion on the interest in freedom from physically damaging contact and from emotionally or intellectually offensive physical contact.[7,p.284] As in other areas, numerous variables in human conduct can lead to charges of battery, but certain characteristics are generally controlling. It must be an intentional act in which some form of physical injury is inflicted or in which the sense of individual dignity is offended by the laying on of hands in a rude or insolent manner.

The law is so jealous of the sanctity of the person that the slightest touching of another, or his clothes or cane, or anything else attached to his person, if done in a rude, insolent or angry manner, constitutes a battery for which the law affords redress.[3]

A charge of liability for battery is not uncommon in medical and nursing practice, since so much of patient care involves physical contact. Ignorance of the legally protected right to privacy would not exonerate the actor if it could be proved that the patient was carelessly draped or that indecent exposure was permitted during a physical examination. The pressure of crowded quarters and numerous patients in outpatient clinics does not constitute a defense. On the other hand, touching to call attention, to offer assistance, or to give most types of physical care is not usually actionable when the dignity of the individual is preserved.

Usually the physician, the hospital, or the nurse is sued for a battery by the patient. However, at times the situation may be reversed:

A registered private-duty nurse sought damages from a patient who was charged with assault and battery when, suffering from delirium tremens, he struck the nurse over the head with a table lamp. The patient's attorney argued that the nurse was aware of the risk in accepting employment. The court did not subscribe to this position and in finding for the nurse said: ". . . a person who is insane or mentally deranged or suffering delusions and hallucinations from a mental disorder from alcohol or any other cause is legally responsible to another person for any injuries or damages caused by assault and battery."[1]

In a similar situation, when an attendant was permitted to recover damages for injuries sustained because of a violent attack by a patient, the court said, ". . . public policy places on one suffering from defective reasoning the same liability for torts of this type as it places on those who are of normal mentality."[11]

Moving from threats of harm and actual physical contact to the legally protected interest in freedom from confinement, this chapter will consider the following hypothetical case:

Patient D is a hyperactive middle-aged woman, pacing the floor of the ward living room. She continually interrupts nurse E who is conversing with patient C. Finally, E becomes annoyed with this interference, knowing that D is overstimulated and in need of seclusion for a period of rest, which D has resisted to this point. This time the nurse suggests to D that they go to D's room so that she may see some art that D is working on. D complies; when they are in the room, the nurse steps out and quickly closes and locks the door. The patient protests, and the nurse tells D that she will be released when she has quieted down. Apart from the issue of betrayed trust in their relationship, does the nurse have a legal defense?

The interest of the patient to move about freely is often a point of conflict between patient and nurse. Sometimes the patient must be confined for his own safety or that of others. Again, confinement may be an essential part of the therapeutic process. When the nurse or attendant takes action to restrain or confine a patient, he should know that he is moving counter to an individual freedom that is a legally protected interest. Any form of restraint is a limitation on freedom; unless it follows legal principles, sanctions may be imposed for false imprisonment.[7, pp. 297-298]

For this reason, most hospitals require by policy that the decision to place a patient in restraints be made by a physician as part of the therapeutic regimen established for the patient. If it is foreseen that the patient's behavior may need to be dealt with frequently by such means, the order should describe the circumstances under which restraints are to be used at the discretion of the nursing staff.

In recent years, tranquilizers and other medications frequently have been referred to as chemical restraints, in that their action on the patient's nervous system lessens desire to perform acts that may be dangerous to the self or others. Is this a restraint within a legal context, or is it a preventive device that inhibits desires that would necessitate restraint?

Demonstrably, skillful interpersonal interventions with disturbed patients may reduce the patient's potential for combative behavior, thereby eliminating the need for restraints. If this view is accepted by the courts, the complexity of the issue concerning the right to freedom of movement is increased. In any situation that *results* in the use of restraints several variables need to be considered:

1. Was the severe disturbance in the patient not mediated by interpersonal intervention?
2. Was there lack of skill on the staff's part as to timing or method of intervening?
3. Is it a reflection of lack of time or interest on the part of the staff?

False imprisonment is loss of freedom of body motion or locomotion. It may occur in an area large or small, at home or in a hospital, but it must have limited boundaries, and the person imprisoned must be aware that he is being detained and must also know that no reasonable means of escape is available and that someone is intentionally preventing him from going to the place or in the direction that he would ordinarily have a right to go. Confinement can take numerous forms: it may be a physical barrier, physical force, or even a threat of physical force.

An employee of a large department store was detained by a private detective under suspicion of taking funds belonging to the store for her own private use. No physical restraint was imposed. However, she was not permitted to call her husband until she had signed a statement admitting her guilt. Following are extracts from the judicial decision in which the store was held liable for the conduct of the detective: ". . . the essential thing to constitute an imprisonment is the restraint of the person, which may be by threats as well as by actual force, and if the words and conduct are such as to induce a reasonable apprehension of fear of force, of disaster, or disgrace, a person may be as effectually restrained and deprived of liberty as by prison walls. . . ." In ordinary practice, words are sufficient to constitute an imprisonment, if they impose a restraint upon the person, and the party is accordingly restrained; for he is not obliged to incur the risk of personal violence and insult by resisting until actual violence be used.[4]

Words may be sufficient to constitute imprisonment, since the person may submit to avoid the threat of a larger harm such as a battery.

Numerous variables and shades of meaning are present in the circumstances surrounding the intent to confine a person. A mistake in identity and confinement of the wrong person is no defense for the one who restricts the freedom. The length of time may be a determining factor as regards damages, although it poses no question concerning legal liability. If the confinement is complete, it is actionable, even if it lasts for only a few moments.

If the one being detained has no means of escape open to him, then the one responsible for detaining him is liable:

The plaintiff accepted a ride home. En route the driver of the car made indecent proposals; when he refused to stop and let her out, she jumped from the car. The defendant was held liable for false imprisonment.[2]

The patient agreed to treatment but on the way to the clinic decided to go home. The staff person refused to stop the car, turn about, and take her home.

Is there a similarity in the legal implications of these two instances? Even though the person does not resist, when it is known that submission is not voluntary, the person can be said to have been illegally confined.

The restraint of an individual may be legally justified under the following conditions: First, if a genuine emergency exists and it is essential to the welfare of the individual or to those around him that he be restrained and confined, such confinement may be imposed for the length of time necessary to deal with the emergency. However, a mere belief on the part of a person, whether nurse, physician, or bystander, that an emergency exists is not sufficient to justify confinement of another; it must be, by an objective standard, clearly an emergency. Second, when formal commitment procedures have been followed, a person may properly be confined for the time limit that such a procedure permits. The time limit and circumstances under which "the right to commit" terminates vary greatly from state to state, and in each case the procedural requirements must be followed to the letter for such commitment to be authorized. A wrongful commitment or attempt to commit a person to, for example, a mental institution can result in legal liability.

How do practitioners avoid liability if these individual basic rights are so definitely protected legally and yet are continually invaded in nursing and medical practice? The law has set up a two-step process in dealing with individual freedoms. On the one hand, the rights are protected from invasion, and, on the other, the means is set forth by which one may relinquish these rights if he chooses or consents to do so in order that some good may accrue. A person taking part in a game such as football manifests willingness to submit to body contact or even injury to have the pleasure of the game. The person in need of medical care or surgery consents to relinquish the freedom from bodily invasion so that some therapeutic benefits may be attained. [8,pp.84-95]

In the absence of an emergency, every patient should be given the option of living with an illness or accepting the necessary treatment and assuming the risks. The legal process for exercising this option requires full disclosure of the risks to enable the patient to give an informed consent. Many medicolegal issues hinge on the meaning of full disclosure leading to an informed consent, often a point of controversy between the practitioners of law and those of medicine. Contrast these two points of view.

Legal view. The law of informed consent could be restructured so as to compel the physician to share critical decision-making power with the patient and to encourage the development of a partnership mode in physician-patient relations to replace the prevalent authoritarian pattern. The doctor's acceptance of the patient as an active decision maker in a partnership will in turn reintroduce a measure of personalization in technical decisions made in the modern medical context and may well stimulate the patient's motivation to accept treatment.[5]

Medical view. Full disclosure could well be considered poor medical practice. To tell the patient of possible unfavorable results of his treatment might run counter to his welfare and interfere with his recovery. The risk of psychophysical response to stress has long been recognized. An essential part of sensitive care is to foresee harm from anxiety-producing therapy and to use the means available to minimize risks.[7,pp.131-134]

To minimize or deny the risk to secure the patient's consent to treatment amounts to a lack of disclosure and nullifies consent, as in the following example:

A patient was admitted to a state mental hospital after a psychiatric examination. Electroshock treatments were advised. As a result of the treatments, the patient claimed to have received injuries consisting of a compression fracture of the spine and a loss of hearing. Claims for damages were based on two counts: First, the physician failed to inform and advise the patient of the dangers involved in electroshock treatments. Second, the physician, under direct questioning by the patient, said that no harmful results could occur. The court stated that failure to disclose or the giving of an untrue answer as to the probable consequences of a treatment constitutes malpractice.[12]

If disclosure is not sufficient to enable the patient to give an intelligent, informed, voluntary consent, then legally no consent has been given.

At the present time the physican has the duty to disclose to the patient the nature of the treatment and any possible adverse effects. As the nurse role expands into increasingly independent practice, the duty of disclosure becomes a cooperative effort on the part of the physician and the nurse or may even be carried out independently by either one. Today the nurse often plays an informal but important role in the process of disclosure. If the patient is anxious and would like to have more information but is loath to question the physician, these are clues to the nurse, who then has a duty to fulfill to both physician and patient so that an informed consent may be executed.

Although the legal steps in disclosure may be the prerogative of the physician, the administrative details of obtaining the patient's consent in writing often fall to the nurse. Without understanding of the concept of consent within the framework of the law, the process might become one of procedure only. This process is an important step in the recognition of the patient's right as a decision maker who must say what will happen to his own body. The seriousness of this decision then takes on added legal meaning. Through the proper execution of the process of consent, litigation may be minimized or avoided. Ideally the conditions of sound consent are as follows:

1. The patient should be competent and free from any condition that might diminish competency, such as an unsound mental condition or being under the influence of drugs.

2. The patient must know that he has the right to refuse consent to the plan of care as proposed and that his compliance is voluntary. If the patient refuses consent, it must be with the knowledge that no consequences will accrue to him other than those of his own act.

3. The patient must understand that he is free to determine the limits of the consent, which may be for a single procedure, such as a blood transfusion, or may be unlimited in the freedom given to the physician or health agency to do whatever is necessary, in their judgment, for his best interests.[7,pp.289-296]

The duty to disclose and the form of consent are so interrelated in medical and nursing practice that, when such issues come before the court, it is difficult to distinguish one from the other. It is plausible to ask whether, if the patient had been informed, he would have given his consent.

Jesús Luna was injured in an industrial accident in which a small piece of metal was flung into his left shoulder. He was hospitalized, had x-ray films taken, and was ordered to bed. The next morning there were external bleeding and swelling at the site of the wound. Surgery was performed, followed by the clawing of two fingers of the left hand from injury to the nerve network in the brachial plexus. It was not established whether the nerve injury occurred at the time of the accident or during surgery.

Luna's attorney effectively contended that the risks incident to surgery should have been disclosed to the patient. The court noted that, notwithstanding the utmost care by the physician, recovery for damages was being allowed because the patient had not given his informed and knowledgeable consent. The physicians appended to their briefs a printed form of consent to surgical procedures that Luna had signed at the time of admission to the hospital. This form was blank regarding the type of surgery covered and thereby was declared not relevant or material to the issue of informed consent.[6]

Following is an early leading case dealing with nurses, physicians, and the act of consent:

The patient alleged that she had told the physician that she did not wish to have surgery. The physician replied that he wished to examine her for a uterine tumor and that this would have to be done under ether. While the patient was anesthetized, a fibroid tumor was removed without the knowledge or consent of the patient. After the operation and because of it, the witnesses testified, gangrene developed in the left arm, some of the patient's fingers had to be amputated, and the suffering was intense. Judge Cardozo, in his decision, made a statement that has been used as legal precedent in numerous litigated cases since that time: "Every human being of adult years and sound mind has a right to determine what shall be done with his own body; and a surgeon who performs an operation without his patient's consent commits an assault for which he is liable in damages."[10] (Note that in this case the term *assault* is used in a broader sense than in its current usage.)

The act of consent may take one of several forms. It may be limited to a single procedure, for example, diagnostic testing such as aortography or encephalography. When a limited consent is given, the patient should know that he is withholding from the physician the means of doing any further diagnostic or therapeutic work. Some patients may consent to surgery but deny consent to a blood transfusion either during or after surgery.

Consent may be implied by the conduct of the patient. A routine physical examination in the physician's office is usually done under implied consent. Hospitals require that a physical examination be done within twenty-four hours of admission. If the patient cooperates, consent is expressed by his conduct, rather than in written form.

Consent may be exceeded and lead to charges of battery against the surgeon.

An action was brought by a patient, her husband, and his insurer for the removal of the patient's reproductive organs without her consent. The issues were those of an unauthorized operation and whether consent, expressed or implied, had been given by the patient or one authorized on her behalf. The surgeon was limited on the consent form to the removal of the appendix. In surgery, both ovaries were found to be cystic, and the surgeon removed them, contending in court that the patient would not have recovered, had such surgery not been performed. The question was not of the surgeon's skill and competence in doing surgery or about the aftercare and recovery of the patient. However, he was found guilty of a battery.[9]

The method used in obtaining the signature of the patient on the consent form may decrease its value. A hastily secured consent, urged on the patient with the explanation that it is just a matter of form, can lead to questions of its legal validity. Medication might so cloud his comprehension that it really is no consent at all.

The legally knowledgeable nurse and other related medical personnel could so implement the process of consent as to protect the patient's basic interests and that of professional personnel, so that legal sanctions would be invoked only on rare occasions.

SUMMARY

A nurse having knowledge of the legally protected interests of patients is in a position to respect and honor those rights and so strengthen the fabric of society. Similarly the nurse can assist physician colleagues and hospital administrators to avoid the invasion of rights, as well as the possibility of expensive and time-consuming litigation.

References

1. *Burrows v. Hawaiian Trust Co.,* 417 P.2d 816 (1966).
2. *Crepliniski v. Severn,* 168 N.E. 722 (1929).
3. *Crosswhite v. Barnes,* 124 S.E. 242 (1924).
4. *Dillon v. Sears-Roebuck Co.,* 253 N.W. 335 (1934).
5. Glass, E. S.: Restructuring informed consent: legal therapy for the doctor-patient relationship, Yale Law J. 79:1533, 1970.
6. *Luna v. Nering and Blanco,* 426 F.2d 95 (1970).
7. Murchison, I. A., and Nichols, T. S.: Legal foundations of nursing practice, New York, 1970, The Macmillan Co.
8. *Restatement of the Law, Torts 2d,* St. Paul, 1965, The American Law Institute.
9. *Rogers v. Lumberman's Mut. Cas. Co.,* 119 So.2d 649 (1960).
10. *Schloendorf v. New York Hospital,* 105 N.E. 92 (1914).
11. *Van Vooren v. Cook,* 75 N.Y.S. 2d 362 (1947).
12. *Woods v. Brunlap,* 377 P.2d 520 (1962).

36

Foreseeability of harm—a legal rationale for decision making

Irene Murchison

Everyday events in nursing practice are those that give rise to litigation. It is knowledge of the law, so clear in its implications for nursing practice, that provides the nurse with the rationale for decision making and a guide for conduct that will prevent litigation.

After a subtotal gastrectomy Mr. Child became restless and confused and suffered from some hallucinatory periods. Medical care included intravenous feeding and suction-syphonage. Because of his disturbed condition, the patient was placed in a private room, with three special nurses in attendance. On the day in question, the physician warned the patient that he must stay in bed. The patient seemed to understand and after his morning care, when he was quiet and dozing, the nurse left him to go to the hospital cafeteria for morning coffee. In her absence, the patient tied two sheets together, lowered himself from the window, and fell two floors, suffering severe and permanent injuries.*

The nurse was found *negligent*. The legal issues that were considered in this decision centered on the *duty* of the nurse to have *foreseen the potential for harm* when consideration was given to leaving the patient and, furthermore, the steps that should have been taken to *eliminate the known risks* attendant on departure. Duty to foresee harm and duty to eliminate or minimize risks are common legal doctrines. They are also easily understood words in nursing practice.

Nurse practitioners who have read summarized reports of litigation such as the one just given have been prone to dismiss them as unfortunate illustrations of poor nursing judgment, which happened somewhere. Not knowing the substantive law on which a decision is based, the reader

finds little if any intellectual challenge in such litigation, and it may even appear threatening. Seldom has this type of litigation been examined constructively for its usefulness as a tool in the improvement of nursing practice.

The nurse has long been aware of the legal responsibilities of professional practice and has had concern for them. Answers have frequently been sought regarding the right to perform certain procedures, and questions have been raised as to the legal boundaries of practice, particularly those dealing with the functional overlap of nursing and medical practice. Both the nurse and the physician know that although their services are complementary, they are not interchangeable either in authority or accountability. For years an orderly transfer of selected responsibilities has taken place. Now, with the present team approach to the delivery of health care, the nurse as a colleague of the physician is engaged in case finding, assessment, and diagnosis in fulfilling the role as a provider of health care, while at the same time working under limited and often remote medical supervision.

Increasingly independent practice brings added legal responsibilities. This should not deter the nurse; rather it should be a challenge to seek knowledge of the law in hitherto unexplored scope and depth.

One way to approach the subject would be to propose two working hypotheses. First, there is a point that can be identified in each litigated case, such as those presented in this chapter at which the quality of nursing care decreased, either on a policy level or on an individual practitioner level. Had this not occurred, no harm would have followed, and litigation could

---

*From *Child v. Vancouver General Hospital*, 67 W.W.R. (N.5) 169 (B.C., C.A., 1968).

have been avoided. Second, through the study of litigated cases and the laws controlling the legal decisions of these cases, the nurse can develop a rationale to guide daily decision making in patient care. The purpose of this chapter is to seek the conceptual framework of law supporting these hypotheses.

Law, in common with other behaviorally oriented disciplines, is a study of the conduct of man. The sanctions that it imposes, although unique to law, are among some of the forms of social control designed to bring about an orderly society. When a person meets with harm and believes that someone else has contributed to this harm, a charge of negligence may be brought and damages sought for reimbursement for the harm that has been incurred. Accusations of the stated harm lead to a legal review of the situation by the court and ultimately to a reasoned legal decision.

A first step in using law as a tool for the improvement of patient care is to study a summary of a case that deals with nursing conduct, such as the one already presented. It is *not* enough to read *what* happened because this is simply a narrative of nursing practice, interesting or disturbing as the case may be. To stop at this point would be a superficial analysis that often is frowned on as *anecdotal law,* and it adds little, if anything, to the nurse's knowledge for future decision making.

Instead, as a case or a summary of a case is studied, it should be considered along three dimensions. First is the *fact pattern,* which is usually a clear running account of what happened.[7, pp. 441] This is important to the nurse as a narrative of nursing practice written by a member of another discipline who is skilled in analysis of human conduct. From the fact pattern emerges the nature of the harm that has occurred and the conduct of the particular person or persons being accused of bringing about the harm. This is a challenging point in case reading, for in some instances it can pose innumerable variables in malpractice charges. Suppose, for example, the patient had suffered an unfavorable reaction to a drug. Who brought about the harm? The nurse who administered the drug? The physician who ordered the drug? The patient's

individual human response, which could not have been predicted?

The nurse who undertakes case reading has to strive for objectivity or analytical reasoning will suffer. All litigation of this type is based on a wrongful act of one or more persons. Loyalty to nursing can get in the way of a dispassionate consideration of what did happen. The case may project an image of a nurse that offends the nurse reader, and it may not reflect favorably what the profession would consider high quality nursing care. Litigation grows out of the errors and faults of others; however, a constructive use can be made of this image. Some litigation casts the nurse in the long outmoded role of handmaiden or fetch-and-carry nurse. Other cases reflect a radical change in social thinking and a new era of responsibility and accountability that can be expected of professional nurses for the future.

The second dimension is the *source of legal authority* related to the charges. In the situation that developed in *Child v. Vancouver General Hospital,* the court focused on the legal duty of the nurse. The reader then should turn to the legal meaning of *duty,* and note the legal implications for nursing practice and its social significance.[7, pp. 120-128]

The third dimension is the *substantive legal meaning of the decision* that coordinates the evidence presented to the court, the law controlling the conduct, and the finding of guilt or innocence for the defendant.

The second and third dimensions will have special emphasis in this discussion, for they are highly significant areas that are most often neglected by nurses in their study of litigation.

The sources of legal authority for nursing conduct flow from statutory and case law. (In Chapter 33 in this section, the distinction between the two is discussed.)

In the American judicial system, case law is judge-made law.[7, p. 13] Common law is a compilation of numerous decisions of individual cases, generally dealing with matters on which the statutes are silent. When the court decides a case, such as *Child v. Vancouver General Hospital,* (1) it settles the dispute between two parties and (2) it establishes a precedent, which means that like situations should and probably will be decided in like ways. In the cases presented in this chapter, it is important to consider the impact of precedent. For example, did the court cast Mr. Child's nurse as a professional practitioner with attendant responsibilities in assessment and decision making, even though she was found wanting?

It is said that case law may be either fixed or fluid, fixed when it follows previous decisions and uses them as precedent, fluid when it departs from precedent and writes "new law." The justification for the latter is that law is sensitive to and follows social change but does not create it. Within the legal system, particularly judge-made law, there are always competing needs, the need for stability and the need for change. In nursing, as in other fields, when precedent is no longer descriptive of current practice, new law may be written, as is illustrated by the following:

An industrial nurse, employed to serve in a first aid station, first saw the plaintiff, Mr. Cooper, when he came to the station for the treatment of a puncture wound to the left side of his forehead brought about by a fellow employee allowing a piece of metal to slip from his hand. According to the employee, the nurse did not probe or examine the wound, just swabbed it and bandaged it. Over a ten-month period Mr. Cooper made repeated visits to the dispensary to call to the attention of the nurse that the wound was not healing properly and was told that if it did not heal, some action would be taken. When the employee finally was referred to a physician for another purpose, the wound was examined. A biopsy was performed, and a diagnosis of basal cell carcinoma was made. Finding the nurse negligent in meeting a professional standard of care, the court stated: "The same degree of responsibility and the same duty of care is imposed upon a nurse in the making of a diagnosis as is imposed upon her in prescribing and administering treatment."[1]

Note the image in which the court cast the role of the nurse—is it in line with present and future goals of the profession?[3]

The third dimension of case reading dealing with the law will now be examined in order to understand the legal decision. In the case of *Child v. Vancouver General Hospital,* the plaintiff charged that the nurse was guilty of negligence. There was little dispute of the facts; the main issues were the duty that the hospital and the nurse owed Mr. Child and whether there had been negligence in carrying out this duty. Two legally sensitive words stand out: *negligence* and *duty.* Their in-depth legal meaning is pertinent to nursing practice. "Negligence is conduct which falls below the standard established by law for the protection of others against unreasonable risk of harm."[8, p.9]

Negligence may be an easily understood word in ordinary conversation, but when it is used as a legal doctrine, it takes on added meaning in which certain definite characteristics have been established. First, negligence is an act of inadvertence, not intent, in which one or more persons have harmed another person or persons. People are often guilty of negligent or careless acts every day, but if no one is harmed, no legal action may be taken. On the other hand, the nurse may have every desire to give the best of patient care, but, if through an error in nursing judgment the patient suffers harm, liability would follow if it could be established that the conduct of the nurse was the cause of the harm.

This introduces a second characteristic of the doctrine of negligence, that of a causal relationship. Merely showing injury and negligent conduct is not enough; the plaintiff must establish a link between the two for the defendant to be held liable. There are times when nursing conduct is so independent that if harm occurs, the causal relationship may be indisputable. At other times, with complex team relationships functions may be blurred and individual responsibility so diffused it is difficult to say who was the one who committed the inadvertent act of negligence.[7, pp.177-182]

One legal test that is used to aid in defining a causal link between the harm and the conduct of the person who may have been a party to the harm is the *but for* test. As applied, it raises the question, but for the conduct of A, would the harm have occurred to B? Applied to Mr. Child's nurse the *but for* test gives a clear answer.[7, pp.173-175]

At times the cause of the harm to a patient is evident (e.g., a sponge left in the abdomen after surgery); other instances are not so clear. When it appears that conduct has fallen short of what society would expect of those dealing with other people, how is such conduct to be measured?

In common law an imaginary man has been created known as the *reasonably prudent man*. No one has ever seen him, he is not a superman or below average in intelligence, judgment, foresight, or skill. The reasonably prudent man behaves according to current standards. For example, he drives his car with average caution, possesses today's knowledge of rules of safe conduct for himself and others, and applies these rules. He knows how to make judgments on the environmental hazards of snow, ice, and slippery streets. When he fails to do so, the law may find him guilty of negligence because he did not act as a reasonably prudent man would have acted under the same or similar circumstances.[7,pp.78-81]

Just as the concept of the reasonably prudent man is used to judge conduct in everyday living, it is also used as a measure of professional conduct, but the focus shifts to another level. When a person professes to have special knowledge and skills, this person is then judged by the standards of conduct of practitioners in the community of specialists to which he belongs and by the possession of the knowledge and skills that one would be expected to use in the practice of the particular profession.[7,pp.81-83]

Although it may seem that nursing is in an unusually difficult situation, undoubtedly practitioners in many scientific fields today face the dilemma of how to keep current with rapidly expanding knowledge and how to apply this knowledge in the development of skills required to practice their particular profession. In nursing, advances in medical science, biomedical engineering, and improved methods in the delivery of health care are making demands of nurses not even known to the practice of medicine a decade ago. What will be the view of the court if harm comes to a patient because of a nurse's lack of knowledge to support the skills necessary for professional practice?

There may be an analogy in the legal decision regarding a surgeon who was on call in the emergency room of a small general hospital. He attempted to set a frac-tured leg, apply a cast, and give aftercare, without calling in an orthopedic consultant, in spite of the steadily deteriorating condition of the patient's leg. The case was first heard in 1964, shortly after the disastrous results of the medical care had occurred. One significant section of the summarized testimony of the surgeon follows:

Dr. Alexander admitted that he could not recall what textbooks on orthopedic procedures he had studied in medical school before graduating in 1927. He could not recall the names of any books on orthopedic procedures that he had studied in the last ten years to update his major orthopedic procedures. He had finished his formal medical studies in 1927. He admitted that medicine had not stood still since then. He acknowledged that important changes and improvements had occurred and that some improvements had been made since then in the treatment of broken bones.[2]

The concept of negligence presupposes that the actor did not know of the risk or ignored it and did not see the potential for harm, else more reasonable conduct would have followed. How much the nurse should *know* in order to assume the risks of acting has long been under discussion by educators. It is hoped this critical inquiry will continue and always remain an open question. The law takes the position that knowledge is essential for risk taking, stating the following:

Knowledge may be defined as consciousness of the existence of fact. . . . If the actor has special knowledge he is required to utilize it, but he is not required to possess such knowledge, unless he holds himself out as possessing it or undertakes a course of conduct which a reasonable man would recognize as requiring it.[8,p.9]

A nurse who holds the title of clinical specialist and, as such, assumes responsibility for the coronary care of one or more patients but does not have the knowledge or skill to deal with a sudden arrhythmia would be liable for failure to know or failure to apply such knowledge, if it were known.

In the *Child v. Vancouver General Hospital* case the nurse was found negligent because of a *breach of duty* in leaving the patient to whom the duty was owed. Just as in negligence, a breach of duty does not of itself invoke liability. It is only when the breach of duty brings about harm to another. The word *duty* as viewed legally means that in certain defined relationships a duty to another is owed and if it is not observed, liability follows.

In daily living most people recognize many common moral, ethical, and legal duties that each owes to the other. These duties so commingle that it is sometimes difficult to decide which duty should have priority. For example, numerous questions have arisen because of advances in biomedical engineering regarding prolonging a human life such as what techniques should be used, for what period of time, and who can or should make the decisions involved —family, physician, or lawyer. Are these primarily moral, ethical, or legal duties?

The law is clear that the exercise of one's legal duty is one measure of the conduct of the reasonably prudent man. When a special relationship exists, as it does between a nurse and a patient, then the measure of that duty is contingent on this particular relationship. In nursing practice there are often conflicts in deciding to whom a first duty is owed—the employer, the physician, or the patient. It might seem that the first two would never be in conflict with the third. To the contrary, at times the nurse must decide to act independently, even though this action runs counter to hospital policy or the physician's orders.

A 21-year-old primipara in active labor was periodically drowsy, lethargic, delerious, and restless. She had made several attempts to get out of bed. Two of the four nurses assigned to the labor room suite were engaged in the delivery room. The head nurse was watching the progress of another patient. The remaining nurse was close to the patient's door making notations on the chart. A physician, not connected with the patient, requested the nurse to accompany him to visit another patient in labor. Because of a hospital rule that a physician could not attend a patient in labor except in the presence of a nurse, the nurse left her patient. She was gone about five minutes, and in that time the patient crawled over the side rail of the bed, fell on the floor, and suffered injuries to her face, arm, and thigh. The nurse was found negligent and liable for the patient's injury.[5]

In this case the nurse was confronted with conflicting duties and through an error in nursing judgment made an unwise

choice. To follow policy does not shield the practitioner if such action brings about a harm.

In other instances, failure to take affirmative action when one has a duty to do so can result in litigation based on charges of misconduct.

The patient, August Valentin, was admitted to the hospital for the repair of a hernia. After several days of uneventful postoperative recovery, the patient's condition showed signs of deterioration, characterized by elevated temperature, tightness in the throat, pain on attempting to open his mouth, and an inability to chew. The patient's physician and surgeon were both out of town. The resident told the nursing supervisor that he suspected tetanus and advised her to call another physician. Because of the supervisor's delay in taking affirmative action, the patient did not receive attention in time to save his life. In commenting on the inaction of the nurse, the court said that ". . . for a supervisory nurse to permit a patient recovering from a major operation to suffer symptoms indicating a growing pathology for three days, without medical care merely because the attending physician was not available is a type of conduct that is negligence."[9]

Compare the nursing conduct in this case with that of *Child v. Vancouver General Hospital.* Each of the nurses had a recognized legal duty, and each was equally culpable. Each nurse was found negligent. In the *Valentin v. La Société Française* case the legal decision discussed the conduct of the nurse as the *proximate cause* of the harm. In the Canadian case the court held the nurse liable for failing to foresee harm and to eliminate known risks. It could be hypothesized that the intellectual components of being able to foresee harm and eliminate known risks add more to the quality of nursing care than some of the factors that might have motivated the nursing supervisor of August Valentin. Or it might be argued that the nurses in both cases failed to foresee harm and eliminate known risks, although the court did not point this out in the Valentin case. Each case set a precedent in patient care that called for a higher level of assessment and accountability on the part of the nurse than that assumed by each of these nurses.

Turning now to the process of decision making and subsequent action that usually follows, foreseeability of harm and elimination of known risks appears to be a two-step process, as viewed within nursing practice. Foreseeability of harm is essentially an act of assessment in which the nurse uses knowledge and skill in applying this knowledge to a given situation. In this process certain variables are identified that offer a potential for harm. Once this step is taken, the nurse takes the second step and decides on a course of action by which risks are eliminated, or at least minimized.

What are the intellectual components of the process of foreseeability? Clearly it is not intuition or an obscure sixth sense, which some gifted people may have. It is not a process of thinking in abstract terms, but rather it is a characteristic that can knowingly be analyzed, and incorporated into the learning process of every professional nurse, based on a body of knowledge and skills.

The ability to acquire knowledge is one intellectual skill and the ability to apply this knowledge to a given situation is another and different skill. If a positive correlation could be assumed for these two skills, it could be concluded that the ability to foresee harm would increase in direct proportion to one's increase in knowledge and thereby the safety of nursing practice would automatically follow. Such is not the case. Directed teaching and practice are necessary to guide the nurse in building a body of knowledge and then in developing the skills necessary to apply this knowledge, as one operational component in the quality of nursing care. Factors that lend themselves to this mental operation are ability to observe or to perceive, ability to remember, and ability to relate knowledge to the skill.

Ability to observe or to perceive. The power of observation is a time-honored phrase in nursing practice. The law is also equally concerned with this skill. What the client is able to report of what was seen may be the evidence sought that could lead to the settlement of litigation. Some characteristics of observation and perception emphasized within the conceptual framework of the law are that what one observes depends on the keenness of the senses, the duration of the sensory impression, and the amount of attention directed toward the event. These could be important characteristics of accurate observation of an accident

that took place on a city street, but in assessing the condition of a patient, there is an added factor. Observation augmented by knowledge should lead to an inference because the nurse sees what is visible and hears what is audible with the trained eyes and ears of a professional nurse, which leads to appropriate conclusion and action. (It may be noted that heavy patient load, long hours, and fatigue offer no legal defense for lowered perceptive ability.)

Mrs. Mildred Mundt was admitted to the Alta Bates Hospital for an intravenous infusion of ACTH. It was decided to do a cutdown on the inner side of the right leg, just above the ankle. The infusion was started; over a forty-eight–hour period the nurses' notes indicated that, although observations were frequently made and recorded, action taken did not indicate clear interpretation of the significance of the findings, although what was recorded showed some knowledge of the risk involved in continuing the treatment. When the patient's leg was twice its normal size and swollen to the knee, the solution was discontinued. A necrosis followed. The physician was sued, and the hospital was also sued for the conduct of its nurses.

In the legal decision supporting the judgment against the hospital, the court stated that it was the duty of nurses to regulate the flow of the catheter and observe the area for swelling, redness, or other signs that the infusion was not running properly. The records indicated that the nurses did observe, but that they failed to be precise in their interpretation and decisive in their communications to the physician.[6]

Ability to remember. Memory is a facet in the utilization of knowledge that contributes to nursing judgment. Legally, important elements of memory that enable the nurse to perceive are (1) *fixation,* by which sensory impressions are fixed in the memory for future use, and (2) *retentiveness,* by which past sensory impressions are retained for future use.[8, p.9] If one has a fixed sensory impression of a thready pulse, cyanosis, dilated pupils, or shallow respiration, knowledge plus perception would enable one to draw inferences concerning the importance of these clinical signs. Knowledge plus memory adds to depth of foreseeability.

Ability to relate knowledge to the skill. The nurse has observed, has the knowledge and memory from previous experiences to know the meaning and importance of clinical observations, and is able to draw inferences and thus foresee the potential for harm and decide on the action to be taken. The crowning point in the entire process of foreseeability of harm and elimination of risks is the decision-making process and the conduct that flows from this decision. It is at this point that quality is added to nursing care, and the care becomes either legally knowledgeable or ineffectual, if not dangerous.

What are some of the areas of knowledge that the nurse draws on daily, in exercise of the duty to foresee harm? There are well-known immediate environmental hazards that the nurse, along with other employees, should be aware of in terms of patient safety, such as improperly positioned wheelchairs, slippery floors, inadequate lighting in bathrooms, and numerous others. But the real measure of the ability of the professional nurse to foresee harm lies in the application of knowledge of physical, biological, social, and behavioral sciences to the patient care situation. The recency of knowledge drawn from these fields and its depth and scope are significant for it is that for which the nurse will be held accountable in the exercise of professional duty. Following are a few illustrations to show how the nurse must draw from an interdisciplinary base of nursing science to foresee harm and eliminate risks as they arise in daily practice:

Knowledge of pathogenic microbiology that gives a rationale for medical and surgical asepsis, ranging from the simplest form of cleanliness to the Laminar Flow technique of bone surgery.

Knowledge that the physiological response to psychological stress may be an increase in the adrenaline output and a resultant increase in blood pressure.

Knowledge of drug reactions, for example, the patient with a thyroid toxicosis may become confused and anxious when given meperidine hydrochloride (Demerol) and diazepam (Valium).

Knowledge of the pathology of occlusion in a myocardial infarction.

Knowledge of the importance of properly grounded electrical equipment for the patient using a pacemaker.

Knowledge of the physiology of circulation, emboli formation, and their movement to vital centers.

Knowledge of the meaning of blood pressure, the body's reaction as reflected in systolic and diastolic pressure, when the vessels are sclerosed and the wall of the aorta has increased in rigidity.

Had Mr. Child's nurse known what she should have known or used what she knew about the etiology of toxic peritonitis, she would have been alert to the fact (1) that the condition did not lend itself to a spontaneous recovery and (2) that periods of lucid behavior did not warrant the conclusion that the hallucinations and delusions from which the patient had suffered would not reoccur. Also complicating nursing clinical assessment was the fact that a Levin tube had been inserted and the patient was receiving fluids by intravenous injection. It may have been irrelevant to the legal issue in question that the nurse left the patient on two other occasions that morning; however, from the standpoint of the quality of care, it reflected a lack of foreseeability of harm that simply compounded the error. The court argued in this case that the real issue was not that of foreseeability of harm, but rather the recognition of known risks and a consequent duty to guard against them.

The intellectual components basic to foreseeing harm have been explored and the process of foreseeing has been discussed as an introduction to the recognition of the existence of risks that often can be minimized. The legal consequences of failure to foresee harm come after the harm has taken place. The knowledgeable nurse, however, will assess the situation, foresee the potential for harm, and then exercise a duty to eliminate all possible risks. The court apparently did not look with favor on intellectualizing about foreseeability as a process in isolation, but it wanted to know how the conduct of the nurse should have been modified and, if the possible danger had been foreseen, what action should have been taken?

Whether all risks can be eliminated in nursing or medical practice is disputable, just as the possibility of eliminating all risks in driving a car or in numerous other daily activities is disputable, whether a professional service is involved or not. The important factor in risk taking is to know the reasonable standard of conduct for the professional nurse and then assume those risks that are inevitable within the framework of this standard. Trace the pattern of nursing care in the following case:

Patient A was injured in an automobile accident with resultant injuries of a crushed chest, dislocated hip, and multiple fractures in the area of the left hip socket and left pelvic region. After a month in another hospital A was transferred to the defendant hospital and placed in a two-bed room. The other bed occupant, patient B, was suffering from a fractured spine and was paralyzed from the waist down. After extensive surgery, A returned to the room shared with B. Several days later B developed an abscess under the right arm. The discharge was cultured, and three days later a positive report of *Staphylococcus aureus* was made.

During the three-day period, while awaiting the return of the laboratory report, the nurses moved from one patient to the other in giving care, changing dressings without washing their hands or in other ways observing sterile technique prescribed by the hospital when an infection is suspected. The day after the positive report the surgical wound of A erupted. The infection entered the bone, requiring further surgery. A sued the hospital on charges of cross infection from B. Circumstantial evidence regarding the quality of nursing care was clear but not conclusive. It was necessary to establish that the same strain of organism was present in the wound of each of the patients before a causal relationship could be established. If the strains were different, the charge of cross infection could not be supported. Extensive medical evidence was used in the proof of a causal relationship, which was confirmed. A was awarded damages.[4]

It should be noted here that the plaintiff might have used expert testimony of a nurse clinican to good advantage. The role of the professional nurse as an expert witness has not been given sufficient recognition by the courts. Professional organizations could well take a position on this nursing function as a public service.[7, pp. 49-54]

As nursing care mounts in complexity, a legal axiom that has increasing significance for the practitioner is that when the gravity of potential harm increases, even though the likelihood of its occurrence diminishes, the law will hold the actor liable if such harm does occur. For example, a nurse caring for a patient with a coronary occlusion relaxes surveillance of the cardiac monitor after several days, when the patient's condition appears to have stabilized. Such action is not defensible if the patient suffers another coronary occlusion with serious sequelae.

Another axiom is that of legal consequence of balancing or minimizing risks, whether it be by taking affirmative action or withholding action. Mr. Child's nurse apparently did not wisely balance the risks in taking the coffee break. Had she waited until a relief nurse could have been sent, it would have prevented harm, avoided the litigation, and indicated a nice balancing of risks in a legally sensitive area of patient care. Balancing risks is a part of everyday nursing practice. In psychiatric nursing the risk of placing a patient in a locked unit may be offset by removing all objects that might be a source of harm and/or increasing staff time to safeguard the patient and give him more freedom.

The boundaries of risk are those that fall within a reasonably foreseeable scope. It is unreasonable to hold a nurse accountable for consequences that are not proximately or closely related to the harm that follows. The nurse did not minimize the risk when leaving a delirious patient in a bed near an open window. It was not foreseeable that the patient would climb out of bed and ring the fire alarm in the hall and that another patient in an adjacent ward would be injured in the rush of evacuating the patients from the area. It is reasonable to limit liability to the consequences that have a reasonably close connection between the defendant's conduct and the harm that it originally threatened.[7, pp. 122-124]

• • •

To summarize, throughout this chapter an attempt has been made to conceptualize the body of law that can be identified and utilized as a tool in clinical decision making and in the implementation of such decisions. It is hoped that it will open the door to the vast body of knowledge that is available to the nurse and will increase awareness of the legal components of daily nursing practice. It is also hoped that it will challenge curriculum planners to include essential legal content on all levels of preparation.

References

1. *Cooper v. National Motor Bearing Co.*, 288 P.2d 581 (1955) 51 A.L.R.2d 963 (1957).
2. *Darling v. Charleston Community Hospital*, 200 N.E.2d 170 (1964).
3. *45 Denver Law Journal* 467 (1968).

4. *Helman v. Sacred Heart Hospital,* 381 P.2d 605 (1963).
5. *Jones v. Hawkes Hospital of Mt. Carmel,* 196 N.E.2d 592 (1964).
6. *Mundt v. Alta Bates Hospital,* 35 Cal. Rptr. 848 (1963).
7. Murchison, I. A., and Nichols, T. S.: Legal foundations of nursing practice, New York, 1970, The Macmillan Co.
8. *Restatement of the Law, Torts 2d, vol. 2,* St. Paul, 1965, The American Law Institute.
9. *Valentin v. La Société Française,* 172 P.2d 359 (1946).

Index